Visual Psychophysics and Physiology

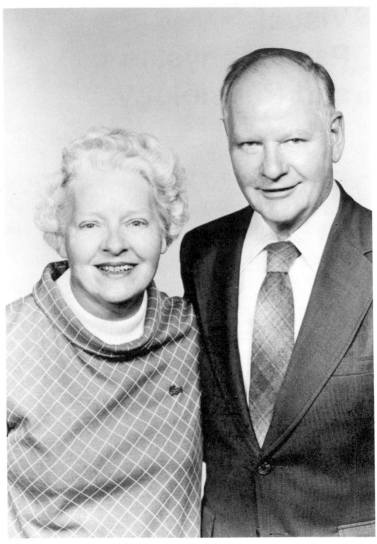

Doris and Lorrin Riggs

Visual
Psychophysics
and Physiology

A Volume Dedicated to
Lorrin Riggs

Edited by

John C. Armington

Department of Psychology
Northeastern University
Boston, Massachusetts

John Krauskopf

Bell Laboratories
Murray Hill, New Jersey

B. R. Wooten

Department of Psychology
Brown University
Providence, Rhode Island

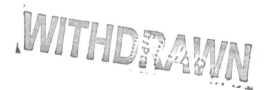

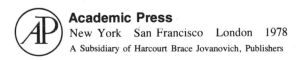

Academic Press
New York   San Francisco   London   1978
A Subsidiary of Harcourt Brace Jovanovich, Publishers

ACADEMIC PRESS, INC.
111 Fifth Avenue, New York, New York 10003

United Kingdom Edition published by
ACADEMIC PRESS, INC. (LONDON) LTD.
24/28 Oval Road, London NW1 7DX

Library of Congress Cataloging in Publication Data

Main entry under title:

Visual psychophysics.

Includes bibliographies.
1. Vision. 2. Psychophysics. I. Armington,
John C. II. Krauskopf, John. III. Wooten, Billy Rex.
QP475.V28   612'.84   78–15974
ISBN 0–12–062260–2

The affection that the members of Lorrin Riggs' academic family have for him was attested to by the attendance at the Symposium of almost all of his students, who came from all over the world. Lorrin's students are indeed a family—a family which skis together, climbs mountains together, and has over the years enjoyed the easy hospitality of Doris and Lorrin Riggs in countless ways.

It is therefore fitting that this book should be dedicated to both heads of the Riggs family: Lorrin and Doris.

Contents

Introduction

Physiological Mechanisms

Sensitivity and Adaptation

Color Vision

Acuity, Contrast, and Movement

List of Contributors

Numbers in parentheses indicate the pages on which the authors' contributions begin.

Alan Adlard (417), University of Cambridge, Cambridge, England

John C. Armington (363), Department of Psychology, Northeastern University, Boston, Massachusetts 02115

James Baker (107), Psychology Department, Brown University, Providence, Rhode Island 02192

Ross Beauchamp (63), Department of Optometry, University of Waterloo, Waterloo, Ontario N2L 3GI, Canada

Robert M. Boynton (193), Department of Psychology, University of California, San Diego, La Jolla, California 92097

Oliver Braddick (417), Psychological Laboratory, University of Cambridge, Cambridge, England

Dwight A. Burkhardt (25), Department of Psychology, Elliott Hall, University of Minnesota, Minneapolis, Minnesota 55455

Thomas W. Butler (373), Department of Physiology–Anatomy, University of California, Berkeley, California 94720

C. R. Cavonius (221), Institut fur Arbeitsphysiologie, Universitat Dortmund, D-46 Dortmund, West Germany

Robert M. Chapman (469), Psychology Department, University of Rochester, Rochester, New York 14627

Tom N. Cornsweet (233), Division of Social Science, University of California–Irvine, Irvine, California 92717

R. H. Day (331), Department of Psychology, Monash University, Clayton, Victoria, Australia

Velma Dobson (385), University of Washington, Seattle, Washington 98105

Marc H. Effron (463), Berman–Gund Laboratory for the Study of Retinal Degenerations, Harvard Medical School, Massachusetts Eye and Ear Infirmary, Boston, Massachusetts 02154

O. Estévez (221), Laboratory of Medical Physics, University of Amsterdam, Amsterdam, The Netherlands

Katherine V. Fite (49), Psychology Department, University of Massachusetts, Amherst, Massachusetts 01003

Kenneth Fuld (245), Walter S. Hunter Laboratory of Psychology, Brown University, Providence, Rhode Island 02912

John G. Gale (129), Institute of Molecular Biophysics, Florida State University, Tallahassee, Florida 32306

Leo Ganz (115), Department of Psychology, Stanford University, Stanford, California 94305

Alan Gibson (107), Psychology Department, Brown University, Providence, Rhode Island 02912

Mitchell Glickstein (107), Psychology Department, Brown University, Providence, Rhode Island 02912

E. Bruce Goldstein (73), Department of Psychology, University of Pittsburgh, Pittsburgh, Pennsylvania 15260

James Gordon (315), The Rockefeller University, Hunter College, City University of New York, New York, New York 10021

A. M. Granda (35), University of Delaware, Newark, Delaware 19711

Guido Hassin* (25), Elliott Hall, University of Minnesota, Minneapolis, Minnesota 55455

Eric G. Heinemann (157), Brooklyn College of the City University of New York, Brooklyn, New York 11210

Mark Hollins (181), Department of Psychology, Davie Hall, University of North Carolina, Chapel Hill, North Carolina 27514

Donald C. Hood (141), Department of Psychology, Columbia University, New York, New York 10027

E. Parker Johnson† (3), Psychology Department, Colby College, Waterville, Maine 04901

M. K. Jory (331), Department of Psychology, Monash University, Clayton, Victoria, Australia

Lenore Katz (245), Walter S. Hunter Laboratory of Psychology, Brown University, Providence, Rhode Island 02912

P. Ewen King-Smith (427), University of Manchester, Institute of Science and Technology, Manchester, England

John Krauskopf (283), Bell Laboratories, Murray Hill, New Jersey 07974

Eilene La Bossiere (107), Psychology Department, Brown University, Providence, Rhode Island 02912

Eleanor H. L. Leung (181), Department of Psychology, University of North Carolina, Chapel Hill, North Carolina 27514

Walter Makous (167), Department of Psychology, University of Washington, Seattle, Washington 98195

Michel Millodot (441), Institute of Science and Technology, University of Wales, Cardiff, United Kingdom

Margaret Moore (245), Walter S. Hunter Laboratory of Psychology, Brown University, Providence, Rhode Island 02912

*Present address: Health Sciences Center, Department of Anatomical Sciences, State University of New York at Stony Brook, Stony Brook, New York 11794.
†Present address: RFD New Vineyard, Maine 04956.

Robert K. Moore (353), Brown University, Providence, Rhode Island 02912

George Mower* (107), Psychology Department, Brown University, Providence, Rhode Island 02912

Floyd Ratliff (299), The Rockefeller University, New York, New York 10021

Farrel Robinson (107), Psychology Department, Brown University, Providence, Rhode Island 02912

Santo Salvatore (397), 521 North Quidnessett Road, North Kingston, Rhode Island 02852

Michael A. Sandberg (463), Berman–Gund Laboratory for the Study of Retinal Degenerations, Harvard Medical School, Massachusetts Eye and Ear Infirmary, Boston, Massachusetts 02154

R. Kevin Sanders (167), Psychology Department, University of Washington, Seattle, Washington 98195

Kenneth L. Schafer, Jr. (93), The Institute of Behavioral Medicine, Providence, Rhode Island 02906

Robert M. Shapley (315), The Rockefeller University, New York, New York 10021

George K. Shortess (85), Department of Psychology, Lehigh University, Bethlehem, Pennsylvania 18015

John B. Siegfried (257), Division of Visual Sciences, Pennsylvania College of Optometry, Philadelphia, Pennsylvania 19141

Samuel Sokol (453), Department of Ophthalmology, Tufts–New England Medical Center, Boston, Massachusetts 02111

L. Spillmann (209), University of Freiburg, Freiburg im Briesgau, West Germany

John Stein (107), Psychology Department, Brown University, Providence, Rhode Island 02912

C. E. Sternheim (209), University of Maryland, College Park, Maryland 20742

C. F. Stromeyer III† (209), University of Freiburg, Freiburg im Breisgau, West Germany

Davida Y. Teller (385), Department of Psychology, University of Washington, Seattle, Washington 98195

Ülker Tulunay-Keesey (341), University of Wisconsin, Madison, Wisconsin 53706

Frances C. Volkmann (353), Department of Psychology, Clark Science Center, Smith College, Northampton, Massachusetts 01063

Keith D. White (267), Department of Psychology, University of Florida, Gainesville, Florida 32611

Theodore P. Williams (129), Institute of Molecular Biophysics, Florida State University, Tallahassee, Florida 32306

B. R. Wooten (245), Walter S. Hunter Laboratory of Psychology, Brown University, Providence, Rhode Island 02912

*Present address: Department of Neurosciences, Harvard Medical School, Children's Hospital Medical Center, Boston, Massachusetts 02115.

†Present address: Division of Applied Science, Harvard University, Cambridge, Massachusetts 02138.

Preface

In recent years remarkable progress has been made in explaining psychological and behavioral phenomena in terms of their physiological substrata. In no area has this interdisciplinary approach been more apparent than in visual science. Visual science is truly interdisciplinary for it draws from many of the ideas as well as from the technologies of physiological optics, psychophysics, electrophysiology, neuroanatomy, biophysics, photochemistry, and other sciences. Furthermore, it is a basic science, but there are many applications of its findings to diverse fields—extending from ophthalmology to child development and human engineering. This book calls attention to all these recent developments by sampling current research in the various subareas that contribute to visual science. Thus, a word concerning organization is in order.

The book intends to illustrate a particular approach to the study of vision, and the contributing authors have been called together with this in mind. The first chapter (and first part, *Introduction*), prepared by E. Parker Johnson, explains the approach, thus providing the philosophical theme for the chapters that follow. The remaining chapters are divided into five parts and present research in ordered sequence that is current in the subdisciplines that together comprise visual science. Examples of comparative and physiological investigations are presented in the second part, *Physiological Mechanisms*. It is well known that distinct visual mechanisms exist for mediating day and night vision, color vision, and movement perception and that these mechanisms are emphasized to varying degrees in different species. Their functioning can be examined directly by combining comparative study with appropriate anatomical, electrophysiological, and photochemical procedures. The second part thus lays the groundwork for the third part, *Sensitivity and Adaptation*, where new research that bears directly upon the classical problems of visual psychophysics is examined. Here, there is an initial concern with measurement, visual sensitivity, scaling, and adaptation. This third part leads to *Color Vision*, where current findings are discussed, and then to *Acuity, Contrast, and Movement*, where some of the factors that contribute to these perceptions are considered. The final part of the book, *Applied Topics*, is concerned with applications of visual science to other disciplines. Specific examples are given that link visual research with ophthalmology, child development, and the investigation of cognitive variables such as meaning, activation, and so forth. In all cases, however, the research interest of these studies goes beyond the specific experimental details to problems of central interest in visual theory.

An essential step for explaining vision in terms of its underlying physiology lies in measurement. Visual processes must be evaluated using acceptable psychophysical procedures, and the physiological processes that are being invoked in explanation must be evaluated on the same scales of measurement. Otherwise, no comparison is justified. The ultimate goal of the work reported here is to deal with vision in these terms—namely, to account for vision in adequate physiological terms. It is not surprising that many of the experiments reported here feature joint psychophysical and physiological measurements. A unique approach to visual science is represented, a complete appreciation of which can only be obtained by reading each chapter in sequence. Although the specific research and ideas may be built upon by continuing research, the general approach is one that is bound to have continuing utility to all visual scientists.

There can be more than one reason for inviting different authors to prepare scientific papers for a single volume. In the present case, two objectives run in parallel. This book celebrates Lorrin Riggs' recent retirement from formal teaching duties. During his teaching career he advised and directed about fifty doctoral and postdoctoral students. The chapters that make up this volume were written by many of these persons, who participated in a celebration symposium held at Brown University in June 1977. Riggs' work has always featured careful experimentation, often exploiting ingenious application of new technologies and consistently giving attention to those physiological variables that are most relevant to psychophysical theory. In fact, his work has gone far toward defining the rapidly developing field of visual science. It is certainly no coincidence that the scientific aims of this collection match Riggs' own interests.

Of course, many persons in addition to those whose names appear at the heads of the individual chapters were involved in its production. There is no way that their efforts can be adequately acknowledged. Yet, in an attempt to do so, the editors express their gratitude to all whose hard work, cooperation, and enthusiasm were essential to the final outcome.

JOHN C. ARMINGTON
JOHN KRAUSKOPF
B. R. WOOTEN

Introduction

1. Light, Mind, and Matter

E. Parker Johnson

I. Objectivity and Subjectivity

A. Inner and Outer Worlds: A Visual Appreciation

The senses—among which vision is preeminent—have been perceived as a bridge between a "real" outer world and an immanent, subjective inner world (Figure 1.1). As Lorrin Riggs indicated, speaking to the American Psychological Association (Riggs, 1976), anyone trying to understand the sense of sight must come to grips with ancient questions about mind and matter—of how the *objective* world of science relates to the *subjective* world of individual experience. How we answer these questions determines our approach to understanding.

The inner world, a reasonably faithful representation of the outer much of the time, strays on occasion through realms of memory, dream, and imagination. The workaday world's persistent recurrence tells us that the dreams and imaginings are not real; so does our communication with other people if we adopt the principle that what is vouched for by others may be considered real. (That this is not an entirely safe principle was noted by Democritus in 420 BC when he said that the senses were sometimes deceptive.) But after allowing for normal or common illusions, it seems that verifiability by others, that hallmark of modern scientific acceptability, initially helped distinguish inner and outer worlds.

Before attention was given to sensory mechanisms, two worlds, an inner and an outer, seemed necessary—and also sufficient. The boundary between them, for vision, was first taken to be the pupils. Scholars later pushed the boundary back to the retina; then, growing cunning in their sophistication, to the "sensorium," wherever that might be.

In defining this sense of vision, which we have called a bridge, we are fortunate that evolution led to a group of organs that we identify without much quibbling as

3

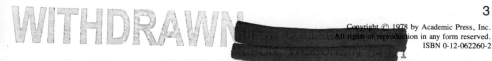

Copyright © 1978 by Academic Press, Inc.
All rights of reproduction in any form reserved.
ISBN 0-12-062260-2

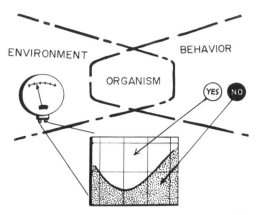

Figure 1.1. An illustration of the psychophysical determination of the visibility function as developed in the text. The meter measures the physical stimulus. "Yes" and "No" mark the energy ranges off as a function of wavelength over which the subject reports that he can or cannot see the stimulus.

eyes. They may vary a little in their ranges and peaks of sensitivity—but only a little—and, this acknowledged, the word *light* can be defined by reference to this family of sensitivity functions, after which we define an *eye* as an organ that receives light and *vision* as capability of response to light.

But both light and sight were conceptualized before man knew about sensitivity functions or the electromagnetic spectrum, because the difference between night and day is noteworthy; so is the difference between having the eyes open or closed. So man early seized on points of agreement between his own capacity for visual discrimination and that of his fellows, and found words to communicate what he saw.[1] In the very existence of these words we recognize an incipient psychophysics of vision. "Bright" and "dim," and "light" and "dark" related to quantity of light. Such terms were objective precisely to the degree that they were useful in communication. Each was an element in a verbal model of the world. Blue, red, green, or white: All could be tied to referents without mention of the spectrum.[2] Other vision-related concepts were conveyed by words such as large and small, near and far, straight, crooked, brief, and prolonged.

In due course these conceptualizations of the world succumbed to *measurement*. And when the physicist measured light in terms of a standard candle at a distance of 1 m, and when he specified points in the spectrum, the way was opened to discovery of the inverse square law, to the "facts" of color mixture, and more.

[1]While communication necessitates agreement on classes and categories, such agreement may be imperfect. The literature on color blindness records not only shifting hue-discrimination boundaries but differences in the number of bounded categories as well. Sheibner and Boynton (1968) note that dichromats see no hue boundaries at 565 nm or 610 nm. Normal individuals do.

[2]Even modern scientific work on color makes use of the fact that people partition the spectrum into categories of hue and do so consistently despite variations in psychophysical method. (See Boynton & Gordon, 1965.)

B. *Approaching the Inner World*

Thus measurement of the outer world was provided for, but what of the inner? Any full account of the sense of sight requires what we know about radiant energy and about the eye to be related somehow to visual *experience*. Therefore, the terms of communication related to sight as experience must be as well developed as possible, otherwise all the precision and regularity of the information about physical energies and about conditions within the visual system will be degraded—and the utility of that information for explaining and understanding vision vitiated—when drawn through the final communications knothole, namely, the attempt to relate that information to our experience.

Experience, however, being subjective in nature, is not communicable in its own terms. To call experience subjective may be tautological, but we shall shortly be discussing the objectivity or subjectivity of psychophysical data. We have used the word *psychophysics* already and will later use it more technically. We emphasize that psychophysics, while related to experience, is not a scheme or set of procedures for directly describing or translating the experiences of one person in terms of those of another. Though related to experience it actually provides objective data regarding sensory discriminations.[3] Psychophysics gives us objective data for comparison with other objective data—physical, physiological, or whatever—in our search and in science's search for relationships. Being public, these psychophysical data are available for anyone to consider in conjunction with his own experience; for just as science develops the structure of public knowledge, each of us compiles an inner knowledge of the world—ordering his own experience into categories and developing a sense of relationships. The data of psychophysics, like the other data of science, serve as additional grist for the private mills that grind out, for each of us, our personal understanding and beliefs.

But if psychophysics is limited in that it reaches not at all into the private realm of experience, its objective character does not confine it to the results of any narrow set of laboratory procedures, that is, to the "psychophysical methods." Looked at broadly, psychophysics embraces whatever is communicable or reportable about the utilization of the senses—anything that reveals the powers of sensory organization and discrimination. Psychophysics provides data. Data are, by definition, communicable. The phrase *subjective data* must constitute, then, a null or empty set. Conversely, the truly subjective is not communicable. (That two hues appear alike is communicable; their actual appearance is not.)

Before turning to a narrower definition of psychophysics let us note that even in that admirably objective science, physics, different statements on the same general theme may vary in precision or utility. The old statement, "The higher they rise, the

---

[3]Ratliff (1962, pp. 417–482), discussing objectivity, says that while science supposedly treats public objects and events external to the mind of the individual, there are no procedures for complete dissociation of observer and object observed, nor by which two persons can observe exactly the same thing. Any one observation, he remarks, is neither more nor less subjective—or objective—than any other, nor any more or less private—or public.

harder they fall," contains significant elements of Newton's fundamental laws of mechanics. This is not to say, however, that folk wisdom fully anticipated Newton.

In the realm of vision, the existence of linguistic categories pointed to commonly shared ranges of sensory discrimination. As in Newton's realm of mechanics, quantification and measurement have served to enhance shared, communicable, scientific understanding. The task of adding scientific precision, of bringing quantification and measurement into the language used to communicate about the senses, has been the function of modern, methodologically sophisticated psychophysics.

II. Psychophysical Procedures

A. Gustav Theodor Fechner: Fame without Fulfillment

Scientific objectivity extends knowledge beyond the framework of individual experience, supplementing what each perceives with reports of what others have observed. All such observations are bound together in an inferential substructure of theory. Thus Newton's observations of light passed through a prism led first to the experience-confounding conception of white light as a compound of hues. A few more observations brought us to the physical concept of wavelength—different colors correlated with different wavelengths. That was in 1704. In 1729, still more than a century before Fechner, Pierre Bouguer (1729, 1760, cited in Fechner, 1860) related differing brightnesses to quantifiable changes in physical intensity. An energy increase of 1 in 64, he said, was just perceptible, a ratio independent of the brightness level.

Newton's and Bouguer's observations relating experience to physical characteristics of light were important. They looked toward an objective, scientific analysis of visual processes.

Fechner's *Elements of Psychophysics* (Fechner, 1860/1966) marks, for some, the beginning of scientific psychology, that is, an attempt to unite the experiential world of the mental philosophers with the material world revealed through physical observation and measurement. His was a simplistic ideal: that relationships initially conceived on two planes, the material and the spiritual, might be reduced to one, the spiritual. This would be effected using one not very complicated formula.

As a physicist, Fechner knew the power and majesty of quantitative measurements simply and elegantly comprehended in "laws." But, as Boring (1966) has said, "He was troubled by materialism. . . . His philosophical solution of the spiritual problem lay in his affirmation of the identity of mind and matter and in his assurance that the entire universe can be regarded as readily from the point of view of its consciousness . . . as it can be viewed as inert matter [p. xiii]."

To make his point Fechner needed quantitative measurements and standards at the "mind" end of the mind–matter relationship. Therefore, in *Elements of Psychophysics,* he outlined the way to produce "elementary laws of the relationship of the material and mental world . . . [p. 6]."

It is difficult to know whether Fechner was a wavering dualist or a wavering monist. He hoped to demonstrate the unity of the mental and physical worlds, and to do so he first acknowledged that they were able to be separately conceptualized. He then sought to demonstrate a linkage. Bouguer, Weber, and others had shown that the successive magnitudes in a series of just noticeable differences (jnds) approximated a geometric series. This led Fechner to his psychophysical law (that the subjective magnitude of the sensation, measured in jnds, is proportional to the logarithm of the physical magnitude of the stimulus). For him this was not an approximate relationship, empirically determined, between two sets of observations; it was the expression of an idealized principle—a glimpse of cosmic truth shining through a screen of imperfect data. And when he had to admit that, despite all refinements of method, the data refused to conform fully to the law, he appealed to future generations to redeem him by showing how intervening sense organs and nerve processes distorted the material world's "message" to some degree before it reached his hypothesized mind–matter interface where the law was presumed to operate.

In developing his argument, Fechner distinguished between outer and inner psychophysics, depending on whether one focused on the relation of the psychic to the body's external aspects or on internal functions to which psychic functions are closely related. "Inner psychophysics has not profited...from painstaking, exact ...investigations. Undoubtedly [it will] one day [and] reach a common meeting ground....We might foresee...that this law will take on for the field of mind–body relations just as general and fundamental meaning as the law of gravitation in the field of celestial movement [Fechner, 1860/1966, p. 57]."

Defending the simple perfection of his law, Fechner fell into the very trap he had earlier derided in a satirical article on the "comparative anatomy of angels," where he had suggested that since the sphere is the most perfect of forms and angels the most perfect of beings, angels must be spherical. His own sophistication was not proof against the same kind of thinking: the establishment of idealized or "canonized" concepts from which any departure must be seen as error or deformity.

In blaming the failure of fit on internal, sensory-afferent processes, Fechner unwittingly called into question the whole concept of two worlds and their interface, since, at that point, in addition to mental and physical worlds, he had conceptualized an interior, physiological world between them. And was this middle, physiological world a single entity? Or was the number of interfaces only a question of how many stations along the way one chose to examine—a question of "how thin you slice it?" That will have to be our problem, however, not Fechner's, and we will return to it.

B. The Methods and the Data

Is it true that psychophysics yields objective data? Psychophysical data are obtained, admittedly, by recording responses that reflect subjective judgments. But what is truly subjective here is any inner experience preceding and accompanying the judgment; and this experience does not get into the data.

One way to be convinced of the objective nature of psychophysical data is to compare how human data are obtained with the way we collect comparable data from animals. (It is generally agreed that animal data are objective; no animal tells you what is on its mind.) Clarence Graham (Graham & Ratoosh, 1962, pp. 483–514) stated that instructions to a human subject or training procedures for animals had the same role in standardizing conditions of measurement as, for instance, control of temperature and pressure in many kinds of physical measurements.

Fechner's best methods typically restricted his human observers to dichotomous judgments such as "more" or "less," "light" or "dark," or "yes" or "no." He then determined the boundaries between conditions leading to a prevalence of one answer as opposed to the other. Thus he might adjust light up or down to determine that level just distinguishable from utter darkness (his absolute threshold) or to find what was just discernibly brighter than a comparison light (a difference threshold or jnd). Or he might find a setting that could not be called brighter *or* dimmer [the point of subjective equality (PSE)]. He restricted his subjects' responses simply by instructions such as, "Say yes if you see it, no if you don't."

Today, when determining a human absolute light threshold, we typically activate a shutter from time to time, presenting the subject with short flashes of light. An optical wedge controls the amount of light in a flash. If the subject says yes when he sees it, no when he does not, we may determine, by repeated trials, what density setting of the wedge produces a flash with a 50% likelihood of eliciting a positive response. This is taken as the threshold.

In the course of dark adaptation, the eye grows more sensitive, and the threshold changes over time. Kenneth Craik (Craik & Vernon, 1941) used a wedge whose position or setting was continuously recorded. During dark adaptation the wedge was frequently adjusted—the light made darker when the subject saw it and backed the other way when he did not. The recording mechanism tracked the threshold over time. Such tracings are probably the most valid representations we have of the progress of dark adaptation in an individual session.

For comparison, let us examine a method of animal psychophysics employed by Ratliff and Blough (1954) and Blough (1956). Their subjects were not instructed, but trained. A pigeon was trained to tap one key when there was a light, another when there was none. The tapping of the keys was then regarded exactly as one would regard a subject's verbal responses, that is, "Yes, I see it," and "No, I don't." Again a wedge controlled the light, and by determining the wedge setting at the 50% response level, the threshold was located. By this procedure the course of adaptation could be traced as precisely as in the human instance. A tap on the "yes" key automatically cut the light down slightly; a tap on "no" increased it. A pen traced the course. The parallel between human subjects and pigeons was complete because Craik too, for human records, dispensed with language in favor of a manual response that directly controlled the movement of the wedge. Here is as clear an illustration as one will find of the futility of trying to distinquish between subjective data, obtained using language, and objective data obtained without it. The human and pigeon results, as discussed, are included in Figure 1.2 (A and B). The dark-adaptation curve for the frog eye, drawn using electrophysiological (not psychophysical) response data, also appears (Figure 1.2C) and will be discussed shortly.

C. Applications

It took only minor development of the Ratliff–Blough technique to extend it also to the determination of spectral sensitivity curves (visibility functions)—still with no need for concern whether words or other kinds of responses were used.

Data such as these are what science turns to for the very definitions of the concepts of dark adaptation or of spectral sensitivity. The physicist, no less than the psychologist, when asked to define light, will exhibit some version of the visibility curve, psychophysically determined.[4] And when we turn to look for electrophysiological or chemical "correlates," or for intermediate mechanisms, that is, for evidence that some process is related to dark adaptation or spectral sensitivity, we ask simply whether anything about these is reminiscent of psychophysical functions which, with their reproducibility and predictability, are as near "bedrock" as the science of vision has come. Psychophysical procedures let us construct, for instance, the scotopic visibility curve, which shows how the amount of radiant energy needed for detection by the dark-adapted eye depends on its frequency or wavelength. Psychophysical research has established this function (incorporated in Figure 1.1 and appearing, in context, in Figure 1.2) as a characteristic of human vision. With this function before us we can reach into the eye and seize upon the photopigment rhodopsin, whose absorption spectrum closely matches the function, as a primary agent determining the responsivity of the eye to light. The fit is good, but not perfect; rhodopsin responds more to the high-frequency end of the spectrum. Science had to keep its fingers crossed until it found the difference accounted for by absorption within the eye.

Thus, we examine the organism—alert for recurrence of the scotopic pattern—for activity similarly linked to the characteristics of the radiant energy entering the eye. Figure 1.2 includes several examples of such findings. Visual scientists are not, of course, limited to this one "clue." If it is not the scotopic or the photopic visibility curve, it may be the dark-adaptation function that serves as our recognition template; or we may artificially brand the sensory input by using flickering light whose oscillations impose an excitation pattern.

---

[4]We continue using psychophysical methods to extend and refine our description of the eye's capabilities. It is an ongoing task. One might suppose that something as basic as the spectral sensitivity of the peripheral retina would have been thoroughly determined long since; but a recent paper by Wooten, Fuld, and Spillman (1975) demonstrates that considerations continue to arise of such a nature that previous data are seen to be inadequate.

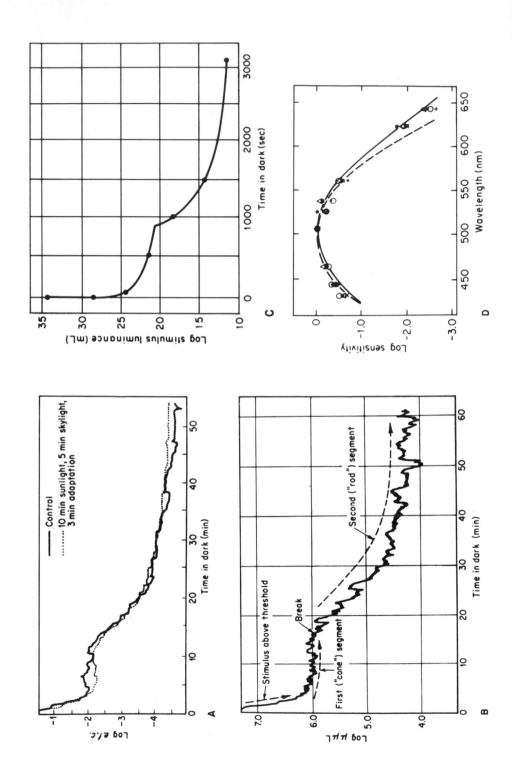

10

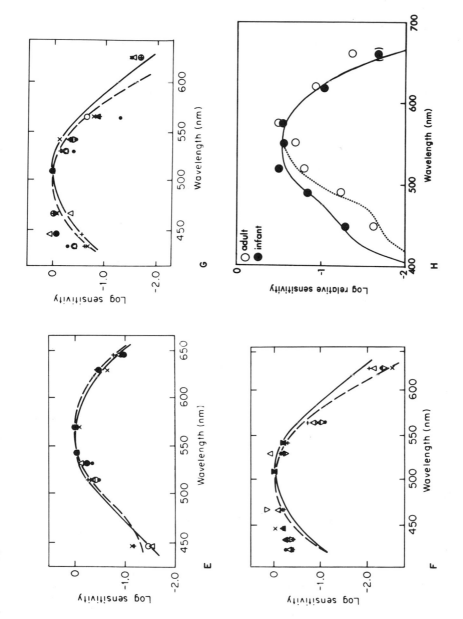

Figure 1.2. Caption appears on page 12.

11

III. Science on the Trail of Coregularities

A. *The Sound of Footsteps*

Science treats regularities, which means there must be more than one of whatever it is before science takes note. But every scientist is aware of Heraclitus' remark that no man can step twice into the same stream. Science seems caught in a paradox. It demands repetition for purposes of verification yet acknowledges that circumstances never repeat absolutely. It employs concepts and laws that assume equivalence and repeatability, knowing that every member of a class differs from every other and that no description fully details the thing or circumstance described. Science's recurrences, then, are partial; instances included under one conceptual head are alike in meeting *some* prescribed definition, but must always be presumed to differ in other characteristics. To assert a law is to acknowledge some looseness, some deviation, the possibility of error. The real question is whether the deviations are tolerable in the light of our purposes. If not, we search for more criteria to revise and refine our categories.

So it is that Percy Bridgman's operationism, pursued to one logical corner, deprives science of categories or generalizations—both of which it must attempt if it is to discover regularities in nature. Its laws are achieved, then, by trading off some degree of precision for some degree of generality. This means that science's greatest scores have been, and will continue to be, "near misses." But any glimpse of organization is better than chaos. Clarence Graham said (Graham & Ratoosh, 1962), discussing one of Hecht's formulations:

> It cannot be maintained that the original Hecht formulation is correct [but] we have used it as an example of a rational account that specifies testable implications and provides a framework for their structuring. . . . It represents experimental results over a considerable range of governing variables [and] a wise scientist will be wary of rejecting it completely until a better account comes along. [It] has the temporary virtue of encompassing more than a single *ad hoc* relation. . . .Few

---

Figure 1.2. (A) Human dark-adaptation curve, presented by Ratliff (1962, p. 470) from data of Craik and Vernon (1941). (B) Dark adaptation in the pigeon, presented by Ratliff (1962) from data of Ratliff and Blough (1954). (C) Dark adaptation in the frog eye as determined by the electrical response of the retina. [From Riggs (1937).] (D)–(G) Psychophysical and electroretinal spectral sensitivity curves compared. [From Riggs, Berry & Wayner (1949).] D shows log spectral sensitivity of the dark-adapted eye, psychophysically determined. E is the same for the light-adapted eye. F is the curve derived from the electroretinogram of the dark-adapted eye, G from that of the light-adapted eye. All stimuli were presented through the same apparatus in a comparable manner. The smooth and the broken curves were taken from the previous literature and represent peripheral rod (for D, F, and G) or (for E) cone sensitivity, psychophysically determined. The various symbols are data points from individual subjects. The conclusion was that the ERG, thus recorded, represented scotopic activity even when the eye was in what was presumed to be a light-adapted state. (H) Spectral sensitivity of the 2-month-old infant as measured by the visually evoked cortical potential. [From Dobson (1976).]

hypotheses are correct beyond a restricted domain. . . . Sometimes it is better to patch than to build anew [p. 510].[5]

And now let me divert you with a fable:

> *Once upon a time (or, for the greater convenience of scientists—who thrive on recurrence—perhaps I should say, "innumerable times"), a billy goat stood on a rocky hill looking down at a lush green meadow, ringed by bushes, on the far side of the river that divided the valley below. "I must run down to that meadow," he said to himself, "and eat some of those delicious bushes!"*
>
> *So down the trail he started: click-clack, click-clack across the ledge he had been standing on; crinch-crunch, crinch-crunch on the gravelly trail; squish-squash, squish-squash through the mud beside a spring-hole near the bottom; thump-thump, thump-thump along the well-trodden path up to the bridge; clip-clop, clip-clop over the bridge itself; then swish, swish through the grass of the meadow until finally, r-r-r-ip, r-r-r-ip, he tore juicy leaves from the first bush.*

If we were assigned the task of following and charting the progress of the goat by sound alone, we might do quite well if conditions were right. We would need facilities for monitoring sounds, wherever they might occur. We would probably be happiest if the world would remain otherwise silent, for then "sound" would equal "goat"—needing only to be detected, then located in time and space. If there *were* other sounds mingled with those of the goat, we might have trouble; but with the adoption of special recognition criteria for the sound of the goat we might still hope for success.

Development of such criteria would be complicated by the fact that the goat does not make exactly the same sound everywhere—a fact likely revealed to us only through sad experience: If we hear the goat start off at the beginning of his run and arrange to accept "click-clack" = "goat," rejecting all other noises, we will lose our animal at the edge of the ledge. So we broaden the range of acceptable sounds in various ways; but as we relax our criteria, we increase the likelihood of "false positives." We must now, as rapidly as we discover our mistakes, elaborate our criteria in ways calculated to maximize correct identifications. We will learn early to discount sounds not close to the latest position of the goat. We may cleverly fashion sound detectors keyed to the rhythm of the gait so that click-clack = crinch-crunch, = squish-squash, and so on, = goat—though before this technique has been perfected we may see research reports alleging that the goat stops upon reaching the meadow, where the swish of his passage through the grass fails to trigger the rhythm-recognition mechanism. Or we may entertain the suspicion that

---

[5]Graham brings this up in the context of his argument that scales purporting to "measure" sensation, whether produced by Fechner or by modern psychophysics, are superfluous: "The concept of intensity of sensation is formally unnecessary if observations are restricted to the variables that must be used to define intensity of sensation [p. 505]."

he has leapt from the bridge into the river when a ca-chug, ca-chug from the reeds along the bank falsely beguiles the goat-detection apparatus. And it may take time before we conceptualize the final rip-rip of leaves being torn from stems as something not a part of the journey itself.

The "goat," the "path," the "journey"—all are abstractions from the data. They have to be put together by the observer, or by science, rather as the five blind men of Indostan, given time and patience, might have created the elephant out of their diverse, but coordinated, observations. It helps, of course, to believe that there *is* a goat and that he moves in a continuous fashion from the hill to the far edge of the meadow.

Just as an individual observer of the world is subject to occasional illusions when discriminatory mechanisms fail, for some reason, to be consistent with other procedures for extracting what should be the "same" information, so scientists are led occasionally to conclusions that leave them happy until they meet the next inconsistency.

We have compared the advancing knowledge of science—public knowledge—with that of the individual. In either case the basis of understanding is the sum and product of the information-gathering and storing apparatus and the cognitive—interpretative processing machinery. These provide the predictive models. The objective remains the same: to maximize recognition and minimize surprise. Neither the individual nor science comprehends past and present fully enough to make predictions except in limited conditions, and with limited success.

B. Taking an Egalitarian Approach to Data

This underlying of inconsistency requires us to take what shall be called an egalitarian approach to data.

It is a truism among those studying vision that illusions provide clues to the way the visual system works. The catalog of visual illusions is a long one—each an acknowledgment that some perception is not fully and directly related to the stimulus or situation. Purkinje is credited with the statement that "deceptions of the senses are the truths of perception."

But confusion leads to knowledge. How much it has helped to know that certain wavelength mixtures may be confused with the white of sunlight! How instructive it is to observe that when the eyes diverge from direct fixation on a point, two such points are seen! It takes but a moment to establish that each eye contributes one, so that one point or the other (take your pick which) is illusory.

If anyone argues that this is not an illusion—because the true stimulus is not the physical point in space, but the image of it on the retina, and that with both eyes open there are in fact two such images—he may simply be asked about the equally puzzling illusion that when both eyes are fixated, the two images are perceived as one! Whether we set the boundary of the organism (where the stimulus impinges) at the cornea, at the retina, or deep within the nervous system, we will always be left with things to explain—and will have to search for principles and mechanisms to explain them. The fact is that as relevant energies are channeled, transmitted, and transmuted, as their effects penetrate and reverberate through the organism, relationships among the components of the signal undergo progressive remodeling. Every relationship that is lost, and every new relationship that is gratuitously imposed by the nature of each successive representational process has the potential of providing a new illusion as we seek unsuccessfully to match parts of earlier with later representations of the same phenomenon, the same message. Although, from a pragmatic point of view, evolution may have kept the inherent "noise" and distortion in the system with tolerable limits, we must be prepared to find protean changes occurring all along the way between any external stimulus and whatever reaction of the organism we propose to trace back to it. For this reason, "curves" or functions obtained with different measuring tools at different points in the system should never be expected to conform perfectly.

Processing of sensory information by the organism begins where the organism begins. From the moment that the physical energy of the outer world first impinges, there is an ongoing succession of energy selection, transformation, and transferral processes. Some of these processes (with how much loss through dissipation as they spread through the organism?) apparently converge (with how much noise, how much organic contamination?) to govern what we designate as the organism's responses or discriminations, that is, the "red," the "blue," the "same," the "different," the "yes," or the "no."

We wish to trace the process. Whether there is a neat chain of definable links or whether the response eventuates from a diffuse matrix is a matter for research. For relevant data we may look anywhere. The responses we are interested in are not electrical, neural, or chemical—not local, not general—not any of these, but all of these. Each level, each mode of observing, is important in its own right as one progresses, temporally or anatomically, from moment to moment or stage to stage. There is no one interface. One starts with the stimulus at one end and ends with the response at the other. Stimulus and response are defined in terms of the organism's interaction with the external world. What happens within the organism is neither—or either—depending on whether we are looking backward or ahead.

A consonant view regarding the status of successive stages was expressed by Hermann Lotze very nearly a full century ago (Lotze, 1886). He spoke not of stimulus and response, however, but of material body and spiritual soul. He addressed the problem of their interface.[6]

> The material body, it is said, would find no point of attachment for its physical forces to the phantom-like soul; but we deceive ourselves if we think we comprehend how reciprocal action takes place. We observe how a machine's parts work on each other. We believe we understand. On reflection, however, we discover we do not understand either the cohesion of its solid parts or the communication of its motion. . . .What we actually observe is but the external scenery which a series of processes runs through—each connected to its successor in a perfectly invisible and incomprehensible manner.

---

[6]Though an effort has been made to preserve the language of the original English translation, this passage has been considerably condensed.

> If we could follow a mechanical series to the point where the physical excitations act on the soul, this last transition would not be in the least degree more incomprehensible than the transition of motion from one material element to another.
>
> Demand is frequently made for some *bond* between body and soul. But we must then say what holds the parts of the bond together. In the end all depends on a perfectly immediate reciprocal action of single elements . . . [pp. 99–101].

Some, he notes, have looked for a point in the brain where sensory nerves unite "to render their messages," and from which the motor nerves issue forth. No such terminal point, says Lotze, has been or appears likely to be found. Today we recognize, as Lotze did, the unique status of each kind of data.

C. Corollary View

If one assumes that the external physical situation is the stimulus and that the recorded evidence of discrimination (e.g., "yes" or "no") is the response, then any move inside the organism for data truncates or segments the process. Is the electroretinogram (ERG) a response? It is not what we have just called *the* response, the recorded judgment. But dark-adaptation and spectral sensitivity curves drawn from ERG measurements show features that correlate with features of the response, as well as those of the stimulus. These suggest involvement with the relevant system.

Work with infants by Lodge, Armington, Barnet, Shanks, and Newcomb (1969) shows the guarded way in which ERG data are characteristically interpreted. An experimenter can tell from the electrical record whether an infant was shown a white or an orange stimulus. Clearly there is, in the retina, a physiological basis for differentiation. May we now assume that the infant organism can, itself, appreciate the difference—extract *from its own retina* the same information as the experimenter? We cannot say. The information *may* penetrate no further. One might still maintain (and some do) that infants are color-blind.

Failure to find any electrical basis for differentiation would not, of course, end hopes of eventually showing that newborns actually do discriminate colors. Riggs and Sternheim (1969) elicited visually evoked cortical potentials (VECPs) from adults by rapidly changing the colors in a pattern of stripes. At the cortex, small (4–7 nm) hue shifts produced measurable potentials. They also produced changes in the perceived hue (psychophysical). But larger (20–25 nm) differences were required to elicit detectable retinal responses (ERGs). Thus electrical recording at the higher level detected what looked to be already lost at the earlier stage; and the subjects' own discriminations surpassed either electrical method. Among these several attempts at discrimination, we find comparability but not equivalence.

IV. The Good Workman Appreciates His Tools

In emphasizing the unique value of each kind of data we have focused largely on sequential events. The goat's progress symbolized succession. But, as we just saw in the work of Riggs and Sternheim, the principle that each set of data stands on its own, resembling but not duplicating other related data, is more general. It applies equally to the way we use collateral information. We are not limited to the use of sounds when we search for goats; and science, looking for regularities and conjunctions, uses every sense and every sort of measure. Good measurements and good measuring tools assist (though they do not ensure) good science.

In our lifetimes, knowledge of sensory mechanisms has leaped ahead through the application of electrophysiological tools. To the traditional five senses we seem to have added a sixth, an electrical sense, one yielding its own realm of information. And, by great good fortune, electrical changes accompany almost all kinds of physiological activity. True, this information must be mediated by meters or other devices that transform it (usually into audible or visible form) for our ready apprehension. But this process is no drawback. We are at home with such transformations. Indeed, given light or sound to record, we often convert these into electrical signals first simply because the apparatus for measuring and recording electrical variations is so much better developed.

Electrical changes are not necessarily the most significant aspect of physiological events. A thorough representation of molecular and chemical events might do more for our understanding; but we lack any methodology to obtain it. Therefore, as there is no way we can directly see, hear, taste, smell, or feel what is happening in a retina or visual cortex, and because other indirect sensors (for chemical, mechanical, or thermal changes) lack simplicity and versatility, electrical data fill what would otherwise be a near void. Some electrophysiological work can even dispense with surgery. Electrodes placed on the scalp record potentials (VECPs) from the underlying cerebral cortex, and electrodes mounted in contact lenses (Riggs, 1941) register the electroretinogram.

A limitation is that from any pair of electrodes we record, unresolved, all the electrical activity within range. To tease out one process may be difficult. One stratagem is to devise a more localized electrode, but for general responses, like the human ERG or VECP, such a stratagem is not feasible. Another approach is to pick conditions that selectively favor one process. As examples we may contrast procedures for recording scotopic as opposed to photopic ERGs, bearing in mind that most flashes of light excite both kinds of activity.

For the purest scotopic responses we (a) dark-adapt the eye; (b) stay in the violet end of the spectrum; and (c) use light flashes of about 100-msec duration. The first two stratagems stem from well-known characteristics of night vision, the third from the fact that the critical duration of the fully dark-adapted, scotopically responding eye is 100 msec. Summation yields an increasingly large scotopic response over this period (Johnson & Bartlett, 1956). Photopic summation is complete sooner. If we want to induce photopic activity we might use a flickering red stimulus (indeed, rapid flicker alone is sufficient) but the responses, while adequately pure, may be so small as to require special recording techniques. Riggs, Johnson, and Schick (1966) used a computer of average transients to record responses as the subject looked at a pattern of rapidly alternating vertical stripes with hues paired from different parts of the spectrum. These aroused responses, identified as photopic, whose magnitudes were consistent with a simple, additive trichromatic theory.

This leads us to a problem we regularly face when we compare psychophysical and electrophysiological data: the question of how to abstract from the electrical record measurements appropriate for comparison with those that produced the psychophysical function. What *is* an electrically determined dark-adaptation curve or spectral sensitivity function?

The psychophysical functions—what we called earlier our templates—are chiefly determined by measuring absolute thresholds or else by low-level matching techniques. We must look, then, for some sort of electrical response threshold, or for a way to equate small responses obtained using different stimulus conditions. But nothing in the electrical record may be accepted, a priori, as the perfect analogue of the sensory threshold. If we specify "a detectable response," the criterion level is determined by happenstance, by the amount of noise in the record. The custom has been to specify some amplitude of response (usually small) as a criterion. Choice of level may then affect the results, that is, the shape of the function found. And the acceptance of any criterion level at all rests on the assumption that amplitude is a uniquely significant aspect of the response—that the psychophysical threshold, regardless of the character of the stimulus or of the state of adaptation of the eye, is associated with a constant, standard change of potential. But even an ERG of standard amplitude is not an altogether standard response. Responses of the same amplitude may vary in latency, duration, and form, suggesting differences in underlying physiological processes.[7]

Reflections of this sort make us wary as we discuss the fit of results obtained in different ways. We make the comparisons but do not demand perfect agreement. We respect the uniqueness of each disparate view of the same process, taking what we have called here the egalitarian approach to data.

But we need not dwell exclusively on the electrical components of physiological activity. Understanding is increased by any development that permits fuller recording. Certainly the history of the development of electrical recording illustrates this point well; but the principle that better measures make possible better science is general. Insights are usually triggered by the clearer pictures of events that flow from better facilities for observation and measurement. To see this principle in action we may look back at the growth of our understanding of the role of eye movements in vision. Eye movements, and feelings of movement, were central in the empiricists' theories of space perception. Investigators limited to uninstrumented observation could not be clear about what was happening. They observed binocular coordination, including vergence movements when distance changed. Johannes Müller (cited in Boring, 1942, p. 230) began pulling together physiological and anatomical facts. Most interest, at first, was in gross movements,

---

[7]Besides amplitude, other characteristics such as latency and implicit time may be used to compare responses, as seen in a paper by Krauskopf (1973) on contributions of chromatic mechanisms to the VECP. All such criteria are subject to similar criticism, however.

but Helmholtz recognized the impossibility of maintaining fixation perfectly—hence the existence of some slight, continuous motion of the eye.

Attempts to record eye movement began with Delabarre's (1898) heroic efforts. The problem was to arrange for freely moving eyes to drive a recording mechanism. Attachments, besides causing discomfort, could affect the movement. A light beam reflected from the cornea was weightless and could be photographically recorded—but the curvature of the cornea distorted the record, making the amount and direction of movement ambiguous. Ratliff and Riggs (1950, Riggs & Ratliff, 1951) mounted a bit of plane mirror of high optical quality in a light, tight-fitting contact lens. This reflected a beam of collimated light. It was found that the unsteadiness of the eye, even under good conditions, is such that "typically the retinal image is carried over a distance corresponding to about 3 min of arc in one sec of time. . . .During a tenth of a sec the typical excursion is 25 sec, approximately the angular subtense of a single cone at the center of fixation [Riggs, Armington, & Ratliff, 1954, pp. 315, 321]." How information so specific would have delighted Helmholtz! Riggs and Ratliff picked out three categories of movement: (a) *slow drift,* (b) *physiological nystagmus*—30- to 70-Hz oscillations covering 15 or 20 seconds of arc, and (c) *saccadic movements*—sudden shifts typically traversing several minutes of arc.

Knowing these details, our next wish is to relate them to underlying physiological mechanisms and to aspects of vision. Do eye movements set limits to some visual capabilities? Do they enhance others? We look for correlations with aspects of the stimulus, and also of the response. Analysis by Cornsweet (1956) suggested that neither drift nor physiological nystagmus was stimulus related, but saccades were, since they were more likely to occur when fixation errors were large, and their size and direction tended to counter the error. Then Krauskopf, Cornsweet, and Riggs (1960) found drift and physiological nystagmus to be independent in the two eyes. Saccades, however, were controlled by the eye that had drifted farthest—the other making a smaller, coincident shift in the same direction.

But neither the drift nor the physiological nystagmus was yet tied to experiential phenomena. No psychophysically determinable functions had been related to them. To know whether they "did" anything it seemed one would need to know what the eye saw with them absent. But they were always there; there was no holding the eye still.

We still cannot immobilize the eye, but we now have a way to simulate the condition—and there are visual consequences. Riggs, Ratliff, Cornsweet, and Cornsweet (1953) adapted the same contact lens–mirror principle first used to detect and measure eye movements and used it to project an image that moved as the eye moved. Seeing eye and seen target were stable with respect to each other. The apparatus, familiar now to all who study vision, is schematically diagrammed in Figure 1.3.

With this development a totally new visual situation was able to be explored. An initial period of clear vision was followed by fading of the target, then by its disappearance. Movement or a change in the light led to restoration of vision—facts

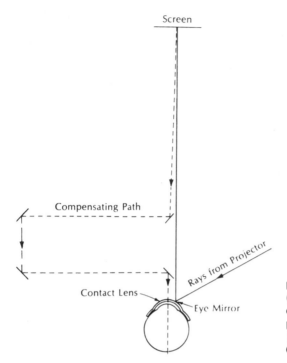

Figure 1.3. Stabilized image apparatus (schematic). The viewing (compensating) path is approximately double the length of the projection path, from the eye to the screen. [From Riggs, Ratliff, Cornsweet, & Cornsweet (1953).]

psychophysically determined by methods analogous to those used for determining other threshold phenomena.

The technique of image stabilization has been seminal, having implications not only with respect to the organization of the retina but to the organization of visual perception and work continues on image regeneration, on the selective disappearance of parts of images, on differences between simple and complex images, and so on.

V. Afterword

We began with consideration of the sense of sight as appreciated by people limited to their own, uninstrumented observations. We looked at advances that accrued when the methodology of science was applied: first those advances that sociated with just "going public"—standardizing and recording conditions of observation and organizing the data for better comparison and communication; then those associated with new instrumentation that extended the senses and the analytic capacity of the investigators. We agreed that instruments increase precision. They also bring new phenomena into view whose meaning or value is realized through pointing out correlations or congruence with previous knowledge.

But mariners who, discovering new lands, tried to fix the positions of their discoveries with respect to the known world ended by reshaping the latter to accommodate their findings. Astronomers, plotting ever more distant galaxies, similarly reshaped their conceptions to encompass all within a unified schema. Visual science is now busy exploring "inner space." It has established templates for recognition of "scotopic vision," "visual cortical potentials," and so on. But as we proceed we must remember that new data are as real as ancient "truth." Ever and again we will find ourselves charting islands on a flat world or locating galaxies in Newtonian space.

Have we ceased our search for the sensorium? Should we? When might the organism be better not regarded as an entity? Who says the ERG and VECP have thresholds? And now, with our technology, we have equipped science with organs that, like those of individuals, are subject to illusions. Purkinje spoke of the illusions of the senses as being the "truths of perception." We note that equivocations that develop during the collection and interpretation of instrumented data easily become the "facts of science."

Our knowledge of the visual process, like our knowledge of the cosmos, is an open system and has no unchallengable "center." Order and understanding are relative. We gather the best data we can and interpret them as intelligently as we can, honoring most those who open ways to new perspectives.

REFERENCES

Blough, D. S. Dark adaptation in the pigeon. *Journal of Comparative and Physiological Psychology*, 1956, *49*, 425–430.

Boring, E. G. *Sensation and perception in the history of experimental psychology*. New York: Appleton-Century, 1942.

Boring, E. G. Editor's introduction. In G. T. Fechner, [*Elements of psychophysics*] (H. E. Adler, trans). New York: Holt, Rinehart and Winston, 1966.

Bouguer, P. *Essai d'optique sur la gradation de la lumière*. Paris: 1729. (*La grande encyclopédie*, Vol. 7. Paris: Lamirault, 1888–1889.)

Bouguer, P. *Traité d'optique sur la gradation de la lumiere*. Paris: M. l'Abbé de la Caille, 1760.

Boynton, R. M., & Gordon, J. Bezold–Brücke hue shift measured by color-naming technique. *Journal of the Optical Society of America*, 1965, *55*, 78–86.

Cornsweet, T. N. Determinations of the stimuli for involuntary drifts and saccadic eye movements. *Journal of the Optical Society of America*, 1956, *46*, 987–993.

Craik, K. J. W., & Vernon, M. D. The nature of dark adaptation. I. Evidence as to the locus of the process. *British Journal of Psychology*, 1941, *32*, 62–81.

Delabarre, E. B. A method of recording eye movements. *American Journal of Psychology*, 1898, *9*, 572–574.

Dobson, V. Spectral sensitivity of the 2-month infant as measured by the visually evoked cortical potential. *Vision Research*, 1976, *16*, 367–374.

Fechner, G. T. [Elements of psychophysics] (H. E. Adler, trans.). New York: Holt, Rinehart and Winston, 1966. [Originally published, 1860.]

Graham, C. H., & Ratoosh, P. Notes on some interrelations of sensory psychology, perception and behavior. In S. Koch (Ed.), *Psychology: A study of a science* (Vol. 4). New York: McGraw-Hill, 1962.

Johnson, E. P., & Bartlett, N. R. Effect of stimulus duration on electrical responses of the human retina. *Journal of the Optical Society of America*, 1956, *46*, 167–170.

Krauskopf, J. Contributions of the primary chromatic mechanisms to the generation of visual evoked potentials. *Vision Research,* 1973, *13,* 2289–2298.

Krauskopf, J., Cornsweet, T. N., & Riggs, L. A. Analysis of eye movements during monocular and binocular fixation. *Journal of the Optical Society of America,* 1960, *50,* 572–578.

Lodge, A., Armington, J. C., Barnet, A. B., Shanks, B. L., & Newcomb, C. N. Newborn infants' electroretinograms and evoked electroencephalographic responses to orange and white light. *Child Development,* 1969, *40,* 267–293.

Lotze, M. [*Outlines of psychology*] (G. T. Ladd, Ed. and trans.). Boston: Ginn, 1886.

Ratliff, F. Some interrelations among physics, physiology, and psychology in the study of vision. In S. Koch (Ed.), *Psychology: A study of a science* (Vol. 4). New York: McGraw-Hill, 1962.

Ratliff, F., & Blough, D. S. *Behavioral studies of visual processes in the pigeon* (Tech. Rep. Contract N5 ori-07663, Project NR 140-072). U.S. Navy, Office of Naval Research, 1954.

Ratliff, 1 ., & Riggs, L. A. Involuntary motions of the eye during monocular fixation. *Journal of Experimental Psychology,* 1950, *40,* 687–701.

Riggs, L. A. Dark adaptation in the frog eye as determined by the electrical response of the retina. *Journal of Cellular and Comparative Physiology,* 1937, *9,* 491–510.

Riggs, L. A. Continuous and reproducible records of the electrical activity of the human retina. *Proceedings of the Society for Experimental Biology, New York,* 1941, *48,* 204–207.

Riggs, L. A. Human vision, some objective explorations. *American Psychologist,* 1976, *31,* 125–134.

Riggs, L. A., Armington, J. C., & Ratliff, F. A. Motions of the retinal image during fixation. *Journal of the Optical Society of America,* 1954, *44,* 315–321.

Riggs, L. A., Berry, R. N., & Wayner, M. A comparison of electrical and psychophysical determinations of the spectral sensitivity of the human eye. *Journal of the Optical Society of America,* 1949, *39,* 427–436.

Riggs, L. A., Johnson, E. P., & Schick, A. M. Electrical responses of the human eye to changes in wavelength of the stimulating light. *Journal of the Optical Society of America,* 1966, *56,* 1621–1627.

Riggs, L. A., & Ratliff, F. Visual acuity and the normal tremor of the eyes. *Science,* 1951, *114,* 17–18.

Riggs, L. A., Ratliff, F. A., Cornsweet, J. C., & Cornsweet, T. N. The disappearance of steadily fixated visual test objects. *Journal of the Optical Society of America,* 1953, *43,* 495–501.

Riggs, L. A., & Sternheim, C. Human retinal and occipital potentials evoked by changes of the wavelength of the stimulating light. *Journal of the Optical Society of America,* 1969, *59,* 635–640.

Sheibner, H. M. O., & Boynton, R. M. Residual red–green discrimination in dichromats. *Journal of the Optical Society of America,* 1968, *58,* 1151–1158.

Wooten, B. R., Fuld, K., & Spillman, L. Photopic spectral sensitivity of the peripheral retina. *Journal of the Optical Society of America,* 1975, *65,* 334–342.

Physiological Mechanisms

2. Retinal Mechanisms of Color Vision[1]

Dwight A. Burkhardt and Guido Hassin

The walleye (*Stizostedion vitreum*) is a highly developed, freshwater teleost that is widely distributed in northern sectors of this continent. Its retina contains a well-formed photopic system. About 30 years ago, Moore (1944) published a paper on the walleye retina which showed that the cones are remarkably large. In fact, they seem to be the largest yet found in vertebrates. When we became aware of Moore's finding several years ago, we decided to begin studies on the electrophysiology of the walleye retina in the hope that it might provide a favorable preparation for intracellular recording and the analysis of mechanisms of color vision. Moore's report gave no inkling that the walleye is among the most difficult freshwater fish to hold in captivity and also rather difficult to obtain—there are few commercial sources and no biological supply houses for walleyes. Unencumbered by such knowledge, we naively proceeded and, to our good fortune, were soon aided by those more sophisticated in its habits and locations. Most of the fish used in our research have been netted by personnel of the Minnesota Department of Natural Resources in the course of their work, performed mostly on frozen lakes in the deep midwinter, to maintain the walleye population and fishing repute of Minnesota waters.

After some travail, we succeeded in recording intracellular responses from walleye cones. A small spot of light evokes a simple hyperpolarizing response whose amplitude is graded with stimulus intensity and may often reach a maximum value in the 10- to 15-mV range (Burkhardt, 1977). Figure 2.1 shows a representative response evoked by a relatively intense flash. When mapped with a small spot of light (25 μm in diameter), the receptive field appears to be quite restricted. Figure 2.2 shows a representative receptive field profile. We have recently confirmed our

[1]This research was supported by Grant EY-00406 from the National Eye Institute and by a grant from the Graduate School of the University of Minnesota.

25

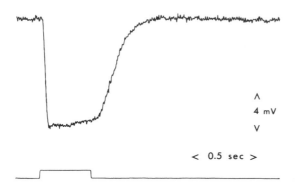

∧

4 mV

∨

< 0.5 sec >

Figure 2.1. Response of a walleye cone to a 100-μm spot of light flashed in the center of the cone's receptive field. Negative (hyperpolarization) is down in this and following figures.

functional criteria for identifying cone responses (Burkhardt, 1977) by using the Procion Yellow dye injection technique (Figure 2.3).

When the receptive field organization is assessed by flashing, centered spots of variable diameter, the cone response increases somewhat as the diameter is increased to 100–250 μm (Figure 2.4A). Most of this increase seems induced by stray light, but there appears to be some true spatial summation as well which may be mediated by fine lateral processes coursing laterally from the cone pedicles (Burkhardt, 1977; Witkovsky & Burkhardt, 1977). When the stimulus diameter is increased beyond 250 μm, the cone of Figure 2.4A shows no appreciable change in response. This result has been found in about 35% of some 100 cones studied. The other 65% show a change in the form of the response when the diameter is increased beyond 250 μm. As shown in Figure 2.4B, the later portion of the response is markedly reduced when the cone is stimulated with a large (2.2 mm) field. Hence,

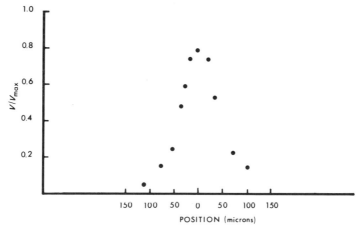

Figure 2.2. Receptive field profile of a walleye cone mapped by flashing a 25-μm spot of constant illuminance at various positions on the retina. The response amplitude evoked at each position is plotted as V/V_{max}, where V is the recorded response amplitude, and V_{max} is the maximum response that can be evoked from the cone by high-intensity flashes.

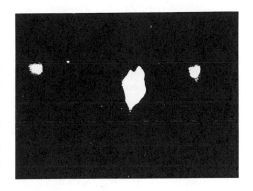

Figure 2.3. A walleye cone injected with Procion Yellow dye. The larger inner segment is filled with dye. The thin proximal process and the cone pedicle are faintly stained. This cone gave responses similar to those shown in Figures 2.1, 2.2, and 2.4A. The small, autofluorescing bodies forming a layer proximal to the cone inner segments are the rod nuclei.

illumination of a large area of retina surrounding the cone induces a delayed depolarizing influence that antagonizes the hyperpolarizing effect of light falling directly on the cone. Cones in the walleye retina thus show evidence for an antagonistic center-surround receptive field organization similar to that previously discovered in turtle cones. There is good evidence in such an organization that the depolarizing surround is mediated by feedback from luminosity-type (L) horizontal cells (Baylor, Fuortes, & O'Bryan, 1971; O'Bryan, 1973). It seems most likely that this is also the mechanism of the antagonistic surround of walleye cones (Burkhardt, 1977).

The finding that cones have an antagonistic center-surround receptive field organization is rather provocative since it contradicts the classic view that cones are organized as a mosaic of functionally independent receptor elements. It is therefore possible that cones may exert considerably more complex influences on retinal information processing than previously believed. It has recently been hypothesized,

Figure 2.4. Responses of two cones, A and B, as a function of the stimulus diameter shown at the left. Cone B shows evidence for center-surround antagonism: The 2.2-mm stimulus evokes a delayed depolarizing influence that counteracts the hyperpolarizing effect of illumination falling directly on the cone. The absolute intensity used in A is about 10 times that used in B so that the maximum responses of each cone are approximately matched at about .9 V_{max}. The calibration marker at the right applies to both cones.

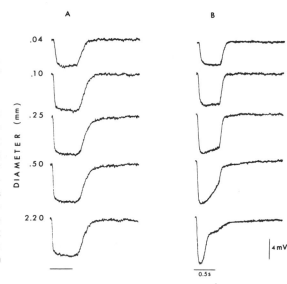

for example, that center-surround antagonism in cones contributes to contour enhancement (O'Bryan, 1973), incremental sensitivity (Burkhardt, 1974), temporal filtering (Marmarelis & Naka, 1973), and opponent color coding (Fuortes, Schwartz, & Simon, 1973; Fuortes & Simon, 1974; Gouras, 1972, pp. 513–530; Stell, Lightfoot, Wheeler, & Leeper, 1975). All these hypotheses still require critical tests. Here we will confine our attention to the role of cones in the elaboration of opponent color coding.

We have studied the spectral properties of about 100 walleye cones in some detail and find that the majority of our recordings (about 90%) are from orange-sensitive cones. The action spectrum of this class of cones is shown in Figure 2.5. It is well fit by the smooth curve which is the absorption spectrum for an A_2 cone pigment absorbing maximally at 605 nm, as specified by the nomogram of Ebrey and Honig (1977).

Horizontal cells in the walleye retina fall into two functional classes, the luminosity type (L) and the chromatic type (C). L cells give hyperpolarizing responses to lights of any spectral composition. The C cells, by contrast, hyperpolarize to short wavelengths and depolarize to long wavelengths. Representative responses of walleye L and C cells are shown in Figure 2.6.

We have studied the spectral properties of nearly 200 L cells and find that the overwhelming majority belong to an orange-sensitive class. We conclude that the

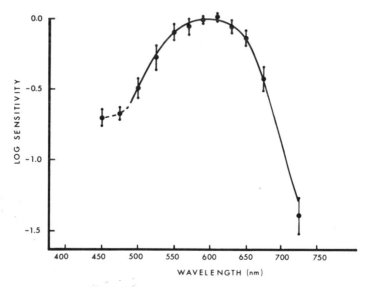

Figure 2.5. Action spectrum of orange-sensitive cones. Sensitivity is the reciprocal of the relative number of photons in the 100-μm flash needed to evoke a constant (criterion) response. The large circles show the mean sensitivity of 11 cones; the small circles and vertical lines indicate the standard deviation. The smooth curve is the absorption spectrum of an A_2 cone pigment which absorbs maximally at 605 nm, as given by the nomogram of Ebrey and Honig (1977). The nomogram does not extend below 487 nm and the dotted curve has therefore been drawn by eye to fit the points at 450 and 475 nm.

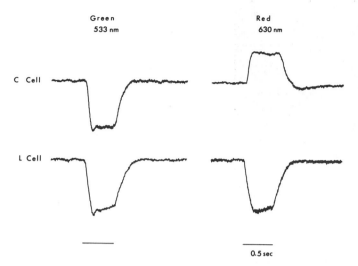

Figure 2.6. Response of L- and C-type horizontal cells evoked by green (530 nm) and red (630 nm) lights. For the L cell, the 530-nm stimulus is about twice as intense as the 630-nm stimulus. For the C cell, the 630-nm stimulus is about three times more intense than the 530-nm stimulus.

majority of L cells receive predominant input from the orange-sensitive cones.

There are three layers of horizontal cells in the walleye retina. Our recent work with Procion Yellow dye injection shows that the L cells lie in the two most distal layers, and the C cells are found in the most proximal layer. Figure 2.7 shows an injected L cell, and Figure 2.8 an injected C cell.

All C cells from which we have recorded in the walleye are the classic, biphasic red–green (R/G) type. Their action spectrum is shown in Figure 2.9. The hyperpolarizing response is maximally sensitive around 530 nm and the depolarizing

Figure 2.7. A horizontal cell which gave an L-type response, filled with Procion Yellow dye. Fine processes extend distally and expand into small feet where they synapse with cone pedicles. This large cell is about 85 μm in lateral extent here and is characteristic of cells that lie in the intermediate layer of horizontal cells.

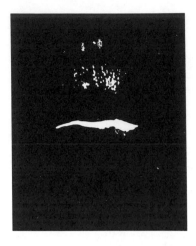

Figure 2.8. A horizontal cell which gave a typical C-type response, filled with Procion Yellow dye. Two fine processes can be seen extending distally, running past more distal horizontal cells toward the cone pedicles. This cell, the nucleus of which was clearly seen in a successive section, is characteristic of the stellate cells that lie in the most proximal layer of horizontal cells.

response is maximally sensitive at about 650 nm. When action spectrum measurements were made in the presence of steady red background fields, the sensitivity of the depolarizing mechanism was depressed. The hyperpolarizing response then showed an appreciable enhancement in the 570- to 610-nm range and the peak sensitivity fell between 530 and 540 nm. This result suggests that the green-sensitive cones of the walleye retina contain a pigment that absorbs maximally in the 530- to 540-nm range. In agreement with this, we have obtained recordings from a few

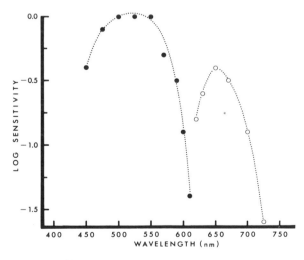

Figure 2.9. Action spectrum of a C-type horizontal cell in the walleye retina. Sensitivity is the reciprocal of the relative number of photons needed to evoke a hyperpolarizing (filled circles) or depolarizing (open circles) response of constant amplitude (4 mV). At lower and slightly higher levels of stimulation, the relative sensitivity of the green- and red-sensitive mechanisms does not change greatly. However, when the stimulus levels are raised more than a log unit above those used here, the red-sensitive mechanism becomes increasingly less sensitive than the green mechanism.

cones that are clearly more sensitive to green (530 nm) than to red (630 nm) light, but we have not been able to hold them long enough to determine their complete action spectrum. Although the green-sensitive cones may be smaller and less susceptible to stable impalement than the orange-sensitive cones, they are also probably much less numerous since the action spectrum of the PIII component of the electroretinogram is predominantly orange-sensitive.

In all our recordings from the walleye retina—these include intracellular recordings from presumptive bipolar, amacrine, ganglion, and pigment epithelial cells as well as extracellular recordings of the proximal negative response and of ganglion cells—we have yet to see evidence of blue-sensitive cones. It thus seems likely that the walleye retina is dichromatic, containing only two classes of cones (green- and orange-sensitive) and only one class of chromatic horizontal cell, the R/G type, as shown in Figure 2.9.

It has been suggested that the chromatically opponent nature of C-cell responses is a consequence of the feedback impressed on cones by L cells (Fuortes *et al.*, 1973; Fuortes & Simon, 1974). In this view, C cells receive their only direct input from green-sensitive cones. Green light hyperpolarizes these cones which in turn hyperpolarize C cells. In contrast, red light has only a weak hyperpolarizing effect on green-sensitive cones but evokes a strong response in red-sensitive cones and hence, in red-sensitive L cells. L cells are, therefore, assumed to feed back a strong depolarizing influence to the green-sensitive cones which in turn depolarize C cells. This hypothesis originated from work with the turtle retina (Fuortes *et al.*, 1973; Fuortes & Simon, 1974) and has also been proposed as the primary mechanism for C-cell responses in fish retinas (Gouras, 1972, pp. 513–530; Stell *et al.*, 1975). Since feedback to cones is the essential basis for the depolarizing response of C cells, it follows that C cells should lose their depolarizing response (and thus their chromatically opponent nature) when feedback to cones is eliminated. In the walleye (and probably in the turtle as well), this feedback can be effectively eliminated by using a 250-μm stimulus, as Figure 2.4B shows. Nevertheless, we have found that such a stimulus is capable of evoking a depolarizing response from walleye C cells. Thus, as Figure 2.10 shows, the chromatically opponent nature of C-cell responses is not fundamentally altered by variations in stimulus diameter that should differentially activate L-cell feedback to cones. This finding argues against a central role for feedback in generating opponent color coding in C cells, as do two further observations:

1. We have obtained several recordings from presumptive green-sensitive cones. Although they show evidence for feedback, they give a net hyperpolarizing response to both small and large spots of red light.

2. The cone feedback is fragile and seems to be absent in isolated retina preparations (Pinto & Pak, 1974). Nevertheless, C cells have been recorded from isolated fish retinas by many investigators, starting with Svaetichin (1956). From the evidence at hand, we thus think it unlikely that the horizontal cell–cone feedback pathway plays a dominant role in the generation of the opponent responses of C cells. The fundamental mechanisms are more likely to reside in postreceptor interac-

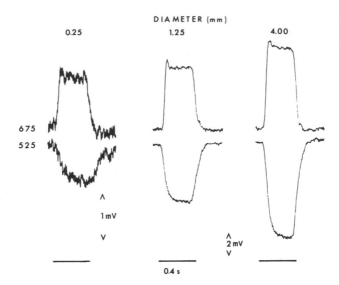

Figure 2.10. Responses of a C-type horizontal cell to red (675 nm) and green (525 nm) lights as a function of stimulus diameter. The C cell is capable of giving a depolarizing response to the small (.25 mm) field of red light even though this stimulus should not significantly activate feedback to cones (see text for further explanation).

tions. It is an important task for future research to specify adequately the nature of these interactions.

ACKNOWLEDGMENTS

We thank W. Diley, K. Nelson, K. Schumann, D. Shodeen, W. Scidmore, E. Tews, R. Weller, and other personnel of the Minnesota Department of Natural Resources for their essential aid in obtaining the fish used in this research.

REFERENCES

Baylor, D. A., Fuortes, M. G. F., & O'Bryan, P. M. Receptive fields of cones in the retina of the turtle. *Journal of Physiology,* 1971, *214,* 265–294.

Burkhardt, D. A. Sensitization and centre-surround antagonism in *Necturus* retina. *Journal of Physiology,* 1974, *236,* 593–610.

Burkhardt, D. A. Responses and receptive field organization of cones in perch retinas. *Journal of Neurophysiology,* 1977, *40,* 53–62.

Ebrey, T. G., & Honig, B. New wavelength dependent visual pigment nomograms. *Vision Research,* 1977, *17,* 147–151.

Fuortes, M. G. F., Schwartz, E. A., & Simon, E. J. Colour dependence of cone responses in the turtle retina. *Journal of Physiology,* 1973, *234,* 199–216.

Fuortes, M. G. F., & Simon, E. J. Interactions leading to horizontal cell responses in the turtle retina. *Journal of Physiology,* 1974, *240,* 177–198.

Gouras, P. S-potentials. In M. G. F. Fuortes (Ed.), *Handbook of sensory physiology (Vol. II/2): Physiology of photoreceptor organs.* New York: Springer, 1972.

Marmarelis, P. Z., & Naka, K. I. Nonlinear analysis and synthesis of receptive field responses in the catfish retina. *Journal of Neurophysiology,* 1973, *36,* 634–648.

Moore, G. A. The retinae of two North American teleosts, with special reference to their tapeta lucida. *Journal of Comparative Neurology,* 1944, *80,* 369–379.

O'Bryan, P. M. Properties of the depolarizing synaptic potential evoked by peripheral illumination in cones of the turtle retina. *Journal of Physiology,* 1973, *235,* 207–223.

Pinto, L. H., & Pak, W. L. Light-induced changes in photoreceptor membrane resistance and potential in gecko retinas. *Journal of General Physiology,* 1974, *64,* 49–69.

Stell, W. K., Lightfoot, D. O., Wheeler, T. G., & Leeper, H. F. Goldfish retina: Functional polarization of cone horizontal cell dendrites and synapses. *Science,* 1975, *190,* 989–990.

Svaetichin, G. Spectral response curves from single cones. *Acta Physiologica Scandinavica,* 1956, *39,* Suppl. 134, 17–46.

Witkovsky, P., & Burkhardt, D. A. Unpublished observations, 1977.

3. Electrophysiological and Psychophysical Determinations of Temporal Integration in Turtle[1]

A. M. Granda

I. Introduction

This chapter is concerned with a simple thesis and some evidence for its support. The thesis is as follows:

1. The photoreceptors, or at least those in the far periphery, set the parametric limits of the visual process.
2. Under controlled conditions, input defined at the periphery is carried without change into displayed behavior.
3. Color information, in a neural code set up by polarity and feedback in the photoreceptor–horizontal cell complex, is also coded by temporal limits that are distinct in photoreceptors, preserved in horizontal luminosity cells and in the ganglion cell discharge, and finally expressed in behavior.

The spectral sensitivity of the visual system in *Pseudemys* is red-light dominated. That fact has been confirmed in a number of studies using a variety of techniques. Spectral sensitivity curves determined from electroretinographic (ERG) records from intact animals show greatest sensitivity to stimulus light at 640 nm. Such a curve appears in Figure 3.1.

The same red sensitivity appears in curves derived from psychophysical data. There we were able to show some years back that red dominance in early dark adaptation gives way to a short-wavelength sensitivity under conditions of prolonged dark adaptation (cf. Figure 3.2). Several spectral processes are obviously present.

Baylor and Hodgkin (1973) showed that several processes were indeed present

[1]This contribution was supported in part by United States Public Health Service Grant EY-01540, National Eye Institute, National Institutes of Health.

35

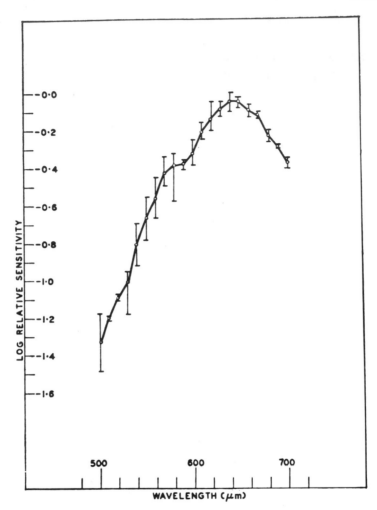

Figure 3.1. Mean spectral sensitivity for *Pseudemys* determined from electroretinograms under dark-adapted conditions. The range for each point from three animals is indicated by vertical lines. [From A. M. Granda, *Vision Research*, 1962, *2*, 343–356.]

with spectral sensitivity maxima at about 460, 550, and 630 nm. They derived these data from intracellular records from individual cones. Figure 3.3 shows their curves and the relative frequencies of the cell types.

The intracellular work accords rather well with microspectrophotometric data in Figure 3.4 gathered by Liebman and Granda (1971) if allowance is made for the presence of intensely colored oil droplets known to exist in the photoreceptors of *Pseudemys*.

In summary, the retina of *Pseudemys* contains three cone pigments based on vitamin A_2. These pigments are housed in individual outer segments with absorption

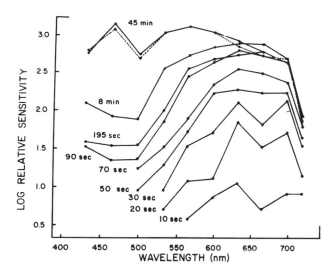

Figure 3.2. Spectral sensitivity functions for one subject (*Pseudemys*). The number placed by each curve indicates the time in darkness at which the curves were defined. [From A. M. Granda, J. H. Maxwell, & H. Zwick, *Vision Research,* 1972, *12,* 653–672.]

maxima at 450, 518, and 620 nm. Because of the presence of red, orange, and yellow droplets uniquely coupled to particular pigment-bearing outer segments, the absorption maxima are shifted to near 540–550 nm for the green-sensitive cones with a yellow droplet, and to 630–640 nm for the red-sensitive cones with red or orange droplets. The blue-sensitive cones are coupled with clear droplets and the absorption maximum of that photopigment remains unchanged. There are double cone arrangements where the two cones, principal and accessory, are electrically coupled. The principal cone has a red-sensitive photopigment coupled with an orange oil droplet; the accessory cone has no oil droplet (Granda & Dvorak,

Figure 3.3. Spectral sensitivities of cones determined from intracellular recordings in photoreceptors. The ordinate is relative quantum sensitivity, the abscissa wavelength. Collected results from 17 cells. Three cells have a peak sensitivity at about 460 nm, six have maxima at about 550 nm, and eight have maxima at about 630 nm. [From D. A. Baylor & A. L. Hodgkin, *Journal of Physiology (London),* 1973, *234,* 163–198.]

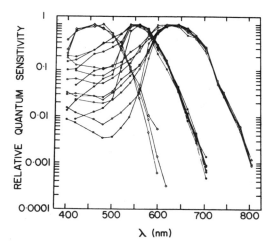

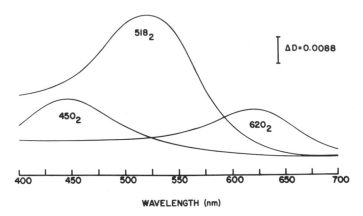

Figure 3.4. Smoothed density spectra for receptor photopigments in *Pseudemys*. [After P. A. Liebman & A. M. Granda, *Vision Research*, 1971, *11*, 105–114.]

1977). A diagrammatic arrangement of retinal cells in *Pseudemys* is shown in Figure 3.5.

There are also rods in this eye whose outer segments contain a 518 pigment. The difference between these receptors and the green-sensitive cones lies in the filtering of light by yellow droplets in the cones. There are no oil droplets in the rods. The three cone processes and the rod processes thus constitute the mechanisms of wavelength information transmission. The codification of this information is of prime interest.

II. Wavelength Coding

Wavelength information is encoded in the photoreceptors as hyperpolarizing electrical responses and these signals are then transmitted to second-order bipolar and horizontal cells. The horizontal cells, classified as chromaticity (C) and luminosity (L) cell types, are similar to those of other vertebrate retinas. In C cells, wavelength is encoded by polarity changes to distinct parts of the spectrum, but in horizontal L cells the responses are all hyperpolarizations whose amplitudes reflect underlying photoreceptor inputs.

A mechanism for encoding wavelength utilizes signals from horizontal cells fed back onto the photoreceptors. These signals appear as delayed inflections of opposite polarity in horizontal cell responses. Biphasic and triphasic horizontal C-cell responses can be explained by this means (Fuortes, Schwartz, & Simon, 1973; Fuortes & Simon, 1974; Yazulla, 1976).

In *Pseudemys* there is yet another mechanism of wavelength encoding that depends on the fact that each cone mechanism has its own characteristic time course. These temporal distinctions are preserved in higher order cells and in the overall visual system.

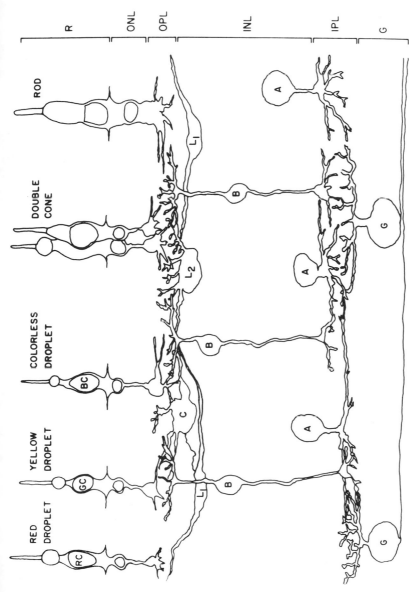

Figure 3.5. Diagrammatic arrangement of retinal cells in the eye of *Pseudemys*. RC, red-sensitive cone; GC, green-sensitive cone; BC, blue-sensitive cone; L_1, luminosity horizontal cell, type 1; L_2, luminosity horizontal cell, type 2; C, chromaticity horizontal cell; B, bipolar cell; A, amacrine cell; G, ganglion cell. The retinal layers are identified at the right side of the figure as follows: R, receptor layer; ONL, outer nuclear layer; OP, outer plexiform layer; INL, inner nuclear layer; IPL, inner plexiform layer; and G, ganglion cell layer. [From A. M. Granda, in M. Harless & H. C. Morlock (Eds.), *Handbook of turtles: Research and perspectives*. Copyright 1978 by John Wiley & Sons, Inc.]

A. Photoreceptors

Baylor and Hodgkin (1973) showed that red-sensitive cones have shorter response times (125 msec, mean value) to peak than green-sensitive cones (165 msec, mean value). In horizontal L cells, where individual cone inputs are not distinguished by polarity changes, it is possible to untangle the separate contributors by measuring summation times to critical durations which differ for the several color mechanisms.

B. Horizontal Cells

Intracellular records from L cells show increased response amplitudes to longer stimulus times until a particular value is reached beyond which increased duration of stimulation has no effect on response amplitude. The growth of the hyperpolarizations are shown in Figure 3.6 for tungsten light stimulation, which mainly excites red-sensitive cones. Stimulus durations vary between 7 and 706 msec. Both the spot diameter of 3.4 mm and the stimulus intensity of 2.3 μW $\times$ cm^{-2} remain constant.

Similar records can be obtained using stimulus lights of 640, 520, and 450 nm. Where the input to horizontal cells is solely from red-sensitive cones, the growth curves plotted in Figure 3.7 will show similar slopes at the two stimulus wavelengths tested, for parametric stimulus-duration values. The displacement along the intensity dimension (abscissa) between the two sets of curves can be accounted for by differing sensitivities of the red-absorbing photopigment to the two lights. However, where there are inputs other than red cones alone, the slopes of curves obtained from responses to differing wavelengths will not be parallel and the curves may not be superimposed by simple displacement along the intensity axis. Figure 3.8 shows data taken from a horizontal cell with blue-sensitive as well as red-sensitive cone input.

In all the curves shown in Figures 3.7 and 3.8, amplitude of response does not increase beyond a certain stimulus duration, the summation time, provided stimulus intensity is held constant and cells are operating below saturation levels. In Figure 3.9 summation time values are plotted for stimulus lights of 640, 520, and 450 nm. At moderate intensities, red light always summates at shorter times than blue or green light at the same quantal intensity. At low light levels, the blue-sensitive mechanism summates over a longer time at levels where red and green do not function effectively. The blue mechanism is capable of summating quanta over longer periods at all light levels. It apparently sacrifices efficiency in terms of time at high-intensity levels to capitalize on its light quanta-gathering abilities at low stimulus levels.

In horizontal L cells mean summation times determined in this fashion are near 125 msec for red light, 140 msec for green light, and a little longer, 150 msec, for blue light at moderate, comparable numbers of quanta (10^{11} quanta $\times$ cm^{-2} $\times$ sec^{-1}).

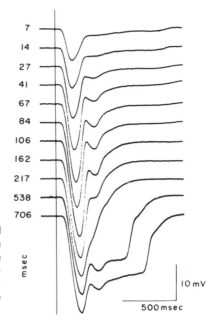

Figure 3.6. Intracellular responses of horizontal L cell in turtle to increases in stimulus durations from 7 to 706 msec. Circular stimulus spot was tungsten light of 2.3 μW $\times$ cm^{-2}. Vertical line indicates stimulus onset. Time (milliseconds) and voltage (millivolts) calibrations are at the bottom right of the figure.

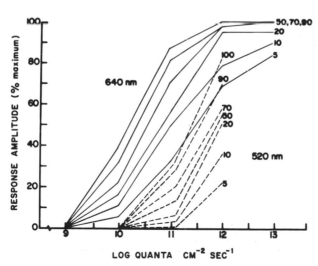

Figure 3.7. Intensity–voltage curves from horizontal L cell in *Pseudemys*. Two sets of curves are shown to stimulus wavelengths 520 (broken lines) and 640 (solid lines) nm. Parameter of stimulus duration is indicated next to each curve.

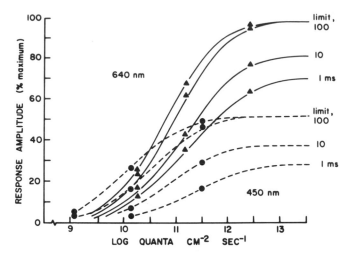

Figure 3.8. Intensity–voltage curves from horizontal L cell in *Pseudemys*. Two sets of curves are shown to stimulus wavelengths 450 (broken lines) and 640 (solid lines) nm. Parameter as in Figure 3.7. Note that these curve sets are not parallel as in Figure 3.7.

C. Ganglion Cells

Together with C. A. Dvorak and J. E. Fulbrook we have pursued this analysis in experiments with ganglion cell unit discharges recorded from the optic nerve via extracellular electrodes. Poststimulus time histograms are shown in Figure 3.10A to equal quantal input of 5.7×10^{11} quanta $\times$ cm^{-2} $\times$ sec^{-1} $\times$ steradian^{-1} at 640-, 520-,

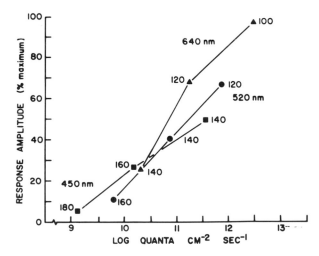

Figure 3.9. Summation time values for red (640 nm), green (520 nm), and blue (450 nm) lights. The points are limiting values beyond which increased duration has no effect on amplitude at the stimulus intensity plotted.

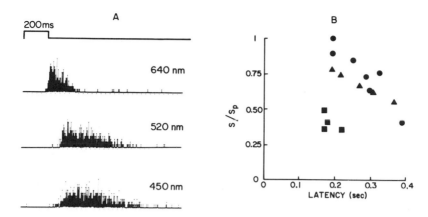

Figure 3.10. (A) Poststimulus time nistograms of ganglion cell unit discharges. Histograms are plotted to equal quantal inputs of 5.7×10^{11} quanta $\times$ cm^{-2} $\times$ sec^{-1} $\times$ steradian^{-1} at 640-, 520-, and 640-nm light flashes of 200-msec duration. (B) Number of spikes (S/S_p) expressed as a fraction of the peak spike output at 450 nm (plotted as unity). See the text.

and 450-nm light flashes of 200-msec duration. This cell is unusual in that it is blue-sensitive. Although the response to 450-nm light is largest, the response latency and time-to-peak of the envelope still remain longest. In Figure 3.10B the number of spikes (S/S_p) is expressed as a fraction of the peak spike output at 450 nm (plotted as unity). For an equivalent spike fraction, 640-nm light (squares) always produces shorter latencies than 450-nm light (circles) or 520-nm light (triangles). For any particular latency, the light required for 450-nm light is very much more intense than for 640-nm light, even though the cell is blue-sensitive and produces a greater number of spikes.

D. Behavioral Psychophysics

A simple head-withdrawal response to threshold lights can be used to measure these same parameters. The appropriate behavior conditioned in this way utilizes the entire visual information-processing system. Figure 3.11 shows a diagram of the apparatus used in these experiments. The method capitalizes on the limited be-havioral repertoire of the animal. Head withdrawal is part of the turtle's natural defense against danger, and discriminative shock applied to the jaw distinguishes stimuli requiring head withdrawal from those that do not. A line attached to the jaw permits the actuation of automatic programming equipment. The animal is then required to pull its head back a small distance in order to signal threshold detection. Stimuli are tracked in a modified up-and-down procedure where the intensity of the next stimulus is determined by the behavioral response to the last. The method concentrates the intensity of stimulation around the threshold, thereby resulting in less variance and more reliability (Maxwell & Granda, 1975).

A

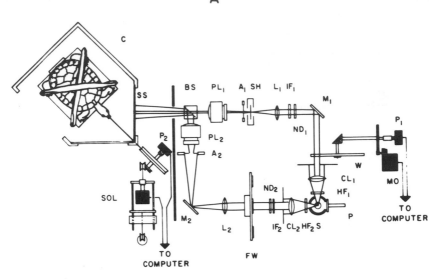

B

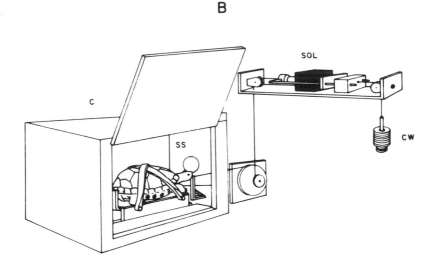

Figure 3.11. Computer-controlled apparatus for head-withdrawal conditioning in turtle. (A) Top view. C, chamber; SS, stimulus screen; PL_1, PL_2, projection lenses; A_1, A_2, apertures; SH, shutter; L_1, L_2, lenses; $1F_1$, $1F_2$, interference filters; ND_1, ND_2, neutral density filters; M_1, M_2, mirrors; HF_1, HF_2, heat filters; S, source; P, photocell; CL_1, CL_2, condenser lenses; P_1, P_2, potentiometers; SOL, solenoid for head positioning; MO, motor; W, wedge; BS, beam splitter; FW, filter wheel. (B) Side view. C, chamber; SS, stimulus screen; SOL, solenoid for head positioning; CW, counterweight.

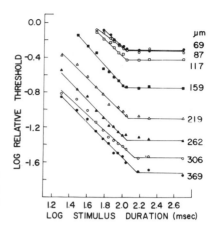

Figure 3.12. Critical duration thresholds as a function of stimulus size: Retinal image diameters ranged from 69 to 369 μm. For increasing stimulus size, critical duration increases.

Applied to problems of temporal integration, the procedures have had good success. Together with J. H. Maxwell, we measured thresholds in order to describe the ability of *Pseudemys* to integrate quanta over time to particular limits. Bloch's law expresses a relationship that defines the domain where integration occurs up to some critical value of stimulus duration for a particular intensity, after which temporal integration ceases and threshold is determined by intensity alone. The point of critical duration is not invariant but differs according to parametric changes in areal extent, adaptational state of the visual system, and color.

In our experiments critical durations increased with larger stimulus diameters over a range of 69–369 μm (Figure 3.12). The slopes approximated −1.0, the value demanded by Bloch's law for complete reciprocity. With increased stimulus duration, a time value, the critical duration, was reached where threshold was no longer affected. The slope of the function became zero at this point. Critical duration values also increased, under otherwise constant conditions, when the animal was dark-adapted from a previous light-adapted state (Figure 3.13).

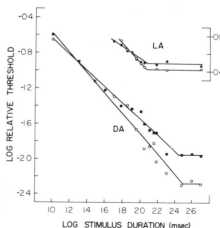

Figure 3.13. Critical duration thresholds as a function of light (LA) and dark (DA) adaptation for two subjects. Ordinate for LA plotted in the right margin. Left ordinate is for DA function.

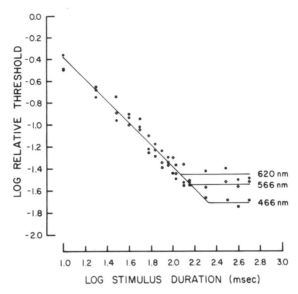

Figure 3.14. Critical duration thresholds for three stimulus wavelengths indicated. Curves are superimposed at integrative portions for comparison. Measured critical duration values (in milliseconds) are 125 for red, 150 for green, and 200 for blue lights at threshold.

Critical durations were also different from different color mechanisms. In Figure 3.14 critical durations to threshold lights at 466, 566, and 620 nm are shown. The curves have been arbitrarily superimposed on the integrative portion of the curves for comparison. The measured critical duration values in milliseconds are 125 for red, 150 for green, and 200 for blue threshold lights.

III. Conclusions

These results, briefly described, are the supporting evidence for a temporal coding of wavelength. Threshold conditions in psychophysics and the suprathreshold dynamic ranges of individual cells are not strictly comparable, of course. But the intensity of stimulus is roughly similar under all conditions, and the order of wavelength critical durations (integration and summation times) is the same at the peripheral receptors, the horizontal and ganglion cell layers, as it is at the level of expressed behavior. The order of response duration magnitudes is likewise similar, in some cases with unusually close numerical values, despite differences in technique and cellular structure or level of wavelength information processing. The similar order of values for temporal summation that results in visual behavior at threshold is apparently determined in the far periphery, in the cones and rods themselves. It may well be the case that behavioral appreciation of color and of certain spatial and temporal parameters will find its limits of operation set largely by the action of the photoreceptors and then transferred to later structural levels with little or no change.

ACKNOWLEDGMENTS

I am grateful to C. A. Dvorak, J. E. Fulbrook, J. H. Maxwell, and T. Ohtsuka for their contributions to various stages of this work. I thank Mrs. C. Groot for skillful editing and typing.

REFERENCES

Baylor, D. A., & Hodgkin, A. L. Detection and resolution of visual stimuli by turtle photoreceptors. *Journal of Physiology (London)*, 1973, *234*, 163–198.

Fuortes, M. G. F., Schwartz, E. A., & Simon, E. J. Colour dependence of cone responses in the turtle retina. *Journal of Physiology (London)*, 1973, *234*, 199–216.

Fuortes, M. G. F., & Simon, E. J. Interactions leading to horizontal cell responses in the turtle retina. *Journal of Physiology (London)*, 1974, *240*, 177–198.

Granda, A. M. Electrical responses of the light- and dark-adapted turtle eye. *Vision Research*, 1962, *2*, 343–356.

Granda, A. M. The eyes of the turtles and their sensitivities to lights of differing wavelengths. In M. Harless & H. C. Morlock (Eds.), *Handbook of turtles: Research and perspectives*. New York: John Wiley and Sons, Inc., 1978 (in press).

Granda, A. M., & Dvorak, C. A. Vision in turtles. In F. Crescitelli (Ed.), *Handbook of sensory physiology* (Vol. VII/5). Heidelberg: Springer-Verlag, 1977. Pp. 451–495.

Granda, A. M., Maxwell, J. H., & Zwick, H. The temporal course of dark-adaptation in the turtle, *Pseudemys*, using a behavioral avoidance paradigm. *Vision Research*, 1972, *12*, 653–672.

Liebman, P. A., & Granda, A. M. Microspectrophotometric measurements of visual pigments in two species of turtle, *Pseudemys scripta* and *Chelonia mydas*. *Vision Research*, 1971, *11*, 105–114.

Maxwell, J. H., & Granda, A. M. An automated apparatus for the determination of visual thresholds in turtles. *Physiology and Behavior*, 1975, *15*, 131–132.

Yazulla, S. Cone input to horizontal cells in the turtle retina. *Vision Research*, 1976, *16*, 727–735.

4. Visual Function in Amphibia: Some Unresolved Issues

Katherine V. Fite

I. Introduction

Major advances in experimental biology frequently occur as a direct consequence of the development of a model system based upon naturally occurring structures and their associated behaviors. For example, the vertebrate visual system has been a particularly valuable and instructive model of peripheral sensory processes, central nervous system (CNS) functioning, and integration within the CNS, and these are ultimately expressed in behaviors that enable adaptation and survival in a complex and challenging environment. Yet vertebrate visual systems exist with many degrees of differentiation, specialization, and complexity. How, then, does one select a particular visual system for analysis? Often an initial choice is based upon pragmatic considerations such as convenience, accessibility, and relative simplicity of the system as well as upon the experimental questions and levels of analysis available to the individual investigator. These, in turn, may depend heavily upon previous research accomplishments.

Many investigators have chosen the visual system of amphibians, particularly of anurans (frogs and toads), for as a group they are extremely dependent upon vision, and, phylogenetically, they occupy an intermediate position between aquatic and terrestrial vertebrates. Furthermore, when compared with other tetrapods, they are less complex both physiologically and behaviorally, with individual experience playing a relatively minor role in visually guided behavior. Studies of the frog visual system have established several fundamental organizational principles of peripheral and central sensory processes and the description of many stereotyped and predictable visually guided behaviors. Several noteworthy examples are the concepts of "receptive field" (Hartline, 1938, 1940), "feature detection" (Barlow, 1953; Lettvin, Maturana, McCulloch, & Pitts, 1959; Maturana, Lettvin, McCulloch, & Pitts, 1960), and the "chemoaffinity" (Sperry, 1963, 1965, pp. 161–186) and

49

"systems matching" (Straznicky, Gaze, & Keating, 1971; Gaze & Keating, 1972) hypotheses of neuronal specificity. A remarkable diversity is found among extant anurans with approximately 20 families and 250 genera recognized by taxonomists (Savage, 1973, pp. 351–445; Blair, 1976, pp. 1–27), but only a small fraction of these have yet been studied by visual scientists. Indeed, relatively little attention has been given to the problem of distinguishing species-specific characteristics and adaptations from the more general organizational principles that characterize vertebrate vision. This chapter describes a few of the many interesting problems that present a challenge to visual neurobiologists, and these are described primarily within the contexts of current knowledge and speculation.

II. Retinal Organization

Studies of the frog retina have revealed a typically laminated arrangement of photoreceptor, three nuclear and two plexiform layers, with a complexity that indicates a substantial degree of neural processing at the periphery. Thus, much of the stimulus selectivity upon which fixed action patterns are based may occur very early in the visual pathway. Synaptic relationships between the inner nuclear and ganglion cell layers have been cited as the anatomic basis for the physiologically demonstrated ganglion cell response selectivity (Dowling, 1968, 1970; Dubin, 1970). However, a great deal of complexity exists at the very beginning of the visual process, and this is only poorly understood at present. Anuran retinas contain five photoreceptor types, including three cone and two rod elements. The cone population is composed of single cones with a pigment whose λ_{max} is 580 nm, double cones containing a principal member (λ_{max} 580 nm) and an accessory member (λ_{max} 502 nm), and a "miniature" cone whose λ_{max} is unknown (Carey, 1975). This latter element may be similar to a new cone type described in goldfish (Marc & Spelling, 1976a, 1976b) which contains a short-wavelength pigment. The rod population in anurans is composed of conventional red (λ_{max} 502 nm) and green rods (λ_{max} 433 nm) whose shorter outer segment and lengthy myoid give them a unique appearance (see Figure 4.1). The obvious questions that arise are: Why are there so many photoreceptor types and what functions do they serve? Electrophysiological studies have established that the majority of ganglion cells in the frog retina are chromatically coded and that many of them receive input from all three photoreceptor pigments (Donner & Rushton, 1959a, 1959b; Chapman, 1961; Reuter, 1969; Reuter & Virtanen, 1972; Bäckström & Reuter, 1975; Scheibner, Hynold, & Bezant, 1975), and from at least two photoreceptor types. In addition, input from a given photoreceptor type may be excitatory and/or inhibitory (Reuter & Virtanen, 1972).

The conspicuous morphological differences between photoreceptors themselves remain unexplained and enigmatic. The green rod is found only in amphibian retinas, and Muntz (1963) has therefore suggested a correlation between these rods and the strong phototaxis to blue light shown by many anurans. However, Donmoyer (1974) has described green rods in species that show photonegative re-

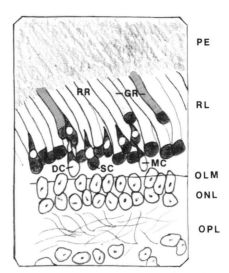

Figure 4.1. Photoreceptors of the anuran retina: DC, double cone; SC, single cone: RR, red rod; GR, green rod; MC, miniature cone; PE, pigment epithelium; RL, receptor layer; OLM, outer limiting membrane; ONL, outer nuclear layer; OPL, outer plexiform layer. Drawn from photograph; 10-μm-thick section.

sponses and found essentially no correlation between the relative number of green rods and phototactic behavior. Indeed, Hailman and Jaeger (1976) have shown that a given species shows either photopositive or photonegative behaviors depending upon the "optimal ambient illumination" for that species. Despite its resemblance to a rod, the green rod shows several photochemical and physiological properties similar to cones (Goldstein & Wolf, 1973; Donner & Reuter, 1962). Physiologically, Bäckström and Reuter (1975) have suggested an opponent color system with green rods versus cones and red rods, since green rods appear to function independently of other photoreceptor types. With respect to double cones, the suggestion has been made that they may be involved in the discrimination of polarized light during migratory orientation. However, Adler and Taylor (1973) have shown that extraocular photoreceptors (probably in the pineal organ) are capable of mediating this behavior. Snyder (1973) has also argued against the double cone as a polarization detection mechanism in teleosts. Saxen (1953, 1954, 1956) has shown that the double cone develops as the result of a fusion between rod and cone receptor elements, and thus appears to be a "hybrid" receptor type. Double cones may be an important adaptation for vision under mesopic and scotopic levels of illumination, since the number of double cones in teleosts has been correlated with the depth of water that each species inhabits (Lyall, 1957; O'Connell, 1963).

Anuran retinas are not homogeneous with respect to distribution of photoreceptor types and ganglion cells. A specialized area of increased cellular density is found near the center of the eye, although the exact location and configuration of this region vary with species and habitat. All photoreceptor types increase in number in this area, with the greatest increase occurring in the cone population. In ranid frogs, single cones show the greatest increase in number, while in bufonid toads double cones increase the most (Figure 4.2) (Fite & Carey, 1973; Carey, 1975). In both

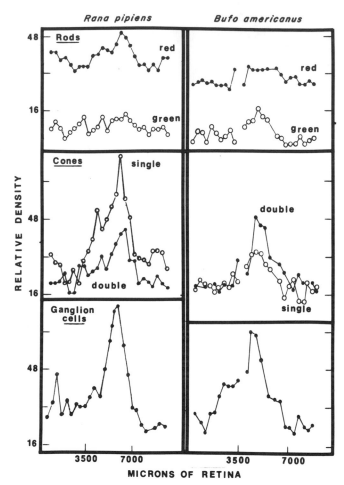

Figure 4.2. Relative cell density counts for photoreceptors and ganglion cells in a 10-μm-thick section taken from the central retina of *Rana pipiens* and *Bufo americanus*.

ranids and bufonids, red rods account for approximately 50% of the total photoreceptor population, despite the fact that toads are more nocturnal than frogs. However, relatively more 502-nm pigment is present in the area of bufonids due to the increased number of double-cone accessory members.

While numerous studies of ganglion cell morphology and physiology have been reported, the displaced ganglion cell is perhaps the least understood. These unusual neurons were described by Cajal (1892/1972) in *Rana pipiens* and are located in the inner nuclear layer along the margin of the inner plexiform layer. Displaced ganglion cells give rise to dendrites that ramify in the inner plexiform layer (first stratum) and an axon joining the optic axon layer. Using horseradish peroxidase (HRP) saturation of the centrally cut optic tract, Scalia and Coleman

(1977) have characterized displaced ganglion cells as both small and large in relation to ganglion cells proper. Furthermore, these investigators have estimated that there may be of the order of five displaced ganglion cells for every 100 ganglion cells proper and that previous studies not utilizing a specific marking technique have greatly underestimated their number (see also Fite & Scalia, 1976, pp. 87–118).

A recent study in pigeon (Karten, Fite, & Brecha, 1977) has also utilized HRP techniques and has demonstrated that displaced ganglion cells project specifically to the nucleus of the basal optic root (nBOR), which is a major component of the accessory optic system. In turn, the nBOR projects directly to the vestibulocerebellum and oculomotor complex (Brauth & Karten, 1977; Brecha, Karten, & Hunt, 1977). The avian displaced ganglion cells are unusually large and are located primarily in peripheral retinal areas. In pigeon, at least, they give rise to a bisynaptic retinocerebellar pathway which may play an important role in oculomotor and orienting reflexes. The accessory optic system is also quite well developed in frogs. Lazar (1972) reported that destruction of either the basal optic tract or the nBOR completely eliminates optokinetic nystagmus in frog. The displaced ganglion cells may thus mediate at least some portion of this field-holding reflex that compensates for movement of the retinal image. Alternatively, displaced ganglion cells may represent the first stage in a visuomotor mechanism that brings an image onto the higher acuity area(s) of the retina and thereby enables fixation. These relationships are yet to be demonstrated in the amphibian visual system.

Another unresolved issue relates to the presence and function of centrifugal fibers (efferents) to the retina. Their presence in anurans is reasonably well documented (Cajal, 1892/1972; Maturana, 1958a, 1958b; Shortess, 1963; Branston & Fleming, 1968), although the source of such efferents has not yet been demonstrated in amphibia. Byzov and Utina (1971) have suggested that centrifugal effects are mediated through amacrine cells, although there is also evidence that centrifugals terminate upon displaced ganglion cells (Maturana & Frenk, 1965; Dowling & Cowan, 1966). Thus, some centrifugals may play a feedback or modulatory role with respect to the excitability and activity of displaced ganglion cells in the frog retina as well. Such a neural circuit may be important in selective attention mechanisms and habituation to stimuli occurring repeatedly at the same retinal locus (Eikmanns, 1955; Ewert, 1970).

III. Central Nervous System Organization

In terms of evolution and phylogeny, amphibians are among the oldest vertebrates possessing the multiple visual pathways found in mammals (Riss & Jakway, 1970; Ebbesson, Jane, & Schroeder, 1970), although the degree of homology and functional significance in behavior of these projections are not entirely clear. The retina projects topographically to four diencephalic and three mesencephalic targets (Figure 4.3). The temporal retinas, which subserve the large frontal and superior binocular field of view, project bilaterally to the anterior thalamic

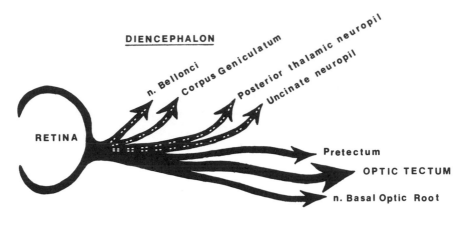

Figure 4.3. Schematic representation of the major retinofugal projections in *Rana pipiens*. Solid and dotted lines indicate, respectively, contralateral and ipsilateral pathways.

neuropils—the neuropil of Bellonci and corpus geniculatum (Scalia & Fite, 1974). Currie and Cowan (1974) have shown that the ipsilateral retinothalamic projections begin developing around the time of metamorphosis when the eyes begin to migrate from a lateral to a more superior, frontally oriented position, thus markedly increasing the size of the binocular field. These relationships suggest that thalamic visual areas may play an important role in binocular vision and depth localization. Monocular enucleation in *R. pipiens* correlates with a marked increase in both the number of prestrike orientations and in prey-catching error rates, both of which appear to be permanent alterations in the frog's visually guided behavior (Fite & Rego, 1974; see also Fite & Scalia, 1976, pp. 87–118). Electrophysiologically, binocular neurons with small receptive fields have been reported in anterior thalamus (Keating & Kennard, 1976; Fite, Carey, & Vicario, 1977), which probably represent the integration of both contralateral and ipsilateral inputs to the thalamus. Collett (1977) has provided behavioral evidence for stereopsis in toads, and it is conceivable that anterior thalamic visual areas may mediate this visual function.

Anterior thalamus has also been implicated in color discrimination behavior in frogs. Many species show a positive phototaxis toward short wavelengths, the so-called "blue preference," which is presumably independent of luminance (Muntz, 1962; Chapman, 1966; Kicliter, 1973; Hailman & Jager, 1974). Muntz (1962) suggested that this behavior is mediated by a blue-sensitive system that projects exclusively to the thalamus. More recently, Kicliter (1973) has shown that lesions of the dorsal anterior thalamus are correlated with a specific loss of the blue preference in frogs and, in some cases, with a loss of flux discrimination as well. Fite and co-workers (1977) have confirmed that the majority of visual units recorded in the area of the neuropil of Bellonci are maximally sensitive to short wavelengths, but many show two sensitivity maxima at short and long wavelengths (433 and 565 nm, respectively), which correspond to the λ_{max} of green rods and the photopic dominator (Figure 4.4).

Recent behavioral studies (Fite, Soukup, & Carey, 1978) indicate that the blue preference may involve more than a simple preference for short wavelengths and possibly include an active "avoidance" of longer wavelengths as well. Muntz (1962) added green to blue light (using broad-band filters) and observed that this combination, when paired with blue, yielded a consistent preference for the blue stimulus, even though the combination of blue and green was more intense (i.e., the frogs preferred blue despite the fact that they generally show a positive phototaxis). These findings were interpreted as a conclusive wavelength discrimination and preference for short wavelengths. However, an alternative interpretation is that the frogs were also actively avoiding, to some degree, the stimulus containing longer wavelengths.

In our study, a series of wratten filters, 76, 75, 74, 73, and 72B (peak wavelength

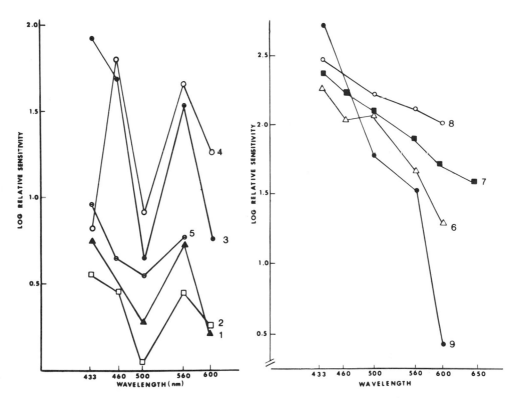

Figure 4.4. Spectral sensitivity curves of nine single units recorded from anterior thalamus of *Rana pipiens*. A threshold criterion response measure and narrow bandwidth filters were used. The various symbols identify the data from the different units. [From Fite, Carey, & Vicario (1977).]

transmissions at 435, 490, 538, 576, and 605 nm, respectively), were paired, each with every other, in a random sequence. Each pair was presented to each of 10 *R. pipiens* a total of 16 times. The average percentage of choice frequency for each filter compared with all the other filters with which it was paired was calculated. As can be seen from Figure 4.5, the 490 (blue) stimulus was chosen significantly more often (75%) than were the other stimuli. However, the 37 and 23% choice frequencies for 576 (yellow) and 605 nm (orange) do not represent nonpreference, which would be close to 50%. Further examination of the data from individual frogs showed that the orange stimulus was chosen less than 50% of the time by *all* subjects, suggesting that the inclusion of the yellow and orange filter may have heightened or exaggerated the apparent preference for short wavelengths.

The anuran blue preference may thus depend partially upon a contrast effect such that the longer the wavelength with which a blue stimulus is paired, the stronger the choice of blue. To test this hypothesis, each chromatic stimulus was paired with a spectrally flat, achromatic, or white light, and the intensity of the achromatic stimulus varied over a range of several log units, including a no-light (dark) stimulus. The photopically equivalent intensity of the achromatic stimulus with each of the chromatic stimuli was determined from the frog photopic luminosity function [based on data presented by Hood and Hock (1973)]. Combined data from 10 subjects revealed that short-wavelength stimuli (471 and 490 nm) were consistently chosen over achromatic stimuli (Figure 4.6), middle-wavelength stimuli (538 nm) were chosen only when substantially brighter than achromatic stimuli, and long-wavelength stimuli (605 nm) were consistently chosen only when paired with no light (Figure 4.7). Thus, *R. pipiens* appear to actively avoid long wavelengths when shorter wavelength stimuli are present in a two-choice discrimination. Chapman (1966) also found an increasing preference for lights of 460 and 540 nm as intensity was increased, but not for a 620-nm stimuli. Teleologically, it is not difficult to

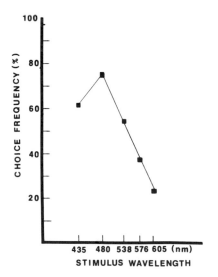

Figure 4.5. Combined data from 10 *Rana pipiens* showing percentage of choice frequency for each of five stimulus wavelengths as compared with all of the other wavelengths with which each was paired.

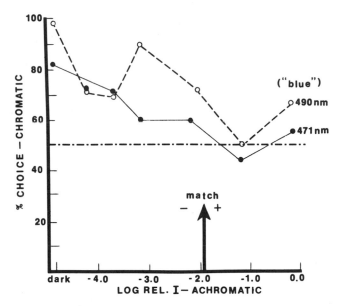

Figure 4.6. Combined data from 10 *Rana pipiens* in a two-choice experiment. Wavelengths of 471 and 490 nm were each paired with an achromatic, white stimulus of various intensities. "Match" indicates the photopic equivalent achromatic stimulus intensity; 0.0 = 2300 cd m^{-2}.

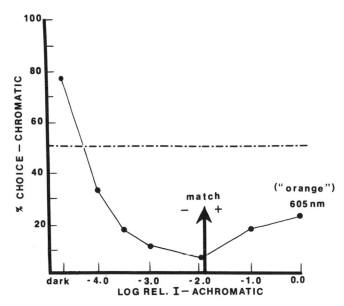

Figure 4.7. Combined data from 10 *Rana pipiens*. A 605-nm wavelength was paired with an achromatic stimulus of various intensities.

imagine why a predominantly green frog would avoid a long-wavelength stimuli background against which it would surely lose the advantage of its natural coloration and camouflage.

While the anterior thalamus receives input from retinal afferents that are particularly sensitive to short wavelengths, information concerning other wavelengths clearly is present in this region. Several other studies describing chromatic coding in retinal afferents that project to the optic tectum and that can be recorded in substantial numbers from the optic tracts have eliminated any expectations that there may be a simple segregation of chromatic information in the frog CNS (Bäckström & Reuter, 1975; Reuter & Virtanen, 1969; Scheibner *et al.*, 1975). The functional significance of the multiple maps of the retina, particularly in the diencephalon, remains a mystery. Whether qualitatively different aspects of retinal information are projected to these and other retinal targets is yet to be resolved.

In another regard, recent evidence and speculation indicate that amphibia may possess the major components of two major visual pathways projecting to the telencephalon, which are well developed in mammals (Kicliter, 1973; Gruberg & Ambros, 1974; Scalia & Coleman, 1975). Studies on the organization of the thalamofrontal tract by Herrick (1925) indicate that the dorsal thalamic cell groups from which the two portions of this tract originate (the lateral and the medial forebrain bundle) are closely associated with the neuropils constituting the terminal fields of retinothalamic and tectothalamic visual projections (see also Fite & Scalia, 1976; Scalia, 1976, pp. 386–406; Kicliter & Ebbesson, 1976). Subsequent studies should provide important new information concerning the functional organization and significance of anuran diencephalic cell groups associated with the thalamotelencephalic pathways. However, bufonid toads may ultimately prove to be a better choice for clarifying these relationships, since both thalamus and telencephalon are larger and more differentiated than in frogs. Behaviorally, toads also appear to show a greater range and diversity of visually guided behaviors that are amenable for measurement and experimental manipulation.

Many important and interesting questions remain for visual scientists to explore in amphibia, not the least of which concerns the modulation of sensory information in the CNS of awake, behaving animals. Future investigations utilizing a behaviorally viable preparation should contribute to major advances in our understanding of many fundamental brain–behavior relationships in vertebrates.

REFERENCES

Adler, K., & Taylor, D. H. Extraocular perception of polarized light by orienting salamanders. *Journal of Comparative Physiology*, 1973, *87*, 203–212.

Bäckström, A. C., & Reuter, T. Receptive field organization of ganglion cells in the frog retina: contributions from cones, green rods and red rods. *Journal of Physiology (London)*, 1975, *246*, 79–107.

Barlow, H. B. Summation and inhibition in the frog's retina. *Journal of Physiology (London)*, 1953, *119*, 69–88.

Blair, W. F. Amphibians, their evolutionary history, taxonomy and ecological adaptations. In K. V. Fite (Ed.), *The amphibian visual system: A multidisciplinary approach*. New York: Academic Press. 1976.

Branston, N. M., & Fleming, D. G. Efferent fibers in the frog optic nerve. *Experimental Neurology*, 1968, *20*, 611–623.

Brauth, S. E., & Karten, H. J. Direct accessory optic projections to the vestibulo-cerebellum; a possible channel for oculomotor control systems. *Experimental Brain Research*, 1977, *28*, 73–81.

Brecha, N., Karten, H. J., & Hunt, S. A visual quickie: A bisynaptic retinal pathway to the vestibula-cerebellum and oculomotor complex. *Neuroscience Abstracts*, 1977, *2*, 554.

Byzov, A. L., & Utina. Centrifugal effects on the amacrine cells in the frog's retina. *Neirofizilogiya*, 1971, *3*, 293–300.

Cajal, R. Y. S. [*The structure of the retina*] (S. A. Thorpe & M. Glickstein, trans.). Springfield, Illinois: Thomas, 1972. [Originally published, 1892.]

Carey, R. G. *A quantitative analysis of the distribution of the retinal elements in frogs and toads with special emphasis on the* areae retinalis. Unpublished master's thesis, University of Massachusetts, Amherst, 1975.

Carey, R. G. The anuran "mystery cone": A new receptor type? Paper presented at the annual meeting of the Association for Research in Vision and Opthalmology, 1976.

Chapman, R. M. Spectral sensitivity of single neural units in the bullfrog retina. Journal of the Optical Society of America, 1961, *51*, 1102–1112.

Chapman, R. M. Light, wavelength and energy preferences of the bullfrog: Evidence for color vision. *Journal of Comparative Physiology and Psychology*, 1966, *61*, 429–435.

Collett, T. Stereopsis in toads. *Nature*, 1977 267, 349–351.

Currie, J., & Cowan, W. M. Evidence for the late development of the uncrossed retinothalamic projections in the frog, *Rana pipiens. Brain Research*, 1974, *71*, 133–139.

Donmoyer, J. E. *Photoreceptor histology and phototactic preferences in amphibians*. Unpublished master's thesis, University of Wisconsin, Madison, 1974.

Donner, K. O., & Reuter, T. The spectral sensitivity and photopigment of the green rods in the frog's retina. *Vision Research*, 1962, *7*, 17–41.

Donner, K. O., & Rushton, W. A. H. Retinal stimulation by light substitution. *Journal of Physiology (London)*, 1959, *149*, 288–302. (a)

Donner, K. O., & Rushton, W. A. H. Rod-cone interaction in the frog's retina analysed by the Stiles–Crawford effect and by dark adaptation. *Journal of Physiology (London)*, 1959, *149*, 303–317. (b)

Dowling, J. E. Synaptic organization of the frog retina: An electron microscope analysis comparing the retinas of frogs and primates. *Proceedings of the Royal Society of London, Ser. B.*, 1968, *166*, 80–111.

Dowling, J. E. Organization of vertebrate retinas. (The Jonas M. Friedenwald Memorial Lecture.) *Investigative Ophthalmology*, 1970, 9, 655–680.

Dowling, J. E., & Cowan, W. M. An electron microscopy study of normal and degenerating centrifugal fiber terminals in the pigeon retina. *Zeitschrift für Zellforschung*, 1966, *170*, 205–228.

Dubin, M. W. 1966. The inner plexiform layer of the vertebrate retina: A quantitative and comparative electron microscopic analysis. *Journal of Comparative Neurology*, 1970, 479–506.

Ebbesson, S. O. E., Jane, J. A., & Schroeder, D. M. On the organization of central visual pathways in vertebrates. *Brain Behavior & Evolution*, 1970, *3*, 178–194.

Eikmanns, K. H. Verhaltensphysiologische Untersuchungen uber den Beutefang und das Bewegungssegen der Erdkrote (*Bufo bufo* L.) *Zeitschrift für Tierpsychologie*, 1955, *12*, 229–259.

Ewert, J. P. Neural mechanisms of prey-catching and avoidance behavior in the toad (*Bufo bufo* L.) *Brain, Behavior & Evolution*, 1970, *3*, 36–56.

Ewert, J. P., & Borchers, H. W. Antworten retinaler Ganglienzellen bei freibeweiglichen Kroten. *Journal of Comparative Physiology*, 1974, *92*, 117–130.

Fite, K. V. The visual fields of the frog and toad: A comparative study. *Behavioral Biology*, 1973, *9*, 707–718.

Fite, K. V., & Carey, R. G. *The photoreceptors of frogs and toads: A quantitative study*. Paper presented at the annual meeting of the Association for Research in Vision and Ophthalmology, 1973.

Fite, K. V., Carey, R. G., & Vicario, D. Visual neurons in frog anterior thalamus. *Brain Research*, 1977, *127*, 283–290.

Fite, K. V., & Rego, M. Binocular vision and prey-catching behavior in the leopard frog *Rana pipiens*. Paper presented at annual meeting of the Society for Neuroscience, St. Louis, Missouri, 1974.

Fite, K. V., & Scalia, F. Central visual pathways in the frog. In K. V. Fite (Ed.), *The amphibian visual system: A multidisciplinary approach*. New York, Academic Press, 1976.

Fite, K. V., Soukup, J. & Carey, R. C. Wavelength discrimination in *Rana pipiens:* A re-examination. (In preparation, 1978.)

Gaze, R. M., & Keading, M. J. The visual system and "neuronal specificity." *Nature (London)*, 1972, *237*, 375–378.

Goldstein, E. B., & Wolf, B. M. Regeneration of the green rod pigment in the isolated frog retina. *Vision Research*, 1973, *13*, 527–534.

Gruberg, E. R., & Ambros, V. R. A forebrain visual projection in the frog *(Rana pipiens)*. *Experimental Neurology*, 1974, *44*, 187–197.

Hailman, J. P., & Jaeger, R. G. Phototactic responses to spectrally dominant stimuli and use of color vision by adult anuran amphibians: A comparative survey. *Animal Behavior*, 1974, *22*, 757–795.

Hailman, J. P., & Jaeger, R. G. A model of photoaxis and its evaluation with anuran amphibians. *Behavior*, 1976, *LVI*, 215–249.

Hartline, H. K. The response of single optic nerve fibers of the vertebrate eye to illumination of the retina. *American Journal of Physiology*, 1938, *121*, 400–415.

Hartline, H. K. The receptive fields of optic nerve fibers. *American Journal of Physiology*, 1940, *130*, 690–699.

Herrick, C. J. The amphibian forebrain. III. The optic tracts and centers of amblystoma and the frog. *Journal of Comparative Neurology*, 1925, *39*, 433–489.

Hood, D. C., & Hock, P. A. Recovery of cone receptor activity in the frog's isolated retina. *Vision Research*, 1973, *13*, 1943–1951.

Karten, H. J., Fite, K. V., & Brecha, N. Specific projection of displaced retinal ganglion cells upon the accessory optic system in the pigeon *(Columbia livia)*. *Proceedings of the National Academy of Sciences*, 1977, *74*, 1753–1756.

Keating, M. J., & Kennard, C. Binocular visual neurons in the frog thalamus. *Journal of Physiology (London)*, 1976, *258*, 69–70.

Kicliter, E. Flux, wavelength and movement discrimination in frogs: Forebrain and midbrain contributions. *Brain, Behavior & Evolution*, 1973, *8*, 340–365.

Kicliter, E., & Ebbesson, S. O. E. Organization of the "nonolfactory" telencephalon. In R. Llinas & W. Precht (Eds.), *Frog neurobiology*. Berlin and New York: Springer Verlag, 1976.

Kicliter, E., & Northcutt, R. G. Ascending afferents to the telencephalon of Ranid frogs: An anterograde degeneration study. *Journal of Comparative Neurology*, 1975, *161*, 239–254.

Lazar, G. Role of the accessory optic system in the optokinetic nystagmus of the frog. *Brain, Behavior & Evolution*, 1972, *5*, 443–460.

Lettvin, J. Y., Maturana, H. R., McCulloch, W. S., & Pitts, W. H. What the frog's eye tells the frog's brain. *Proceedings of the Institute of Radio Engineers*, 1959, *47*, 1940–1951.

Lyall, H. G. Cone arrangement of teleost retinae. *Quarterly Journal of Microscopic Science*, 1957, *98*, 101–110.

Marc, R. E., & Sperling, H. G. Color receptor identities of goldfish cones. *Science*, 1976, *191*, 487. (a)

Marc, R. E., & Sperling, H. G. Chromatic organization of the goldfish cone mosaic. *Vision Research*, 1976, *16*, 1211–1224. (b)

Maturana, H. R. The fine structure of the optic nerve and tectum of anurans: An electron microscope study. Unpublished doctoral dissertation, Harvard University, Cambridge, Massachusetts, 1958. (a)

Maturana, H. R. Efferent fibers in the optic nerve of the toad *(Bufo bufo)*. *Journal of Anatomy*, 1958, *92*, 21–27. (b)

Maturana, H. R , & Frenk, S. Synaptic connections of the centrifugal fibers in the pigeon retina. *Science,* 1965, *150,* 359–361.

Maturana, H. R., Lettvin, J. Y., McCulloch, W. S., & Pitts, W. H. Anatomy and physiology of vision in the frog *(Rana piniens). Journal of General Physiology,* 1960, *43* (Supplement 2), 129–175.

Muntz, W. R. A. Microelectode recordings from the diencephalon of the frog *(Rana pipiens)* and a blue-sensitive system. *Journal of Neurophysiology,* 1962, *25,* 699–711.

Muntz, W. R. A. Phototaxis and green rods in Urodeles. *Nature (London),* 1963, *199,* 620.

O'Connell, C. P. The structure of the eye of *Sardinops caerulea, Engraulis mordax.* and four other pelagic marine telcosts. *Journal of Morphology,* 1963, *113,* 287–330.

Reuter, T. Visual pigments and ganglion cell activity in the retinae of tadpoles and adult frogs *(Rana temporaria). Acta Zoologica Fennica,* 1969, *122,* 1–64.

Reuter, T. & Virtanen, K. Border and colour coding in the retina of the frog. *Nature (London),* 1972, *239,* 260–263.

Riss, W., & Jakway, J. S. A perspective on the fundamental retinal projections of vertebrates. *Brain, Behavior & Evolution,* 1970, *3,* 30–35.

Savage, J. M. The geographic distribution of frogs: Patterns and predictions. In J. L. Vial, (Ed.), *Evolutionary biology of the anurans.* University of Missouri Press, Columbia, 1973.

Saxen, L. An atypical form of the double visual cell in the frog *(Rana temporaria* L.). *Acta Anatomica,* 1953, *19,* 190–196.

Saxen, L. The development of the visual cells. Embryological and physiological investigations on amphibia. *Annales Academiae Scientiarum Fennicae,* 1954, *23,* 1–93.

Saxen, L. The initial formation and subsequent development of the double visual cells in amphibia. *Journal of Embryology and Experimental Morphology,* 1956, *4,* 57–66.

Scalia, F. The optic pathway of the frog: Nuclear organization and connections. In R. Llinas & W. Precht (Eds.), *Frog neurobiology.* Berlin: Springer-Verlag., 1976.

Scalia, F., & Coleman, D. Identification of telencephalic-afferent thalamic nuclei associated with the visual system of the frog. *Neuroscience,* 1975, Vol. 1 (abstr.).

Scalia, F., & Coleman, D. Unpublished observations, 1977.

Scalia, F., & Fite, K. A retinotopic analysis of the central connections of the optic nerve in the frog. *Journal of Comparative Neurology,* 1974, *158,* 455–478.

Scheibner, H , Hunold, W , & Bezant, M. Colour discrimination functions of the frog optic tectum *(Rana esculenta). Vision Research,* 1975, *15,* 1175–1180.

Shortess, G. K. Binocular interaction in the frog retina. *Journal of the Optical Society of America,* 1963, *53,* 1423–1429.

Sperry, R. W. Chemoaffinity in the orderly growth of nerve fiber patterns and connections. *Proceedings of the National Academy of Sciences,* 1963, *50,* 703–710.

Sperry, R. W. Embryogenesis of behavioral nerve nets. In R. L. De Hann & H. Ursprung, (Eds.), *Organogenesis.* New York: Holt, Rinehart and Winston, 1965.

Straznicky, K., Gaze, R. M., & Keating, M. J. The retinotectal projections after uncrossing the optic chiasma in *Xenopus* with one compound eye. *Journal of Embryology and Experimental Morphology,* 1971, *26,* 523–542.

Synder, A. W. How fish detect polarized light. *Investigative Opthalmology,* 1973, *12,* 78–79.

5. Color Vision in Goldfish: A Comparison of Psychophysical and Neurophysiological Findings[1]

Ross Beauchamp

I. Introduction

Analysis of color vision in neural terms is simplified in the goldfish by the fact that its three cone pigments have widely separated absorption maxima at 625, 530, and 455 nm (Marks, 1965; Liebman & Entine, 1964; Harosi & MacNichol, 1974). Therefore the cone mechanisms contributing to a neural response anywhere along the visual pathway can be identified by noting the location of peaks in the spectral sensitivity curve. For example, the spectral sensitivity curves of many single optic fibers have a prominent peak at 455 nm with the same shape as the difference spectra of the blue-absorbing cone pigment. The 455-nm peak indicates that these optic fibers are activated by blue-sensitive cones (Beauchamp & Lovasik, 1973). The wide separation of cone absorption maxima also permits the effective use of chromatic adapting backgrounds to reduce the sensitivity of one or more of the cone processes. A bright yellow adapting background, for example, will reduce the sensitivity of green- and red-sensitive cones, allowing the blue-sensitive cones to dominate the response over a wider-than-normal range of the spectrum. Chromatic adapting backgrounds are also useful for identifying interactions between two cone processes. Green- and red-sensitive cones are normally mutually antagonistic in color-coded ganglion cells (Wagner, MacNichol, & Wolbarsht, 1960; Daw, 1968; Beauchamp & Lovasik, 1973). However, the activity of red-sensitive cones alone can be examined by selectively lowering the sensitivity of the green-sensitive cones with a bright blue–green adapting background which bleaches a good deal of green-absorbing but very little red-absorbing pigment.

For a number of years, my students and I have used chromatic adapting techniques to analyze the neural basis of color vision in curarized goldfish. The

[1]Supported by the National Research Council, Canada, and the Medical Research Council, Canada.

63

curarized preparation has the advantage of being suitable both for single cell record-ing (Beauchamp & Daw, 1972; Beauchamp & Lovasik, 1973; Beauchamp, 1974; Beauchamp, 1977) and for psychophysical determination of color vision in the intact animal (Beauchamp & Rowe, 1977). Since preparation and stimulus condi-tons are comparable for single cell and psychophysical measurements, there is justification for relating the two sets of observations.

II. Method

Goldfish were immobilized with curare, respired, and supported so that one eye faced a back projection screen (Figure 5.1). Color backgrounds and superimposed spot stimuli were projected onto the back projection screen. Animals in psychophys-ical experiments were fitted with external heart rate monitor electrodes and shock electrodes. A conditioned fear response to light, inhibition of heart beat, was used to establish thresholds to monochromatic lights (Beauchamp & Rowe, 1977). Animals in neurophysiological experiments had their viewing eye located at the center of a hemisphere filled with water so that receptive fields anywhere in the visual field could be mapped. The optic nerve was exposed by drilling a small hole in the cranium and removing overlying fluid and cartilage. The procedure left the eye and brain intact and the nerve in air for purposes of microelectrode recording (Beauchamp & Lovasik, 1973).

III. Three Components of the Spectral Sensitivity Curve

Psychophysical measurements of increment-threshold spectral sensitivity against a 1.2 log ft-L tungsten-white background gave a spectral sensitivity curve with three components: a peak at 460 nm, a shoulder at 520 nm, and a peak at 660 nm (Figure 5.2A). The shape of the spectral sensitivity curve was the same for noncurarized and curarized animals although the curves of curarized animals were on the average approximately .5 log unit higher in sensitivity than those of noncurarized fish.

Spectral sensitivity curves of the receptive field center of single optic fibers mea-sured against white backgrounds were more variable in shape than psychophysically determined curves but they always had a long-wave peak at 620–660 nm and often a short-wave peak at about 460 nm (Figure 5.2B). Evidence for an additional medium-wave component was seen for some fibers. The long- and short-wave peaks were seen also in on–off cells (Figure 5.2C) where on and off phasic re-sponses occurred at wavelengths across the spectrum.

The presence of more than one class of optic fiber, each having the potential of carrying threshold responses to the brain, necessitates careful stimulus specification when reporting spectral sensitivity curves (Northmore & Muntz, 1974). Stimulus parameters such as size and movement may influence which fiber class mediates the threshold response at a given wavelength with consequent changes in the shape of

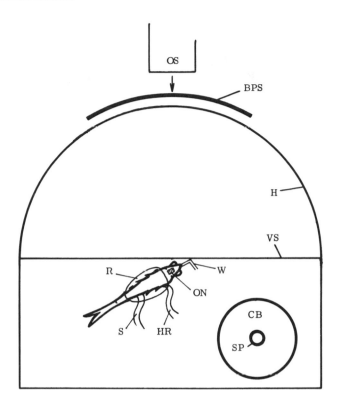

Figure 5.1 Top view of apparatus used for stimulation of goldfish eye. A curarized fish, held in a restrainer (R) and respired with aerated water (W), is fitted with external shock electrodes (S) and heart rate electrodes (HR). The fish's left eye is at the center of a hemisphere (H) filled with water and supported by a vertical plastic sheet (VS). The fish views a back projection screen (BPS) illuminated by an optical system (OS). The stimulus seen by the fish, a monochromatic spot (SP) superimposed on a chromatic background (CB), is illustrated in the inset. In experiments where single fiber recordings are made from the optic nerve, the optic nerve is exposed by drilling a hole (ON) in the cranium, and raising the water level to cover the eye but not the hole in the cranium.

spectral sensitivity curves. For example, on–off fibers are particularly sensitive to small moving stimuli and, in free-swimming measurement situations where the eye may move relative to the stimulus, as in studies by Yager (1967, 1969, 1970, 1974), Yager and Thorpe (1970), and Thorpe (1971), on–off fibers may respond first to threshold stimulation and thereby determine the shape of the spectral sensitivity curve. Because on–off fibers seem to have less antagonistic input from the three cone mechanisms (Beauchamp, 1974), the shape of the on–off fiber-dominated psychophysical curve may be quite different from the curve obtained for stimulus conditions in which color-coded units predominate, as when a stationary stimulus is used.

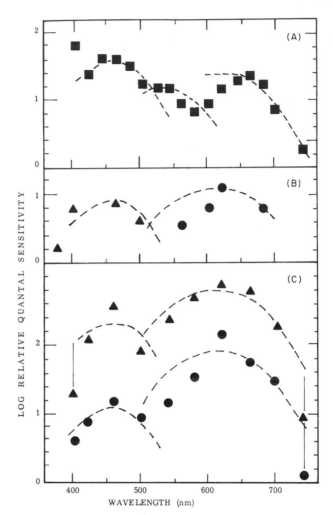

Figure 5.2. Goldfish spectral sensitivity measured against a tungsten-white adapting background. (A) Mean curve for seven fish using a conditioned heart rate procedure and a 1.2 log ft-L background. Here, and in panels below, the components of the curve are fitted with photopigment nomograms with peak sensitivity at 455, 530, and 625 nm (Ebrey & Honig, 1977). (B) Curve from the receptive field center of a single, color-coded optic nerve fiber using a 2 log ft-L background. Triangles represent off responses, circles on responses. (C) The curve for the on response (circles) and the off response (triangles) of a single, on–off, non-color-coded optic nerve fiber using a .1 log ft-L background. Curves have been displaced on the ordinate for clarity.

IV. The Blue Mechanism Response

About 25% of goldfish cones contain blue-absorbing photopigment (Stell & Harosi, 1976; Marc & Sperling, 1976) and spectral sensitivity curves measured against a tungsten-white background are characterized by a prominent short-wave peak (Figure 5.2). In the psychophysically determined curve, the short-wave peak is the most sensitive of the three components (Figure 5.2A). It is particularly notice-able when using a yellow adapting background (Figure 5.5A). Since the short-wave peak has the same shape and peak location as the absorption spectrum of the blue-sensitive pigment, there is little doubt that it originates in activity of blue-sensitive cones.

V. The Red and Green Mechanism Responses

The long-wave component of the psychophysically determined spectral sensitiv-ity curve peaks at 660 nm, about 35 nm above the 625-nm absorption maximum of the red-absorbing photopigment, while the midspectral component peaks a little below the absorption maximum of the green-absorbing photopigment (Figure 5.2A). Both shifts can be accounted for by antagonistic interaction between red- and green-sensitive cones when both are simultaneously stimulated at wavelengths be-tween 500 and 600 nm (Wagner *et al.*, 1960; Daw, 1968; Beauchamp & Lovasik, 1973). If green mechanism antagonism is reduced by application of a blue–green adapting background, the long-wave component peaks at 625 nm and fits the ab-sorption spectrum for the red-absorbing cone pigment (Figure 5.3A). In addition, neural activity originating from beta band absorption by red-sensitive pigment be-comes apparent (Figure 5.3B). It is not clear how beta band activity peaking at 400–

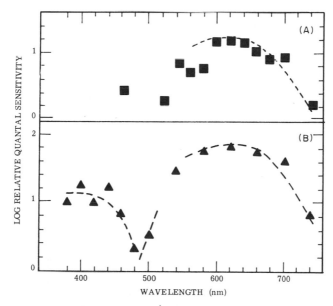

Figure 5.3. Spectral sensitivity against a blue–green adapting background designed to re-duce blue–green antagonism on the red-sensitive cone response. (A) Psychophysically deter-mined thresholds using a 550-nm short-pass filter in a 2.9 log ft-L beam. (B) Red-off-center re-sponse of a single optic fiber measured against a blue–green background using a 550-nm short-pass filter in a 2 log ft-L beam.

420 nm influences the sensitivity of blue-absorbing cones responding at the same wavelengths. However, short-wave peaks may have been mistakenly attributed to blue-sensitive cones when in fact they originated in beta band absorption by red-sensitive cones (Spekreijse, Wagner, & Wolbarsht, 1972).

VI. High Aberrant Short-Wave Sensitivity

As with previous investigators (Yager, 1967; Muntz & Northmore, 1970), we have noted psychophysically determined sensitivities at the short end of the spectrum that are higher than predicted from the pigment absorption curve. Against a 1.2 log ft-L white background, only the 400-nm point is affected (Figure 5.2A). We wondered if red mechanism beta band activity might be responsible for this high 400-nm point. To test this explanation we added a yellow adapting background to the white background to depress red-sensitive cone activity. Red mechanism sensitivity was indeed depressed, but the high aberrant sensitivity at 400 nm remained (Figure 5.4). We concluded that activity in red- and green-sensitive cones could not

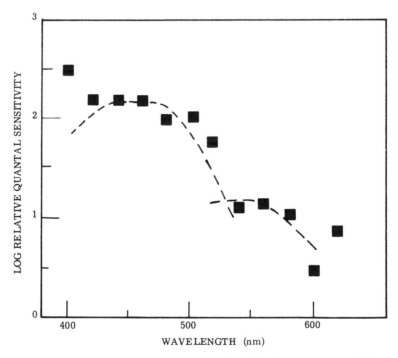

Figure 5.4. Spectral sensitivity against a 1.2 log ft-L white background to which is added a bright yellow background to selectively depress the red mechanism sensitivity (550-nm long-pass filter in a 2.9 log ft-L beam). Note that high aberrant sensitivity at 400 nm remains.

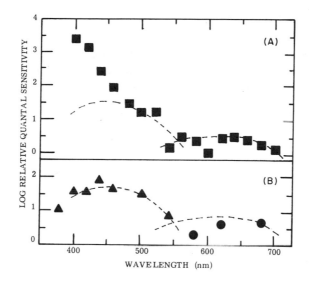

Figure 5.5. Spectral sensitivity against a yellow background. (A) Psychophysical measurements using a 550-long-pass filter in a 2.9 log ft-L beam. (B) Receptive field center response using a 550-long-wave pass filter in a 1.5 log ft-L beam; circles represent on responses; triangles, off responses.

account for high aberrant short-wave sensitivity (Rowe, 1975; Beauchamp & Rowe, in preparation). An observation of some interest was the absence of prominent aberrant high blue sensitivity in optic fiber spectral sensitivity curves when using a tungsten-white adapting background (Figure 5.2B).

VII. Yellow Adapting Background

Against a yellow background alone, the psychophysically determined curves for some fish showed high aberrant sensitivity not just at 400 nm but at all wavelengths below 460 nm (Figure 5.5A). In other fish, only sensitivity at 400 nm was high, as in Figure 5.4. Similarly, yellow adapting conditions for a single optic fiber did not lead to aberrant high sensitivity (Figure 5.5B). Why there should be prominent, psychophysically determined high blue sensitivity in some fish and not others is somewhat of a puzzle. A possible explanation could be the presence of scattered light that extended into the far retinal periphery. Curves for single optic fibers were not affected because the adapting backgrounds used, which were approximately 100° in diameter, were large enough to adapt the total receptive field. However, in the psychophysical experiments, a ring of about 40° or so of peripheral retina remained relatively dark-adapted, and hence sensitive to scattered blue light.

VIII. Conclusion

A comparison of spectral sensitivity curves obtained psychophysically from intact animals and electrophysiologically from single optic fibers has provided insights into goldfish color vision. Current experiments extending the use of colored adapting backgrounds (Beauchamp, Rowe, & O'Reilly, in preparation) and suprathreshold work related to wavelength discrimination (Beauchamp, 1977) may further broaden our understanding of color vision.

ACKNOWLEDGMENTS

John Rowe was responsible for gathering and interpreting psychophysical data as part of a thesis (1975). John Lovasik collaborated in the neurophysiological work, and Betty Wilkinson typed the manuscript.

REFERENCES

Beauchamp, R. D. Cone mechanisms initiating response of on–off goldfish optic fibers. *Nature*, 1974, *249*, 668–670.

Beauchamp, R. D. Action potential patterns are a code for color in goldfish optic fibers. Papers presented at the Spring meeting of the Association for Research in Vision and Ophthalmology, Sarasota, 1977.

Beauchamp, R. D., & Daw, N. W. Rod and cone input to single goldfish optic nerve fibers. *Vision Research*, 1972, *12*, 1201–1212.

Beauchamp, R. D., & Lovasik, J. V. Blue mechanism response of single goldfish optic fibers. *Journal of Neurophysiology*, 1973, *36*, 925–939.

Beauchamp, R. D., & Rowe, J. S. Goldfish spectral sensitivity: A conditioned heart rate measure in restrained or curarized fish. *Vision Research*, 1977, *17*, 617–624.

Beauchamp, R. D., & Rowe, J. S. Aberrant high blue sensitivity in goldfish spectral sensitivity curves. (In preparation.)

Beauchamp, R. D., Rowe, J. S., & O'Reilly, L. Goldfish spectral sensitivity II: Isolation of cone mechanisms using chromatic adapting backgrounds. (In preparation.)

Daw, N. W. Color-coded ganglion cells in the goldfish retina: Extension of their receptive fields by means of new stimuli. *Journal of Physiology (London)*, 1968, *197*, 567–592.

Ebrey, T. G., & Honig, B. New wavelength dependent visual pigment nomograms. *Visual Research*, 1977, *17*, 147–151.

Harosi, F. I., & MacNichol, E. F. Visual pigments of goldfish cones. *Journal of General Physiology*, 1974, *63*, 279–304.

Liebman, P. A., & Entine, G. Sensitive low-light-level microspectrophotometer: Detection of photosensitive pigments of retinal cones. *Journal of the Optical Society of America*, 1964, *54*, 1451–1459.

Marc, R. E., & Sperling, H. G. Color receptor identities of goldfish cones. *Science*, 1976, *191*, 487–489.

Marks, W. B. Visual pigments of single goldfish cones. *Journal of Physiology (London)*, 1965, *178*, 14–32.

Muntz, W. R. A., & Northmore, D. P. M. Vision and visual pigments in a fish *Scardinius erythrophthalmus* (the rudd). *Vision Research*, 1970, *10*, 281–298.

Northmore, D. P. M., & Muntz, W. R. A. Effects of stimulus size of spectral sensitivity in a fish (*Scardinius erythrophthalmus*) measured with a classical conditioning paradigm. *Vision Research,* 1974, *14,* 503–514.

Rowe, J. S. Goldfish spectral sensitivity: A classical conditioning measure. Unpublished masters thesis, University of Waterloo, 1975.

Spekreijse, H., Wagner, H. G., & Wolbarsht, M. L. Spectral and spatial coding of ganglion cell responses in goldfish retina. *Journal of Neurophysiology,* 1972, *35,* 73–86.

Stell, W. R., & Harosi, F. I. Cone structure and visual pigment content in the retina of the goldfish. *Vision Research,* 1976, *16,* 647–657.

Thorpe, S. A. Behavioral measures of spectral sensitivity of the goldfish at different temperatures. *Vision Research,* 1971, *11,* 419–433.

Wagner, H. G., MacNichol, E. F., Jr., & Wolbarsht, M. L. The response properties of single ganglion cells in the goldfish retina. *Journal of General Physiology,* 1960, *48,* 45–62 (suppl.).

Yager, D. Behavioral measures and theoretical analysis of spectral sensitivity and spectral saturation in the goldfish *Carassius auratus. Vision Research,* 1967, *7,* 707–727.

Yager, D. Behavioral measures of spectral sensitivity in the goldfish following chromatic adaptation. *Vision Research,* 1969, *9,* 179–186.

Yager, D. Spectral sensitivity with the freely moving eye. *Vision Research,* 1970, *10,* 521–523.

Yager, D. Effects of chromatic adaptation on saturation discrimination in goldfish. *Vision Research,* 1974, *14,* 1089–1094.

Yager, D., & Thorpe, S. Investigations of goldfish color vision. In W. Stebbins (ed.), *Animal psychophysics.* New York: Appleton-Century-Crofts, 1970.

6. Cone Pigment Regeneration in Frogs and Humans[1]

E. Bruce Goldstein

The research reported in this chapter describes how I have used the early receptor potential (ERP) to study the regeneration of visual pigments in frogs and humans. This research began with the observation that when a frog's retina that has been separated from the pigment epithelium and removed from the eyecup is bleached so that its ERP is reduced to about 30% of its dark-adapted amplitude, the ERP subsequently recovers to almost its original dark-adapted amplitude as the retina sits in the dark following the bleach. This result, shown in Figure 6.1, was surprising because many people had shown that when the retina is isolated from the pigment epithelium little rhodopsin regenerates (Kuhne, 1879; Zewi, 1939; Baumann, 1965). I confirmed this lack of appreciable rhodopsin regeneration by extracting rhodopsin from retinas after bleaching and then allowing time for pigment regeneration. After 10 min in the dark, less than 5% of the rhodopsin regenerates, while the ERP recovers to over 80% of its dark-adapted amplitude.

The conclusion that rhodopsin regeneration could not explain the ERP's recovery in the dark still left open the possibility that one of the frog's other pigments might be responsible, and the ERP action spectrum of the fully dark-adapted retina shown in Figure 6.2 indicates that this is the case. The curve in this figure peaks at about 580 nm and falls close to Liebman and Entine's (1967) microspectrophotometric measurements, published almost simultaneously with the ERP results, of the pigment of the frog's principal cones that absorb maximally at about 580 nm.[2] The conclusion that this 580-nm pigment regenerates in the isolated retina is supported by the fact that the ERP action spectrum measured in a bleached retina which has been allowed to recover for 30 min still peaks at 580 nm and matches the original action spectrum (Goldstein, 1967, 1968a).

[1]Supported by United States Public Health Service Grant EY-00135.

[2]Liebman and Entine (1968) call this pigment a 575-nm pigment, although the density spectrum in Figure 16 of their paper peaks slightly above 580 nm.

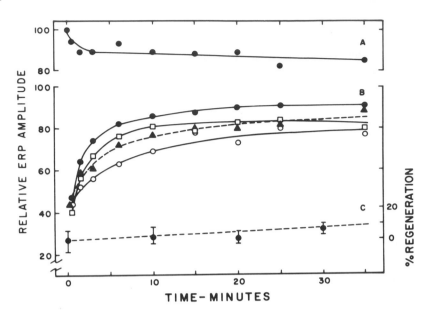

Figure 6.1. (A) Control. ERP responses generated by a series of white test flashes. No bleaching flash presented. (B) Recovery of the ERP of the isolated frog retina at 23°C (Goldstein, 1967, 1968a). The procedure for determining these curves is as follows: A dim test flash that elicits a response of 30–70 μV is presented to the dark-adapted retina, and this flash is followed by a high-intensity white flash that bleaches about 75% of the rhodopsin. The bleaching flash is followed by a series of test flashes identical to the one presented to the dark-adapted retina. The amplitudes of the responses generated by these test flashes are expressed as a percentage of the response to the test flash presented prior to the bleaching flash. Each curve is for a test flash of a different wavelength: $\bigcirc$ = 380 nm; $\blacktriangle$ = 490 nm; $\square$ = 630 nm; $\bullet$ = white. Each point is the average of from four to eight experiments. (C) Regeneration of rhodopsin in isolated frog retina at 23°C. The points are rhodopsin concentrations determined by extraction with hexadecyl-trimethylammonium bromide. Concentration is expressed in relative units (left ordinate) with the concentration in the dark-adapted eye being set at 100. The concentration can also be read as percentage regeneration from the scale on the right ordinate. Percentage regeneration = 100 $(D_t - D_0)/(D_d - D_0)$ where D_t = pigment density at time t, D_0 = density immediately after the bleaching flash (t = 0), and D_d = density in the dark-adapted eye. Each point is the mean of from three to seven experiments. Brackets indicate ranges. The dashed line is a plot of the percentage of rhodopsin regeneration versus time, adapted from Zewi's (1939) measurements on isolated frog retina. [From E. B. Goldstein, Early receptor potential of the isolated frog (*Rana pipiens*) retina. *Vision Research*, 1967, *7*, 837–845.]

Two aspects of these results are surprising. First, the fact that the 580-nm cone pigment generates most of the frog's ERP is surprising since this pigment accounts for only about 1% of the total visual pigment in this retina. In the rod-dominated rat retina, ERP amplitude is proportional to the number of visual pigment molecules excited by a flash (Cone, 1964, 1969, pp. 187–200). In the duplex frog retina, however, it appears that rhodopsin, which accounts for about 93% of the pigment in

Figure 6.2. Action spectrum of the ERP of the isolated frog retina (Goldstein, 1967, 1968a, 1968b). Sensitivity is the reciprocal of the number of photons per test flash needed to elicit a constant amplitude of ERP (20–40 μV). Average of 10 retinas. The dashed line is the absorption spectrum of the frog's principal cone pigment measured by Liebman and Entine (1968). The correspondence between the peaks of the principal cone pigment absorption spectrum and the ERP action spectrum indicates that the principal cone pigment generates most of the ERP in this retina. The higher sensitivity of the ERP action spectrum at short wavelengths compared to the absorption spectrum is due to the response generated by the frog's 502- and 433-nm pigments.

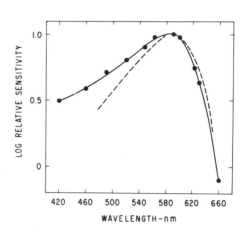

the retina, makes only a small contribution to ERP.[3] A rough calculation indicates that a molecule of 580-nm cone pigment results in a response approximately 250 to 300 times larger than the response of a molecule of 502-nm pigment.[4]

The second surprising aspect of these results is the regeneration of the 580-nm cone pigment in the isolated retina. Somehow, most of the cone pigment manages to regenerate under conditions that keep most of the rhodopsin in the bleached state. I will return to this result later, but first will consider some experiments on the cone dominance of the ERP.

Evidence that cone domination of the ERP is not restricted to the frog is provided by the action spectrum of the live monkey, shown in Figure 6.3 (Goldstein, 1969). The curve in Figure 6.3 is located far to the right of the absorption spectrum of the monkey's rod pigment ($\lambda_{max} = 502$ nm), which indicates that at least half of the monkey's ERP is generated by its long-wave absorbing cone pigments ($\lambda_{max} = 535$ and 575 nm). This conclusion is supported by the fact that in the live monkey the

---

[3]"Rhodopsin" is used here to refer to the 502-nm pigment that Liebman and Entine (1968) found in both the frog's red rods and accessory cones. Although the red rods contain 93% of the visual pigment in the retina compared to only .5% for the accessory cones, the possibility cannot be ruled out that part or all of the ERP generated by the 502-nm pigment may come from the accessory cones.

[4]This is calculated from the results of selective bleaching experiments reported in Figure 3 of Goldstein and Wolf (1973). These results indicate that the relative amplitudes of response to a 440-nm test flash are 30.7, 23.7, and 45.6 for the 580-, 502-, and 433-nm pigments, respectively. When these responses are corrected for the relative extinction of each pigment at 440 nm the relative response of each pigment becomes 153 (580), 40.9 (502), and 46.1 (433). The division of these responses by the relative concentrations of each pigment (580 = 1.25%, 502 = 93.3%, 433 = 5.5%; Liebman & Entine, 1968) indicates that each molecule of 580-nm pigment results in a response about 280 times larger than each molecule of 502-nm pigment and that each molecule of 433 pigment results in a response about 20 times larger than each molecule of 502-nm pigment. A similar conclusion can be reached by the fact that 75–80% of ERP elicited by a white flash is due to the 580-nm cone pigment (Goldstein, 1968b).

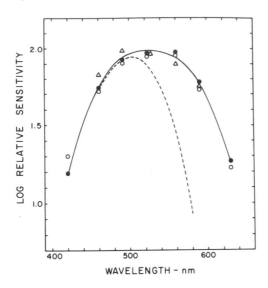

Figure 6.3. Action spectrum of the monkey ERP. △ = live monkey; ● = whole excised eye; ○ = peripheral retina. Sensitivity is the reciprocal number of photons per test flash needed to elicit a constant amplitude ERP (about 50 μV). Each point is the average of from five to eight experiments. [From E. B. Goldstein, Contribution of cones to the early receptor potential in the rhesus monkey. *Nature*, 1969, *222*, 1273–1274.]

ERP recovers in the dark with a half-time of 2 min, a rate slightly slower than the rate of psychophysically measured cone recovery, but much faster than the 5-min half-time of rod recovery (Goldstein, 1969). Similarly, E. Berson and I found that the human ERP recovers at the same rate as psychophysical cone recovery, as shown in Figure 6.4 (Goldstein & Berson, 1969), and Carr and Siegel (1970) later showed that the action spectrum of the human ERP peaks at 560 nm. Human and monkey cone pigments, which account for only 1–2% of the total visual pigment in these retinas, generate most of the human and monkey ERP.

The cone dominance of the human ERP enabled us to use this response to measure cone pigment regeneration in patients with retinitis pigmentosa (Berson & Goldstein, 1970a, 1970b, 1970c). Figure 6.5 shows the results of experiments on two siblings with dominantly inherited retinitis pigmentosa. The ERP in these patients recovers over three times as fast as the ERP of normal subjects. This result is consistent with Alpern's (1977) and Pearlman's (1977) fundus reflectometry measurements which indicate that rhodopsin regeneration is accelerated in humans with retinitis pigmentosa and in rats with hereditary retinal distrophy.

The use of fundus reflectometry by Alpern and Pearlman raises an interesting question. If pigment regeneration can be measured using fundus reflectometry, why use the ERP? One answer to this question is that it is desirable to be able to use more than one method to measure the same phenomenon; but there is a more important reason for using the ERP. When a flash of light elicits an ERP, the response comes from all the receptors that are stimulated. Since our stimulating flash covers an area of about 60°, we are stimulating both foveal and peripheral cone pigments, and since over 99% of the cones in the human retina are peripheral cones (LeGrand, 1957), the ERP generated by our stimulus flash is therefore a measure of peripheral cone activity. When we consider the fact that fundus reflectometry can-

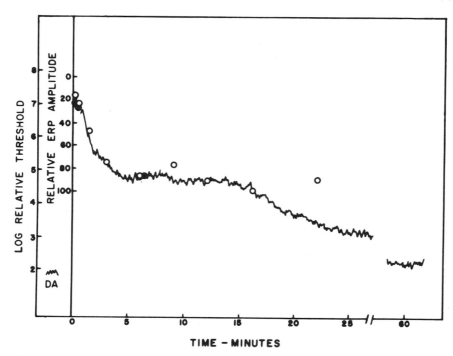

Figure 6.4. Comparison of human ERP recovery and psychophysical dark adaptation. Both the psychophysical curve and the ERP recovery were measured after presentation of a 30-msec long-wavelength ($\lambda > 500$ nm) bleaching flash at $t = 0$. Psychophysical adaptation was measured with an 11° white flash located 8° above the fovea. The ERP test flashes covered an area of 60° and were centrally fixated. The ERP amplitudes have been scaled along the ordinate to fit the psychophysically measured dark-adaptation curve and are expressed relative to the response recorded from the dark-adapted eye prior to bleaching (dark-adapted response = 100). Recovery measured with white test flashes is indicated by open circles, and red ($\lambda > 620$ nm) test flashes with filled circles. Each point is the average of from three to four experiments on a single subject. The record marked DA is the dark-adapted threshold measured before bleaching. [From E. B. Goldstein & E. L. Berson, Cone dominance of the human early receptor potential. *Nature*, 1969, *222*, 1272–1273.]

not be used to measure peripheral cone pigments due to the abundance of rods in the periphery, we can appreciate the importance of ERP as a tool for measuring these pigments. The ERP is the only method now available to measure peripheral cone pigments *in vivo* in retinas such as the human which contain many more rods than cones.

The ERP holds a similar advantage over microspectrophotometry, a method that has yielded impressive results when measuring pigments in excised human and monkey retinas (Brown & Wald, 1963, 1964; Marks, Dobelle, & MacNichol, 1964), but that cannot at present measure pigments in intact human or monkey retinas. A similar situation exists in the frog. Liebman and Entine's (1967, 1968) measurements of the absorption spectra of frog cones were done on cones isolated from the retina and placed on a coverslip. Microspectrophotometric measurements

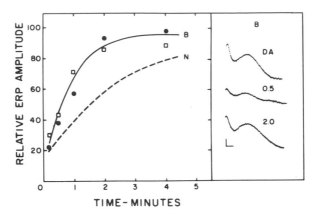

Figure 6.5. ERP recovery for two siblings with dominantly inherited retinitis pigmentosa after a 30-msec long-wavelength (λ > 500 nm) bleaching flash presented at t = 0. ERP amplitudes for each subject are expressed relative to the response recorded from the dark-adapted eye prior to bleaching (dark-adapted response = 100). Data points are the averages of from two to four responses for each subject. The solid line is an exponential curve with a half-time of 35 sec. The dashed line, which is the average recovery curve for four normal subjects, is an exponential function with a half-time of 165 sec. Representative responses for one subject with retinitis pigmentosa (dark adapted and .5 and 2.0 min after the bleaching flash) are illustrated on the right. Calibration symbol indicates .5 msec horizontally and 50 μV vertically. [From E. L. Berson & E. B. Goldstein, Recovery of the human early receptor potential during dark adaptation in hereditary retinal disease. *Vision Research*, 1970, *10*, 219–226.]

of cones in the intact frog retina are precluded by the size and abundance of the rods surrounding the cones.

In addition to providing information about the regeneration of cone pigments, the ERP has provided some information about a very conelike rod pigment: the green rod pigment of the frog (λ_{max} = 433 nm). Exposing the frog's isolated retina to wavelengths greater than 550 nm selectively bleaches the frog's principal cone pigment and rhodopsin while leaving the green rod pigment. If, while the long-wave bleach is present, we present a white bleaching flash to bleach the green rod pigment and then present dim 440-nm test flashes, we find that the response generated by these test flashes increases in the dark with a rate equal to or greater than the rate of cone pigment regeneration in the isolated retina. In addition, the action spectrum of this recovered response matches the absorption spectrum of the frog's green rod pigment (Goldstein & Wolf, 1973). Thus, the frog's green rod pigment, like the principal cone pigment, but unlike the rod pigment rhodopsin, regenerates in the isolated retina. Other investigators have also observed that the frog's green rods have conelike properties. For example, Dartnall (1967) has shown that the frog's green rod pigment, like many cone pigments, is destroyed by hydroxylamine, while rhodopsin is not, and Reuter (1966, 1969) has found that the green rod pigment regenerates faster than rhodopsin and has many other conelike properties.

It is obvious from the preceding that the ERP provides an excellent tool for measuring difficult-to-measure pigments. But we are still left with two questions: First, why do the cones generate such a large ERP compared to the rods? Second, what is the mechanism responsible for cone and green rod pigment regeneration in the isolated frog retina?

Neither of these questions has been answered adequately. One answer that has been proposed to the first question is that the large cone ERP is due to the fact that the pigment-containing lamellae of the cone outer segments are open to extracellular space whereas the rod lamellae are not (Moody & Robinson, 1960; Nilsson, 1963; Lettvin, 1965; Cohen, 1969; Cone, 1969, pp. 187– 200; Cone & Pak, 1971). This hypothesis runs into difficulty, however, when we remember that the ERP generated by the rod-dominated rat retina, which has closed rod lamellae, is as large as the ERP generated by the all-cone retina of the ground squirrel (Cone, 1964; Pak & Ebrey, 1966).[5]

The second question is very important because the answer might help us to understand the process of visual pigment regeneration in general. One of the problems facing the biochemists, who will, I hope, eventually discover the mechanism of visual pigment regeneration, is to determine exactly what happens in the pigment epithelium during regeneration. It is generally accepted that migration of a product of bleaching from the retina to the pigment epithelium and back to the retina is an important step in the regeneration of rhodopsin (Wald, 1934, 1935a, 1935b; Hubbard & Wald, 1952; Hubbard & Coleman, 1959; Reuter, White, & Wald, 1971). The fact that cone pigments can regenerate in the isolated retina means, however, that migration to the pigment epithelium is not a *necessary* condition for cone pigment regeneration. Whatever substance is necessary to catalyze cone pigment regeneration is either contained within the receptor or is nearby, perhaps deposited there by the absent pigment epithelium.[6]

That this regeneration in the absence of the pigment epithelium does not occur only for frog cone pigment has been demonstrated by Cone and Brown (1969). They found that rhodopsin will regenerate in an isolated rat retina placed inside a small, moist chamber. These demonstrations of both cone and rod pigment regeneration in the absence of pigment epithelium does not mean, however, that we should ignore the pigment epithelium in our search for the mechanism of pigment regeneration. When pigment regeneration does occur in the absence of the pigment epithelium it is much slower than the regeneration occurring when the pigment epithelium is present. The rhodopsin regeneration observed by Cone and Brown in the isolated rat retina takes about 3 hr whereas rhodopsin regenerates in the live animal within 90 min (Dowling, 1960). Similarly, cone pigment regenerates more rapidly in the live frog or excised eye than in the isolated retina (Taylor, 1969; Price, 1977). Figure

---

[5]Cone (1969, pp. 187–200) and Govardovskii (1975) have suggested a way out of this dilemma by hypothesizing that the rat's rod lamellae may be connected to the extracellular space by small tubules that are broken during fixation and are therefore not seen in electron micrographs. While this is a possible explanation, it is unsatisfying in the absence of any evidence.

[6]The fact that the principal cone pigment and green rod pigment regeneration occurs in the isolated retina following a 1-msec flash or a long-wave bleach eliminates the possibility that this regeneration is due to the photoisomerization of a short-wave absorbing photoproduct of bleaching, as described by Baumann (1970) and Frank (1969).

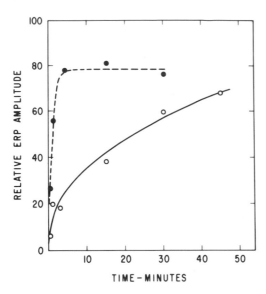

Figure 6.6. ERP recovery after a 5-min bleach at 23° C for the excised opened eye cup (●) and isolated retina (○) (Price, 1977).

6.6 compares cone pigment regeneration in the isolated frog retina to regeneration measured in the excised open eye, both after 5-min bleaches (Price, 1977), and shows that the presence of the pigment epithelium in the excised eye preparation greatly increases the rate of cone pigment regeneration.

Another difference between pigment regeneration in the isolated retina and in the live animal is that, in the isolated retina, regeneration is slowed by repeated bleaches, as shown in Figure 6.7 (Goldstein, 1968a), or by longer bleaches (Goldstein & Price, 1975; Price, 1977), while regeneration in the live animal is maintained for the lifetime of the animal. Whatever substance is responsible for pigment regeneration in the isolated retina is apparently used up by repeated or long bleaches.

Where does all of this leave us? Some mechanism for pigment regeneration exists in the outer segments and this mechanism is either greatly enhanced or augmented by a mechanism residing in the pigment epithelium. I had planned to end this chapter by discussing an experiment designed to investigate the relationship between cone pigment regeneration and the pigment epithelium. Unfortunately, the experiment is yet to be completed, due partially to the coldness of the winter of 1977 and the resulting short supply of frogs. However, I would like to describe the experiment anyway since it provides another example of how the ERP is useful in studying visual pigments.

My proposed experiment is based on that of Reuter et al. (1971). They showed that in the bullfrog retina, rhodopsin, a vitamin A_1 pigment, is segregated in the ventral retina, and porphyropsin, a vitamin A_2 pigment, is segregated in the dorsal retina, as shown in Figure 6.8A. They further showed that vitamins A_1 and A_2 migrate to the pigment epithelium during bleaching and migrate back to the retina during regeneration. This was demonstrated by first light-adapting a frog for 2–3 hr, then decapitating the frog, dissecting the retina from the pigment epithelium, rotat-

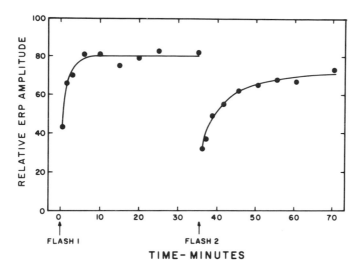

Figure 6.7. ERP recovery in the isolated frog retina measured with a white test flash after 1-msec white bleaching flashes presented at $t = 0$ and $t = 35.5$ min. Mean of three experiments (Goldstein, 1968a).

ing the retina 180°, and replacing it on the pigment epithelium. Thus when rotated, the ventral retina contacts the dorsal pigment epithelium and the dorsal retina, the ventral pigment epithelium, as shown in Figure 6.8C. Reuter *et al.* then allowed time for pigment regeneration to take place. They found that rhodopsin regenerated in the dorsal retina (which previously contained porphyropsin) and porphyropsin regenerated in the ventral retina (which previously contained rhodopsin). Vitamins A_1 and A_2 had migrated to the pigment epithelium during bleaching, as shown in Figure 6.8B, and then back to the rotated retina during regeneration, as shown in Figure 6.8D, thereby reversing the location of rhodopsin and porphyropsin in the retina.

The questions that we plan to ask with the aid of the ERP are: (*a*) Is A_1 cone pigment ($\lambda_{max} = 580$ nm) segregated in the ventral retina and A_2 cone pigment ($\lambda_{max} = 620$ nm) in the dorsal retina? (*b*) Do the cone pigment retinals migrate to the pigment epithelium and back during bleaching and regeneration? We plan to answer these questions by repeating Reuter *et al.*'s experiments, but instead of measuring rod pigments by extraction, as they did, we will measure cone pigments with the ERP. We will answer the first question by measuring the action spectra of the ERP in the dorsal and ventral parts of dark adapted retinas and the second, by measuring action spectra after bleaching the retina, rotating it on the pigment epithelium, and allowing time for regeneration. If, in fact, the A_1 and A_2 cone pigments switch positions in the rotated retina, as did the rod pigments in the experiments of Reuter *et al.*, then we will have shown that although cone pigments can regenerate in the absence of the pigment epithelium, the cone retinals will migrate to the pigment epithelium and back to the retina if the pigment epithelium is

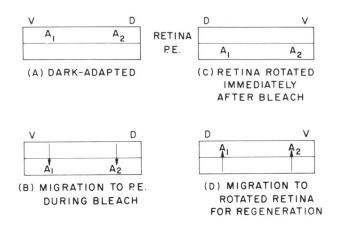

Figure 6.8. The Reuter *et al.* (1971) experiment. (A) The dark-adapted retina contains rhodopsin, a vitamin A_1 pigment, in the ventral retina (V) and porphyropsin, a vitamin A_2 pigment, in the dorsal retina (D). (B) The retina is bleached and vitamins A_1 and A_2 migrate to the ventral and dorsal pigment epithelium, respectively. (C) Near the end of bleaching, the retina is lifted from the pigment epithelium, rotated 180°, and replaced on the pigment epithelium. The dorsal retina then contacts the ventral pigment epithelium (containing A_1) and the ventral retina contacts the dorsal pigment epithelium (containing A_2). (D) A_1 and A_2 migrate back to the retina during dark adaptation and regenerate rhodopsin in the dorsal retina and porphyropsin in the ventral retina.

present. If, on the other hand, the A_1 and A_2 cone pigments do not switch positions in the rotated retina we will have demonstrated an important difference between rod pigment regeneration and cone pigment regeneration.

REFERENCES

Alpern, M. Personal communication, 1977.

Baumann, C. Die Photosensitivitat des Sehpurpurs in der isolierten Netzhaut. *Vision Research,* 1965, *5,* 425–434.

Baumann, C. Regeneration of rhodopsin in the isolated retina of the frog (*Rana esculenta*). *Vision Research,* 1970, *10,* 627–637.

Berson, E. L., & Goldstein, E. B. Recovery of the human early receptor potential during dark adaptation in hereditary retinal disease. *Vision Research,* 1970, *10,* 219–226. (a)

Berson, E. L., & Goldstein, E. B. The early receptor potential in dominantly inherited retinitis pigmentosa. *Archives of Ophthalmology,* 1970, *83,* 412–420. (b)

Berson, E. L., & Goldstein, E. B. The early receptor potential in sex-linked retinitis pigmentosa. *Investigative Ophthalmology,* 1970, *9,* 58–63. (c)

Brown, P. K., & Wald, G. Visual pigments in human and monkey retinas. *Nature,* 1963, *200,* 37–43.

Brown, P. K., & Wald, G. Visual pigments in single rods and cones of the human retina. *Science,* 1964, *14,* 45–52.

Carr, R., & Siegel, I. M. Action spectrum of the human early receptor potential. *Nature,* 1970, *225,* 88–89.

Cohen, A. I. New evidence supporting the linkage to extracellular space of outer segment saccules of frog cones but not rods. *Journal of Cell Biology*, 1969, *37*, 424–444.

Cone, R. A. Early receptor potential of the vertebrate retina. *Nature*, 1964, *204*, 737–739.

Cone, R. A. The early receptor potential. In *Processing of optical data by organisms and machines*. New York: Academic Press, 1969.

Cone, R. A., & Brown, P. K. Spontaneous regeneration of rhodopsin in the isolated rat retina. *Nature*, 1969, *221*, 818–820.

Cone, R. A., & Pak, W. L., The early receptor potential. In W. R. Lowenstein (Ed.), *Handbook of sensory physiology* (Vol 1). New York: Springer Verlag, 1970.

Dartnall, H. J. A. The visual pigment of the green rods. *Vision Research*, 1967, *7*, 1–16.

Dowling, J. E. Night blindness, dark adaptation, and the electroretinogram. *American Journal of Ophthalmology*, 1960, *50*, 875–887.

Frank, R. N. Photoproducts of rhodopsin bleaching in the isolated, perfused frog retina. *Vision Research*, 1969, *9*, 1415–1433.

Goldstein, E. B. Early receptor potential of the isolated frog (*Rana pipiens*) retina. *Vision Research*, 1967, *7*, 837–845.

Goldstein, E. B. Early receptor potential of the isolated frog (*Rana pipiens*) retina. Unpublished doctoral dissertation, Brown University, 1968. (a)

Goldstein, E. B. Visual pigments and the early receptor potential of the isolated frog retina. *Vision Research*, 1968, *8*, 953–963. (b)

Goldstein, E. B. Contribution of cones to the early receptor potential in the rhesus monkey. *Nature*, 1969, *222*, 1273–1274.

Goldstein, E. B., & Berson, E. L. Cone dominance of the human early receptor potential. *Nature*, 1969, *222*, 1272–1273.

Goldstein, E. B., & Price, T. M. Temperature dependence of cone pigment regeneration in the isolated frog retina following flash and continuous bleaches. *Vision Research*, 1975, *15*, 477–481.

Goldstein, E. B., & Wolf, B. M. Regeneration of the green rod pigment in the isolated frog retina. *Vision Research*, 1973, *13*, 527–534.

Govardovskii, V. I. The sites of generation of early and late receptor potentials in rods. *Vision Research*, 1975, *15*, 973–980.

Hubbard, R., & Coleman, A. D. Vitamin-A content of the frog eye during light and dark adaptation. *Science*, 1959, *130*, 977–978.

Hubbard, R., & Wald, G. Cis-trans isomers of vitamin A and retinene in the rhodopsin system. *Journal of General Physiology*, 1952, *36*, 269–315.

Kühne, W. Chemische Vorgänge in der Netzhaut. In Herman, L. (Ed.), *Handbuch der Physiologie* (Vol. 3). Leipzig: Vogel, 1879. Pp. 235–239.

LeGrand, Y. *Light, Colour and vision*. London: Chapman and Hall, Ltd., 1957.

Lettvin, J. Y. General discussion: Early receptor potential. *Cold Spring Harbor Symposia of Quantitative Biology*, 1965, *30*, 501–502.

Liebman, P. A., & Entine, G. Cyanopsin, a visual pigment of retinal origin. *Nature*, 1967, *216*, 501–503.

Liebman, P. A., & Entine, G. Visual pigments of frog and tadpole (*R. pipiens*). *Vision Research*, 1968, *8*, 761–775.

Marks, W. B., Dobelle, W. H., & MacNichol, E. F. Visual pigments of single primate cones. *Science*, 1964, *143*, 1181–1183.

Moody, M. F., & Robertson, J. D. The fine structure of some retinal photoreceptors. *Journal of Biophysical and Biochemical Cytology*, 1960, *7*, 87–91.

Nilsson, S. E. G. The ultrastructure of the receptor outer segments in the retina of the leopard frog (*Rana pipiens*). *Journal of Ultrastructural Research*, 1965, *12*, 207–231.

Pak, W. L., & Ebrey, T. G. Early receptor potentials of rods and cones in rodents. *Journal of General Physiology* 1966, *49*, 1199–1208.

Pearlman, I. *In vivo kinetics of rhodopsin in RCS and normal rats*. Paper presented at the annual meeting of the Association for Research in Vision and Ophthalmology, 1977.

Price, T. The role of the pigment epithelium in cone pigment regeneration in the frog retina. Unpublished doctoral dissertation, University of Pittsburgh, 1977.

Reuter, T. The synthesis of photosensitive pigments in the rods of the frog's retina. *Vision Research,* 1966, *6,* 15–38.

Reuter, T. Visual pigments and ganglion cell activity in the retinae of tadpoles and adult frogs *(Rana temperaria* L.). *Acta Zoologia Fennica,* 1969, *122,* 1–64.

Reuter, T. E., White, R. H., & Wald, G. Rhodopsin and porphyropsin fields in the adult bullfrog retina. *Journal of General Physiology,* 1971, *58,* 351–371.

Taylor, J. W. Cone and possible rod components of the fast photovoltage in the frog eye: a new method of measuring cone regeneration rates *in vivo. Vision Research,* 1969, *9,* 443–452.

Wald, G. Carotenoids and the vitamin A cycle in vision. *Nature,* 1934, *134,* 65.

Wald, G. Carotenoids and the visual cycle. *Journal of General Physiology,* 1935, *19,* 351–368. (a)

Wald, G. Pigments of the retina, I. The bullfrog. *Journal of General Physiology,* 1935, *19,* 781–795. (b)

Zewi, M. On the regeneration of visual purple. *Acta Societatis Scientiarium fennical.,* 1939, N.S. B, 1–57.

7. Some Comments on the Functional Significance of Centrifugal Fibers to the Vertebrate Retina

George K. Shortess

I. Introduction

These comments will be concerned with the general significance of neurons whose cell bodies are in the central nervous system, and which synapse with retinal neurons, and by this means, influence the neural processing of retinal cells in vertebrates.

It is generally agreed that at least in certain avian species there exists a well-defined system of centrifugal fibers to retinal neurons, whereas there has been considerably less agreement that such a system exists in other vertebrates (e.g., Cowan, 1970; Ogden, 1968, pp. 89–109; Rodieck, 1973, pp. 673–689; van Hasselt, 1972/1973). Comments will therefore be directed toward two questions: First, what function does the centrifugal fiber system seem to serve in avian species? Second, what evidence is there that this system is of general significance for understanding visual function? In attempting to answer these questions, I will try to make two points. First, based on existing evidence, centrifugal fibers appear to be a supplemental system for increasing sensitivity in certain avian species. Second, there is no evidence yet to support the idea that centrifugal fibers are a general system of major significance for understanding vertebrate visual processes.

II. The Avian System

In the visual system of pigeons and chickens, it is well established with both anatomic and physiological evidence that the cell bodies of centrifugal fibers to the retina are located in the isthmo-optic nucelus (ION), with cell axons forming the isthmo-optic tract (IOT). [Cowan (1970) has provided an extensive review of this earlier literature.] By way of summary, the major input to the ION is from the ipsilateral optic tectum (OT), which is the major terminal nucleus for ganglion cells from the contralateral retina. Thus a feedback loop exists from retina to OT to ION and back to the retina. Moreover, it has been shown that the integrity of the two-dimensional visual space, as projected on the retina, is preserved throughout the feedback system, at least in a general way. While feedback characteristics of the system have been emphasized in the literature, it should be pointed out that there are parallel pathways within the system and that it is not closed.

Such parallel pathways and interactions with structures outside the feedback system have not yet been examined sufficiently to allow any statements concerning their possible significance. The main effort at functional analysis has been to manipulate the ION or IOT and observe retinal or behavioral effects. It has been found that electrical stimulation of the ION or IOT results in sensitization or potentiation of ganglion cell responses to light stimulation such that these cells respond more readily and to a wider range of stimuli (Ertchenkov, Gusselnikov, & Zaborskis, 1972; Miles, 1970, 1972b; Galifret, Condé-Courtine, Repérant, & Servière, 1971). Furthermore, cooling the IOT (Miles, 1972c; Pearlman & Hughes, 1976) has the opposite effect, of reducing the sensitivity of ganglion cells. Pearlman and Hughes (1976) have shown that a cold block applied to fibers efferent from the ION reduced sensitivity in about 75% of various types of ganglion cells. However, this figure may be a little high since about half the cells were lost before retesting after cooling, and any general deterioration during the process would probably have resulted in lowered sensitivity. For all cells tested, apart from overall reduced sensitivity, there was no change in the general character of the stimulation to which the cells were sensitive. Pearlman and Hughes suggest that efferent activity normally inhibits inferred inhibitory amacrine cells and thus enhances ganglion cell sensitivity, primarily by disinhibition. Whether all types of synaptic input to amacrine cells are involved is still unknown.

These electrophysiological results are consistent with the behavioral consequences of lesions in the IOT and ION. Rogers and Miles (1972) reported that ION-lesioned chicks had more difficulty discriminating grain from pebbles against a dark background than unlesioned controls, but both groups did equally well against white backgrounds. The ION-lesioned birds also had difficulty detecting moving targets in the peripheral visual field. In a more detailed study, Shortess and Klose (1977) reported that IOT-lesioned pigeons were not different from controls in their ability to discriminate vertical from horizontal black and white gratings at high contrast levels, but the two groups differed when the contrast was close to the level at which discrimination was no longer possible. However, the difference between them at lower levels of contrast was small. These results are also consistent with the report of Hodos and Karten (1974), who found no performance deficits on suprathreshold discrimination tasks for birds with ION lesions.

Taken together, the evidence supports the hypothesis that activity in the efferents increases the general sensitivity in the retinal ganglion cells. Furthermore, one can hypothesize that a dimming of the field might be a triggering stimulus condition. This was, in fact, the suggestion made by Miles (1972c) in developing the hypothesized mechanism he referred to as "dynamic adaptation." He proposed that this mechanism operated to help the bird detect food in darkened areas of the ground. This suggestion is also consistent with the finding that the anterior–inferior visual field seems to be more heavily represented in the ION (Holden & Powell, 1972).

Another source of ION stimulation is suggested by the receptive field properties of the ION cells. Holden and Powell (1972), working with pigeons, and Miles (1971, 1972a), working with chicks, both reported that most ION cells were particularly responsive to movement and that a majority were directionally selective. The directionally selective cells tended to be most responsive to vertical or anterior movement through the receptive field. This would suggest that head movements in a normal contrasting visual environment would generate activity in the ION cells, which would facilitate food-searching behavior of these species. But whether dynamic adaptation is the best descriptive term is not clear.

Two additional hypotheses, not necessarily inconsistent with the above idea, are (a) that ION cells have some involvement with response habituation to novel stimulation, and (b) that they play a role in the control of visually guided motor responses.

In a test for habituation to novel visual stimulation, Shortess and Klose (1977) could find no difference between IOT-lesioned and control birds. Furthermore, in several pilot studies, both optokinetic movements and key-pecking accuracy were recorded among IOT-lesioned and control pigeons. No differences were found that could be attributed to the effects of centrifugal fibers (Shortess, Klose, & Seech, 1974–1975). In preliminary observations with the optokinetic drum, birds followed moving suprathreshold vertical black and white stripes with both head and eye movements. They did about equally well whether they had lesions in the centrifugal system or not. For key-pecking accuracy, a plate was placed around the response key in a typical operant key-pecking situation and was arranged so that small pressures would activate a counter. The birds were videotaped and scored for pecking that failed to activate either the key or the plate. On the videotapes, general behavior was also examined. Again no effects attributable to the loss of centrifugal control was found. In some birds with lesions that included neighboring structures there were deficits, but these deficits could not be attributed exclusively to IOT damage. It is certainly possible that the techniques used in these pilot studies may not have been sensitive enough or did not measure the correct response, but in several attempts it was not possible to demonstrate involvement of the centrifugal fiber system with the mechanisms controlling the accuracy of these visually guided motor responses.

Rogers and Miles (1972) and Shortess and Klose (1977) reported some response latency increases when lesions of the centrifugal system were present, as compared to nonlesioned birds. Shortess and Klose (1977) also demonstrated partial compensation of this latency deficit within the test sessions. Whether the increase in latency was simply a manifestation of the sensitivity change or involved some other interaction was not clear. An examination of the possible involvement of inputs at the optic tectum and the isthmo-optic nucleus, as well as the functional significance of the parallel pathways, might provide answers.

III. The General Significance of Centrifugal Fibers

Since the results thus far described have involved either the pigeon or the chicken, the extent to which the centrifugal fiber system exists in other species is of interest. Among avians, the ION has been described as well differentiated in a number of orders other than those already mentioned (reviewed in Shortess & Klose, 1975). However, the ION apparently does not exist in the kiwi (*Apteryx australis*) (Craigie, 1930). Furthermore, it is poorly differentiated or nonexistent in the ibis (*Mycteria americana* Linn.) (Showers & Lyons, 1968), the American kestral (*Falco sparverius*), and the red-tailed hawk (*Buteo jamaicensis*) (Shortess & Klose, 1975).

This information suggests that the centrifugal fiber system might not be best characterized as an avian system, but rather as a more specialized adaptation in certain avian species. For example, the known species distribution of the well-defined ION is consistent with ground-searching and feeding behavior occurring in dimly illuminated areas, as proposed by Miles (1972c).

The main question, however, concerns the general importance of the centrifugal fiber system for understanding the visual function of vertebrates. What evidence is there that centrifugal fibers exist in nonavian vertebrates? A complete review of this literature will not be attempted here. However, several examples from recent reports follow to illustrate the types of problems that have plagued this work.

Witkovsky (1971) described relatively large diameter fibers within teleost and elasmobranch retinas, which appeared to enter the retina with the optic nerve and to terminate on amacrine and bipolar cells. On the basis of the general similarity of these fibers to those described in avians, he identified them as centrifugal, but conceded the possibility that they could be looping colaterals from ganglion cell axons. This same problem of interpretation applies to the reports of Honrubia and Elliott (1968) on the human retina and Goldberg and Galin (1973) on the mouse.

As another example, Halpern, Wang, and Colman (1976) recently identified the contralateral nucleus of the ventral supraoptic decussation as the apparent location of cell bodies having fibers terminating in the globe of the garter snake. These cells accumulated horseradish peroxidase (HRP) by retrograde transport after injection of HRP in the vitreous body of the globe, while they failed to do so when the HRP was injected outside the globe. Further, after injecting HRP into the nucleus, Wang and Halpern (1977) observed orthograde transport in the contralateral optic nerve. However, it is apparently not yet known where in the globe these fibers might terminate, whether on nerve cells, blood vessels, glial cells, or other structures in the globe.

As a third example, it apparently has been possible to record amacrine cell responses in a number of vertebrates as a result of electrical stimulation of the optic nerve. Byzov and Utina (1971) have suggested that amacrine cell responses which they recorded from frog retina were the result of the activation of centrifugal fibers reaching the retina as part of the optic nerve. Marchiafava (1976) has also recorded intracellular potential changes in presumed amacrine cells in the turtle retina in response to electrical stimulation of the optic nerve, and has attributed these changes to a centrifugal fiber system. Optic nerve stimulation seemed to enhance ganglion cell responses to low level light stimulation, which is similar to the effects of electrical stimulation of centrifugal cells in the pigeon and chick (Cervetto, Marchiafava, & Pasino, 1976).

However, other interpretations of these results are possible. Matsumoto (1975) has reported similar effects of optic nerve stimulation on intracellular recordings from frog amacrine cells. He has proposed that his effects resulted from retinal ganglion cells, which were antidromically invaded, acting back on the amacrine cells. Another possible interpretation is that some form of amacrine cell interaction with Müller cells took place. Recently, Miller, Dacheux, and Proenza (1977) reported that antidromically activated retinal ganglion cells can depolarize Müller cells in axolotl. Similar alternative suggestions can be made for claims of electrophysiological demonstrations of centrifugal fiber systems in the perciform teleost *Eugerres plumieri* (Vanegas, Amat, & Essayag-Millán, 1973) and in the trigger fish *Hemibalistes chrysopterus* (Sandeman & Rosenthal, 1974). Thus there are problems of interpretation for much of the data discussed and for further results not reviewed here.

However, techniques exist to select among competing interpretations of the significance of centrifugal fibers in species where data are not conclusive. It seems reasonable, therefore, to ask the next question: What is the best estimate of the significance of centrifugal control of the vertebrate retina?

One approach is to examine the relative numbers of fibers and terminals both in well-documented systems and in some of those that have been proposed. Overall the numbers do not appear large. In the pigeon and chicken, isthmo-optic fibers constitute less than 1% of the optic nerve (Rodieck, 1973; Binggeli & Paule, 1969). In other avian species, with less well-developed systems, this percentage may be considerably smaller (Shortess & Klose, 1975). In nonavians, Witkovsky and Stell (1973) have indicated that the centrifugal fibers and terminals described by Witkovsky (1971) in dogfish retinas are "few in number compared to the number of amacrine cell processes [p. 149]." Furthermore, the number of cell bodies identified by Halpern *et al.* (1976) in the garter snake does not appear large. Others who have described fibers in a variety of species have all reported relatively few (e.g., Brooke, Downer, & Powell, 1965; Noback & Mettler, 1973; Rubinson, 1968). In some cases, interpretation can be questioned and in others the terminus in the eye is unknown. However, even if those reported are truly centrifugal fibers, as defined here, the number of fibers appears small.

The argument concerning numbers, by itself, is of course not completely convincing since relatively few fibers could exert a disproportionately large effect.

Functionally, however, deficits produced by lesions of the centrifugal system in pigeons and chicks are relatively small, and are significant primarily at low levels of contrast and in detecting peripheral stimuli (Rogers & Miles, 1972; Shortess & Klose, 1977). The effects on ganglion cells of stimulating and blocking isthmo-optic fibers seem to show that these fibers do not make a major impact on retinal function, but provide a supplemental system for modulating sensitivity (Galifret *et al.,* 1971; Miles, 1970, 1972b, 1972c; Pearlman & Hughes, 1976). In other avian species with fewer centrifugal cells, their functional significance would apparently be less. Further, in the turtle, if it is assumed that Marchiafava (1976) is correct in his interpretation of the significance of the centrifugal fiber system, then the influence of the system appears predominantly at low levels of illumination (Cervetto *et al.,* 1976). An interesting suggestion consistent with these data and worth developing is that the function served by the centrifugal system to the retina in avians is accomplished in mammals by lateral geniculate neurons acting on other central nervous system structures (Swanson, Cowan, & Jones, 1974).

In conclusion, there is no evidence yet to support the hypothesis that direct centrifugal control of retinal neurons is a general system of major significance for understanding visual processing in vertebrates. This is not to deny a real functional role for centrifugal fibers in those species with a clearly defined system, particularly among nonmammals. However, it would appear that there are more significant visual problems which require attention before it is necessary to answer the remaining unanswered questions concerning the centrifugal fiber system. A number of other contributions to this volume point them out.

One is reminded of Brindley's comments (1960, pp. 107–115, 1970, pp. 105–110) in which he argued that centrifugal fibers, if they exist, are probably supplemental in function and of relatively little importance, especially for human vision. There is a risk in this conclusion, of course, since it is always possible that no one has yet made the appropriate measurements that would show that this type of centrifugal control is of more general significance. However, existing information does not seem to point in that direction, although additional data will, of course, be the final test.

REFERENCES

Binggeli, R. L., & Paule, W. J. The pigeon retina: Quantitative aspects of the optic nerve and ganglion cell layer. *Journal of Comparative Neurology,* 1969, *137,* 1–18.

Brindley, G. S. *Physiology of the retina and the visual pathway.* London: Edward Arnold, 1960.

Brindley, G. S. *Physiology of the retina and the visual pathway* (2nd ed.). Baltimore: Williams & Wilkins, 1970.

Brooke, R. N. L., Downer, J., & Powell, T. P. S. Centrifugal fibres to the retina in the monkey and cat. *Nature,* 1965, *207,* 1365–1367.

Byzov, A. L., & Utina, I. A. Centrifugal effects on amacrine cells in the frog's retina. *Neurophysiology,* 1971, *3,* 219–224.

Cervetto, L., Marchiafava, P. L., & Pasino, E. Influence of efferent retinal fibres on responsiveness of ganglion cells to light. *Nature,* 1976, *260,* 56–57.

Cowan, W. M. Centrifugal fibres to the avian retina. *British Medical Bulletin,* 1970, *26,* 112–118.

Craigie, E. H. Studies on the brain of the kiwi (*Apteryx australis*). *Journal of Comparative Neurology*, 1930, *49*, 223–357.

Ertchenkov, V. C., Gusselnikov, V. I., & Zaborskis, A. A. On efferent effects upon responses of the pigeon retina ganglion cells. *Sechenov Physiological Journal (USSR)*, 1972, *58*, 385–392.

Galifret, Y., Condé-Courtine, F., Repérant, J., & Servière, J. Centrifugal control in the visual system of the pigeon. *Vision Research* (Supplement No. 3), 1971, 185–200.

Goldberg, S., & Galin, M. Response of retinal ganglion cells axons to lesions in the adult mouse retina. *Investigative Opthalmology*, 1973, *12*, 382–385.

Halpern, M., Wang, R. T., & Colman, D. R. Centrifugal fibers to the eye in a nonavian vertebrate: Source revealed by horseradish peroxidase studies. *Science*, 1976, *194*, 1185–1188.

Hodos, W., & Karten, H. J. Visual intensity and pattern discrimination deficits after lesions of the optic lobe in pigeons. *Brain, Behavior & Evolution*, 1974, *9*, 165–194.

Holden, A. L., & Powell, T. P. S. The functional organization of the isthmo-optic nucleus in the pigeon. *Journal of Physiology (London)*, 1972, *223*, 419–447.

Honrubia, F. M., & Elliott, J. H. Efferent innervation of the retina. *Archives of Ophthalmology*, 1968, *80*, 98–103.

Marchiafava, P. L. Centrifugal actions on amacrine and ganglion cells in the retina of the turtle. *Journal of Physiology (London)*, 1976, *255*, 137–155.

Matsumoto, N. Responses of the amacrine cell to optic nerve stimulation in the frog retina. *Vision Research*, 1975, *15*, 509–514.

Miles, F. A. Centrifugal effects in the avian retina. *Science*, 1970, *170*, 992–995.

Miles, F. A. Visual responses of centrifugal neurones to the avian retina. *Brain Research*, 1971, *25*, 411–415.

Miles, F. A. Centrifugal control of the avian retina. II. Receptive field properties of cells in the isthmo-optic nucleus. *Brain Research*, 1972, *48*, 93–113. (a)

Miles, F. A. Centrifugal control of the avian retina. III. Effects of electrical stimulation of the isthmo-optic tract on the receptive field properties of retinal ganglion cells. *Brain Research*, 1972, *48*, 115–129. (b)

Miles, F. A. Centrifugal control of the avian retina. IV. Effects of reversible cold block of the isthmo-optic tract on the receptive field properties of cells in the retina and isthmo-optic nucleus. *Brain Research*, 1972, *48*, 131–145. (c)

Miller, R. F., Dacheux, R., & Proenza, L. Müller cell depolarization evoked by antidromic optic nerve stimulation. *Brain Research*, 1977, *121*, 162–166.

Noback, C. R., & Mettler, F. Centrifugal fibers to the retina in the rhesus monkey. *Brain, Behavior & Evolution*, 1973, *7*, 382–399.

Ogden, T. E. On the function of efferent retinal fibres. In C. von Euler, S. Skogland, & U. Söderberg (Eds.), *Structure and function of inhibitory neuronal mechanisms*. New York: Pergamon Press, 1968.

Pearlman, A. L., & Hughes, C. P. Functional role of efferents to the avian retina. II. Effects of reversible cooling of the isthmo-optic nucleus. *Journal of Comparative Neurology*, 1976, *166*, 123–131.

Rodieck, R. W. *The vertebrate retina*. San Francisco: W. H. Freeman, 1973.

Rogers, L. J., & Miles, F. A. Centrifugal control of the avian retina. V. Effects of lesions of the isthmo-optic nucleus on visual behavior. *Brain Research*, 1972, *48*, 147–156.

Rubinson, K. Projections of the tectum opticum of the frog. *Brain, Behavior & Evolution*, 1968, *1*, 529–561.

Sandeman, D. C., & Rosenthal, N. P. Efferent axons in the fish optic nerve and their effect on the retinal ganglion cells. *Brain Research*, 1974, *68*, 41–54.

Shortess, G. K., & Klose, E. F. The area of the nucleus isthmo-opticus in the American kestral (*Falco sparverius*) and the red-tailed hawk (*Buteo jamaicensis*). *Brain Research*, 1975, *88*, 525–531.

Shortess, G. K., & Klose, E. F. Effects of lesions involving efferent fibers to the retina in pigeons (*Columba livia*). *Physiology & Behavior*, 1977, *18*, 409–414.

Shortess, G. K., Klose, E. F., & Seech, M. Unpublished observations, 1974–1975.

Showers, M. J. C., & Lyons, P. Avian nucleus isthmi and its relation to hippus. *Journal of Comparative Neurology*, 1968, *132*, 589–616.

Swanson, L. W., Cowan, W. M., & Jones, E. G. An autoradiographic study of the efferent connections of the ventral lateral geniculate nucleus in the albino rat and the cat. *Journal of Comparative Neurology*, 1974, *156*, 143–163.

Vanegas, H., Amat, J., & Essayag-Millán, E. Electrophysiological evidence of tectal efferents to the fish eye. *Brain Research*, 1973, *54*, 309–313.

van Hasselt, P. The centrifugal control of retinal function. *Ophthalmic Research*, 1972/1973, *4*, 298–320.

Wang, R. T., & Halpern, M. Afferent and efferent connections of thalamic nuclei of the visual system of garter snakes. *Anatomical Record*, 1977, *187*, 741–742.

Witkovsky, P. Synapses made by myelinated fibers running to teleost and elasmobranch retinas. *Journal of Comparative Neurology*, 1971, *142*, 205–221.

Witkovsky, P., & Stell, W. K. Retinal structure in the smooth dogfish *Mustelus canis:* Electron microscopy of serially sectioned bipolar cell synaptic terminals. *Journal of Comparative Neurology*, 1973, *150*, 147–168.

8. Receptor Sensitivity and Pigment Migration to Ionizing Radiation and Light in the Noctuid Moth[1]

Kenneth L. Schafer, Jr.

I. Introduction

Shortly after the discovery of X rays, experimental studies and clinical reports began to accumulate which suggested that ionizing radiation could give rise to visual sensation. Lipetz (1953) cites dozens of studies dating back to 1898 which describe visual sensations from ionizing radiation emitted by radium packs, X-ray tubes of all descriptions, and sources of gamma and beta radiation. These data indicated that the human visual system as well as the visual systems of many vertebrate and invertebrate species were quite sensitive to ionizing radiation. For instance, Newell and Borley (1941) found that an X-ray beam producing a 1-mm^2 spot on the retina with an exposure rate of 8 mR sec^{-1} was sufficient to obtain a visual sensation in humans. Pape and Zakovsky (1954) employed X-ray stimulation of the whole eye and found that threshold sensitivity was as low as 1.6 mR sec^{-1} for long exposures, and for short (20 msec) exposures to the whole retina, .5 mR total dose was sufficient to obtain a visual sensation.

In addition to behavioral studies, a large number of electrophysiological studies have been conducted on a wide variety of species to determine the effect of ionizing radiation on visual processes, and these studies of sensitivity confirm behavioral thresholds. For example, in a study utilizing the electroretinogram (ERG) in humans, Elenius and Sysimetsa (1957) found that X-ray exposure of 25 msec for a total dose of .5 R was sufficient to produce a criterion b-wave response. Noell (1962) demonstrated that 10 mR for 100 msec of 2 MeV X-ray irradiation could produce a measurable "on" response in the rabbit eye. Lipetz (1955) employed 75 kVp X rays

[1]This research was supported jointly by Grant AT-(40-1)-2903 from the Division of Biology and Medicine, United States Atomic Energy Commission to Dr. James C. Smith, and a research fellowship, 1 F01 MH-40, 593-01 PS, from the National Institute of Public Health to the author.

to evoke an ''off'' discharge from a single ganglion cell of the frog retina. Nerve spikes could be obtained with as little as 156 mR at an exposure rate of .78 R sec^{-1}. Bachofer and Wittry (1962) used the ERG from the frog's eye as a dependent measure and found that a criterion response (b wave) could be obtained with 7 mR at an exposure rate of 162 mR sec^{-1} from a 150 kVp X-ray source. Baldwin and Sutherland (1965) reported that total doses of .09 mR from a 300-kVp X-ray source were sufficient to produce an ERG in the cockroach *Blaberus giganteus*. These investigators found that the amplitude of the response to X rays was directly related to the total dose of the stimulus pulse and not to the exposure rate. Since the stimuli employed in this study were quite short (less than the latent period of the eye), these data suggest that the cockroach eye obeys the Bunsen–Roscoe law for X-ray pulses under the critical duration.

Electrophysiological investigations have also been conducted with beta and gamma sources of radiation. Pogasyan, Trunova, and Tsypin (1961) found that 1 mR sec^{-1} for a total dose of 4 mR gamma irradiation from a ^{60}Co source was sufficient to produce an ERG in a dark-adapted frog. Smith and Kimeldorf (1964) determined visual thresholds for various noctuid moths using beta radiation from a ^{90}Sr source. By measuring the ERG elicited with the stimulus flickering at a rate of 11 Hz, they obtained threshold responses with exposure rates as low as 20 mR sec^{-1} for a total dose of .25 mR in some of the noctuid species tested.

II. Experiment I: Effects of Background Gamma Radiation on the Moth ERG

In this series of experiments, the ERG produced by stimulating the moth's eye with white light is recorded in the presence of both diffuse white light and gamma (^{60}Co) radiation backgrounds. Essentially the experiment consists of measuring the reduction in amplitude of the ERG response to $(I + \Delta I)$ where I consists of either gamma radiation or diffuse white light.

Using gamma radiation as a background stimulus offers one distinct advantage over the more generally employed method of comparing similarities between light and ionizing radiation by direct elicitation of the ERG with these stimuli. When these stimuli are presented as background energy to the system the shape of the stimulus pulse becomes relatively unimportant because the effect of the background stimulus is measured as a steady-state reduction in the ERG instead of as a dynamic ERG response to a stimulus pulse. This is extremely important in situations where it is difficult to equate the rise and decay time of a light and an ionizing radiation stimulus due to presentation of the radiation which must, as in this experiment, be controlled by a device such as an elevator.

A. Materials and Methods

The moths used in all experiments were *Heliothis zea* of the family Noctuidae which were obtained commercially in the pupa stage. When pupae were received they were placed immediately in individual wire chambers where glucose and water were available after emergence. The specimens were not segregated by age or sex, but the date of emergence was recorded on the cage for each moth. Specimens were selected for the experiments by age, typically 2–4 days after emergence.

In this group of experiments, the intact moth was placed in a small Plexiglas restraining block, shown in detail in Figure 8.1. The front of the block had a brass yoke attached to it which permitted the experimenter to restrain the insect by securing the body between the head and the thorax. The restrained moth was then placed on a platform equipped with several micromanipulators which were used to insert electrolytically tapered, stainless steel electrodes with tip sizes of about 25 μm. All recordings were conducted with the active electrode inserted about .5 mm under the corneal layer of the compound eye. The indifferent electrode was passed through the exoskeleton in the posterior portion of the head just behind the antenna adjacent to the eye from which recordings were being made. Both direct- and capacitor-coupled recordings were utilized, and all responses were fed into a computer of average transients for analysis and comparison of waveforms. Averaged responses were also recorded on an x–y plotter for later data analysis.

The light stimulus consisted of a white light flash from a glow modulator tube controlled by electronic timers. The light stimulus passed through a beam splitter where it was combined with the background light stimulus and transmitted to the eye via a plastic (Crofon) fiber optic system. The plastic fiber optics were not

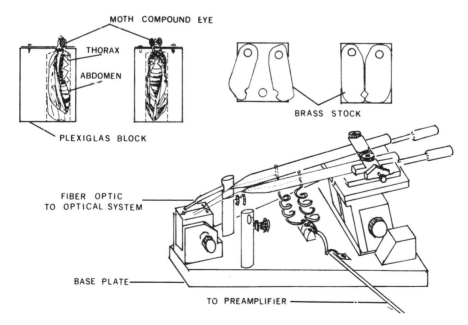

Figure 8.1. Apparatus for restraint of the moth during electrode placement and electrical recording. The fiber optic from the optical system attaches to the restraining platform and is positioned as shown in the diagram. Note the brass stock which immobilizes the moth's head when secured around the neck.

discolored by the radiation as in the case of glass optical fibers. The intensity of the background light stimulus was controlled via a 4 log-unit neutral density wedge mounted in front of a tungsten projector bulb. The fiber optic system that transmitted the light to the eye was attached to the block holding the preparation, and the whole apparatus was inserted into the port of the ^{60}Co (Gamma Beam 150, Atomic Energy of Canada Limited) source. The transmission of both the I and ΔI light stimuli through the same fibre optic system ensured that the $(I + \Delta I)$ light was stimulating the same receptor population.

The intensity of the background gamma radiation was varied by moving the preparation with respect to the source. Lead plugs inserted into the port were also employed to attenuate the intensity of the gamma radiation. The exposure rate from the gamma source was monitored and calibrated with a Philips dosimeter calibrated from 60 kV to 3 MeV. Light measurements were made with a Salford Electronics Exposure Photometer and a "standard white" magnesium carbonate reflective surface. In certain experiments the temperature of the preparation was monitored via a thermocouple placed in the contralateral eye.

B. Changes in the Photically Evoked ERG as a Function of Background Light and Gamma Radiation

In this experiment the eye was stimulated with 250-msec flashes from the glow modulator tube at a rate of one flash every 2 sec. The eye was permitted to reach a steady state of dark adaptation under these conditions before the effects of background intensity were tested. The stimulus flash was weak enough (6.3 fc at the cornea) so that the preparation was well dark-adapted, and eye-shine measurements (cf. Hoglund, 1963) indicated that the pigment migrated to the extreme distal position under these conditions.

When a steady state of dark adaptation had been reached, the eye was exposed to 35 R sec^{-1} background gamma radiation. Eight ERG responses were averaged by the computer while the ionizing radiation was present, and the response was then compared to a control measurement taken just before the radiation background was initiated. When baseline sensitivity was recovered (usually only seconds after the background was removed) the reduction in ERG amplitude and change in waveform during gamma radiation background were matched by presenting the background light stimulus. The optical wedge was adjusted until the amplitude and waveform of the ERG evoked by the $(I + \Delta I)$ stimulus corresponded to that obtained with background gamma radiation. When a match was obtained, the intensity of both background light and ionizing radiation were reduced by a log unit, and the process was repeated to determine whether the correspondence between light and gamma radiation backgrounds was maintained over the log-unit range of intensities.

Figure 8.2 shows the data obtained from a typical preparation under the conditions just described. One can easily see that the reduction in amplitude and change in waveform of the photically evoked ERG produced by a gamma radiation background can be matched perfectly with a given intensity of white light. It is also clear from these data that the effect of a change in the intensity of either background

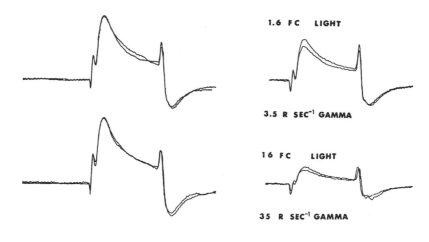

Figure 8.2. Matching effects of background light and gamma radiation on the photically evoked ERG. The control waveforms represent the average of eight stimulus flashes previous to initiation of either light or gamma radiation background. The waveforms on the right show the reduction and changes in waveform during the background stimulus as labeled in the figure. Flash intensity was 6.3 fc with a duration of 250 msec. The upward deflection shows negative electrical potential, and the peak negative deflection of the control waveform represents 1.5 mV. All bioelectric responses were direct-coupled to the preamplifiers and recording equipment.

stimulus can be matched by a corresponding change in the intensity of the other. This relationship was maintained over the entire range of background intensities employed in this study, which was limited only by the maximum exposure rate obtainable from the gamma source. In certain preparations where discrepancies were observed between the effects of the two background stimuli, differences could be traced to two sources. In some cases the distal-shielding pigment in the eye was observed to migrate toward the proximal position, which reduced the effect of the background light stimulus. Since the gamma radiation background was not attenuated by the shielding pigment, a proportionally greater reduction in ERG was obtained with radiation background compared to light background to which the ERG was originally matched.

The second source of error was found to be the result of the failure of the stimulus light in stimulating a large number of the photoreceptor population. If the fiber optic system was not placed in a manner that permitted fairly uniform stimulation of the entire compound eye, differences in waveform between light and radiation backgrounds were observed. Since ionizing radiation does not depend upon optical structures of the eye for transmission to receptor sites, gamma stimulus produces uniform excitation of the total receptor population. The waveform of the ERG depends greatly on the number of photoreceptive elements stimulated as well as on the intensity of stimulation. Therefore, it would be expected that if the total population of photoreceptive units were not stimulated by the light stimulus in a manner analogous to the excitation provided by the radiation background, the waveforms would indeed be different. When the eye is in the dark-adapted state and the shielding pigment is in the extreme distal position, there seems to be enough scattering of light to produce uniform stimulation of the receptor layer. However, when the eye is in the light-adapted state with the shielding pigment restricting transmission of light from extreme angles, large waveform discrepancies are often observed.

In an additional experiment the effects of superimposing the gamma and light backgrounds upon the photically evoked ERG were tested. Details of the experiment are identical to those in the previous study, except that after a reduction in the ERG response was obtained by presenting one of the background stimuli, the other background stimulus was also initiated and subsequently produced an additional reduction in the response to the light flash. As seen in Figure 8.3 the sequence of presentation was not a critical variable, and the two backgrounds were mutually additive in their effect. On the basis of these two experiments it seems quite clear that at some point in the photoreceptive process ionizing radiation acts in a manner quite similar to light stimulation in producing excitation of the visual processes.

III. Experiment II: Visual Sensitivity and Pigment Migration during Dark Adaptation

Surrounding the ommatidia of the compound eye of many insects, including the noctuid moth, is an accessory shielding pigment that migrates as a result of light stimulation (Exner, 1891; Day, 1941; Jahn & Wulff, 1941). In the light-adapted state the distal pigment surrounds the translucent structure that forms the ommatidia, thus making the retinula cells directionally sensitive to light entering parallel to the ommatidial axis. During dark adaptation this pigment retracts to the distal extremes of the ommatidial structure permitting light from angles oblique to the ommatidial axis to reach the retinula cells. The stimulation of retinula cells by oblique rays of light in addition to light parallel to the ommatidial axis obviously increases the total amount of light available to the eye, but at the same time the directional properties of the receptor system are compromised.

When dark-adaptation functions are plotted for some species of moths (i.e., *Cerapteryx graminis*) there appear to be two distinct phases of dark adaptation (Bernhard & Ottoson, 1960). Bernhard (1963), Bernhard, Hoglund, and Ottoson (1963), and Bernhard and Ottoson (1964) have suggested that the second, slower phase is mediated by migration of the distal pigment, and it was noted in a number of studies that the initiation of pigment migration marked the break between phases of adaptation while termination of pigment migration correlated quite well with the asymptotic sensitivity of the eye. In preparations where the pigment failed to migrate due to injury, the second phase of dark adaptation was invariably absent.

Smith and Kimeldorf (1964) obtained dark-adaptation curves for various species of noctuid moths using both light and beta radiation as visual stimuli. These investigators found that the function for beta radiation reached its maxima after 4–5 min

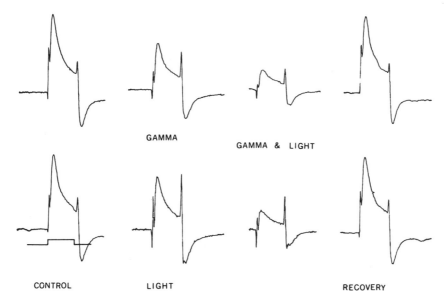

GAMMA

GAMMA & LIGHT

CONTROL   LIGHT   RECOVERY

Figure 8.3.   Addition of light and gamma radiation backgrounds. The reduction and change in the waveform during different combinations of backgrounds are shown for 13 R sec^{-1} gamma background and 8 fc light background. Control and recovery waveforms represent the average of eight stimulus flashes without background radiation. The marker on the lower left control waveform shows the stimulus duration, which was the same as Figure 8.2. Stimulus flash intensity and details of the ERG recording are also the same as Figure 8.2.

while the function obtained for light stimulus did not reach its terminal value for over 30 min. The authors suggested that this difference in time course was due to the fact that the pigment shields surrounding the ommatidia were transparent to beta radiation. Therefore, the dark-adaptation function obtained for beta radiation reflects only the photochemical adaptation of retinula cells, while the curve obtained for light is the result of an initial photochemical adaptation followed by the second phase where shielding pigment migrates toward the distal end of the ommatidia. In preparations where the eye was bleached with an intense zenon flash in several microseconds, dark-adaptation curves for beta and light were identical. The intense flash of short duration did not permit the shielding pigment to move from the distal position in this experiment, which suggests that the difference in light and beta radiation function is indeed due to pigment migration during dark adaptation.

Hoglund (1966) has provided additional evidence for the idea that the second phase of dark adaptation is due to movement of the shielding pigment. This investigator placed a single light-transmitting fiber under the cornea to a depth that permitted stimulation of retinula cells directly without shielding from most of the accessory pigment. By plotting visual sensitivity as a function of time in the dark for light transmitted directly to retinula cells and for light entering from outside the cornea, Hoglund was able to separate changes in sensitivity due to adaptation in retinula cells as opposed to increased sensitivity as a result of more light reaching retinula cells during pigment migration. Post and Goldsmith (1965) have reached similar conclusions from the study of pigment migration during light adaptation and its contributions to visual sensitivity in the moth *Galleria mellonella.*

In the present experiment light and beta radiation were employed as stimuli during dark adaptation to determine the relative contributions of photochemical adaptation and pigment migration to the increase in visual sensitivity for the noctuid moth *Heliothis zea.*

Latency and rate of pigment migration as a function of intensity and duration of the bleaching light were determined by comparing differences between light and beta radiation functions for different preadapting parameters.

A. Materials and Methods

Preparations utilized in this experiment were identical to those employed in the gamma radiation experiment, except that the moth was placed in front of a one-eighth inch steel disc which served as a radiation shield and shutter for the beta (50 mCi of ^{90}Sr) source. The sectored disc was then rotated with a constant speed motor to provide brief pulses of beta radiation. The adapting and stimulus light in this experiment were provided by the same 2-channel system described in Section I, A, 1. Placement of electrodes was also the same as in the previously described experiments except that an optical electrode was employed as the subcorneal active electrode. This electrode consisted of a single optical fiber that transmitted light past the migrating accessory pigment layer directly to the photoreceptor cells. A thin coating of silver epoxy permitted bioelectric responses from the fiber tip to be fed into a Grass P5 preamplifier with a frequency bandpass of from .1 to 1000 Hz. The light source for the fiber optic electrode was a General Electric 217 zenon photoflash tube with a discharge time of .5 msec in conjunction with a 4 log-unit neutral density optical wedge. All ERGs were measured on a Fairchild 701 persistent trace oscilloscope and preserved by simultaneous strip chart recording.

B. Dark-Adaptation Functions for Infrapigment, Transpigment, and Beta Stimuli

In this series of investigations the infrapigment function referred to ERG response to a stimulus presented to the eye via the single optical fiber electrode, while the transpigment function resulted from stimulation external to the eye which had to cross the accessory shielding pigment. As Hoglund (1966) has demonstrated, a comparison of infrapigment and transpigment response thresholds before and after pigment migration permits one to determine the amount of increase in visual sensitivity due to retinular cell adaptation as opposed to migration of distal-shielding pigment granules. In this study infrapigment and transpigment responses were recorded simultaneously with responses to beta radiation pulses throughout the course of dark adaptation. The results of infrapigment stimulation were compared to functions obtained with beta radiation since the two techniques presumably were measuring receptor sensitivity during the adaptation process. These functions were in turn compared with the transpigment function to determine the contribution of the migrating pigment granules and also their latency and rate of movement.

Figure 8.4 is a typical set of curves for a preparation demonstrating infrapigment, transpigment, and beta dark-adaptation functions obtained after a 15-min bleach with 3.8 log fc of white light. It is obvious that the infrapigment and beta function are quite different. Receptor sensitivity appears to be at asymptotic levels after about 28 min as judged by beta and infrapigment functions, but transpigment adaptation is not complete for nearly an hour. Note also that the transpigment response appears to level off during the time from Minutes 8–14. However, after Minute 15 there is a sharp and almost linear increase in the response for the next 15 min. It is this late phase of dark adaptation that presumably results from the migration of the shielding pigment, while the earlier rise may be attributed to the same increase in receptor sensitivity seen in the beta and infrapigment functions. When the intensity of the bleaching light is reduced to 2.8 log fc for the same duration the functions similar to the curves seen in Figure 8.5 are produced. There is little difference in the infrapigment and beta functions when compared with the 3.8 log fc bleach except that the curves seem to reach asymptote somewhat earlier. The transpigment curve is also quite similar, but the plateau effect is less prominent and the second phase of adaptation is initiated about 6 min earlier. The pigment migration in the case of the 2.8 log fc bleach seems to involve the same amount of time as when the stronger bleach is used, but the longer bleach increased the latency of the migration in this preparation. There is considerable variation in the functions obtained with identical adapting intensities and durations from different preparations,

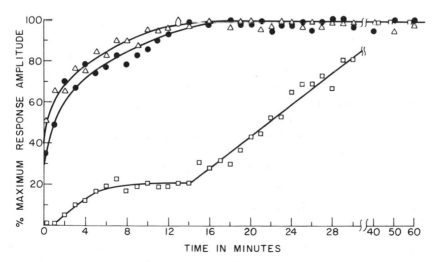

Figure 8.4. Percentage of maximum b-wave response amplitude for transpigment (□), infrapigment (●), and beta (△) stimuli as a function of time in the dark after a 15-min light adaptation with 3.8 log fc of white light.

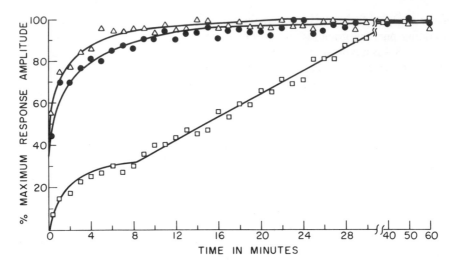

Figure 8.5. Percentage of maximum b-wave response amplitude for transpigment (□), infrapigment (●), and beta (△) stimuli as a function of time in the dark after a 15-min light adaptation with 2.8 log fc of white light.

causing difficulty in determining the exact effect of adapting parameters on the latency or rate of pigment migration. When durations shorter than 15 min were used for the bleach the pigment was often not in the fully light-adapted position when checked for appearance of a well-defined pseudopupil. When dark-adaptation functions were obtained after such a bleach, the transpigment function was usually monophasic, indicating that the two adaptational processes were occurring simultaneously.

In several preparations the infrapigment response was found to increase to its maximal level in about 10 min and then decline over the next 20–30 min. Figure 8.6 shows all three response functions for such a preparation, and it is obvious that the decline in the infrapigment threshold is initiated at about the same time the transpigment function is beginning the second phase. Further investigation showed that vertical displacement of the fiber placing its tip near the corneal surface was responsible for the function obtained. With the fiber tip in this position the migrating granules increased in density around the stimulus source, thus reducing the effective stimulus intensity as dark adaptation proceeded.

C. Control Studies with Transpigment and Beta Stimulation

The control studies employed involved the use of a rapid photochemical bleach using the zenon flash technique described by Smith and Kimeldorf (1964). These investigators demonstrated that the pigment shield in the eye of the noctuid moth does not migrate from the extreme distal position during a rapid light bleach, so the subsequent dark-adaptation function represents only increases in receptor sensitiv-

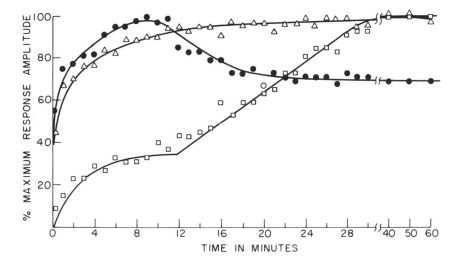

Figure 8.6.   Percentage of maximum b-wave response amplitude for transpigment (□), infrapigment (●), and beta (△) stimuli as a function of time in the dark after a 15-min light adaptation with 3.1 log fc of white light. The optical fiber for infrapigment stimulation was placed with its tip in the corneal area opposite the point of electrode entry.

ity. Under these conditions one would expect that dark-adaptation functions for beta radiation and transpigment stimulation would be identical since the pigment migration mechanism is not activated.

In the present study the completely dark-adapted eye was bleached in .5 msec with two intensities of light from a zenon flash tube, and the subsequent dark-adaptation functions for transpigment and beta stimulation were recorded. As seen in Figures 8.7 and 8.8 the recovery of sensitivity after both flash intensities was identical, which suggests that the difference between the two functions after an extended bleach is due to migration of the shielding pigment.

D. Locked Pigment Control

The most convincing control procedure was made possible when it was found that the shielding pigment could be "locked" in the proximal position by injecting approximately 100 μl of $10^{-4} M$ nicotine alkaloid into the optic lobe of the insect's visual system. With the migration mechanism inactivated it was possible to bleach the eye with normal adapting parameters and measure transpigment, infrapigment, and beta dark-adaptation functions with respect to receptor sensitivity alone. Figure 8.9 shows the data obtained from such a preparation, and one can easily see that the three functions are the same with respect to (*a*) time in the dark necessary for asymptotic sensitivity and (*b*) the general shape of the curve approaching asymptotic response levels. Thus, it would appear that under these conditions all three response functions reflect the gain in sensitivity due to adaptation of the photoreceptor elements. Further evidence for this statement comes from the reversibility of the locked

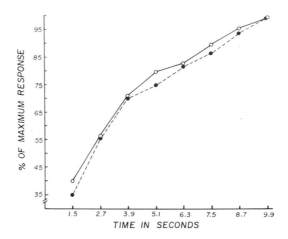

Figure 8.7. Percentage of maximum response amplitude for beta (O———O) and light (●--●) stimuli as a function of time in the dark after a low intensity, .5-msec bleach with a zenon photoflash tube.

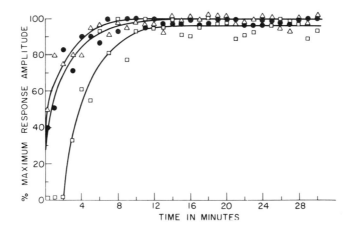

Figure 8.8. Amplitude of ERG b-wave for beta (●--●) and light (O———O) stimuli as a function of time in the dark after a high intensity, .5-msec bleach with a zenon photoflash tube.

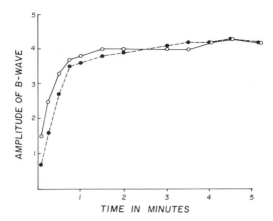

Figure 8.9. Percentage of maximum b-wave response amplitude for transpigment (□), infrapigment (●), and beta (△) stimuli as a function of time in the dark after a 15-min light adaptation with 2.2 log fc of white light. The pigment migration mechanism was locked for the duration of the dark adaptation shown in this figure with an injection of nicotine alkaloid into the optic lobe of the eye.

pigment preparation. The nicotine injection is usually effective in blocking pigment movement for only 2–3 hr. After this period eye-shine measurements indicate that the pigment does move toward the cornea, and when this migration takes place, a corresponding increase is also seen in the amplitude of the transpigment response. The effectiveness of the drug has no corresponding influence on infrapigment or beta response levels, which again suggests that the increase in sensitivity is indeed associated with movement of the shielding pigment in the case of light passing through the dioptric media.

The results of this study suggest that the increase in transpigment visual sensitivity during dark adaptation is associated with outward pigment migration and subsequent decrease in light attenuation by the screening pigment consistent with the findings of Bernhard and Ottoson (1960), Bernhard (1963), Bernhard et al. (1963), Bernhard and Ottoson (1964), and Post and Goldsmith (1965). The data obtained from these experiments also support the conclusion reached by Smith and Kimeldorf (1964) that the difference in adaptation functions to light and beta radiation are due to the fact that light sensitivity is affected by both receptor threshold and pigment screening, while beta radiation functions are dependent only on receptor sensitivity.

Baldwin and Sutherland (1965) suggest that the temporally extended dark-adaptation functions for *Blaberus* to X-ray stimuli result from pigment migration. However, there were no measurements of pigment migration included in their report, and the results of the present series of experiments with beta and gamma radiation strongly suggest that screening pigments are completely transparent to ionizing radiation of widely different quantal energies. It is possible that in the cockroach eye X-ray stimulus produces internal fluorescence which is filtered differentially as the screening pigment migrates. However, this possibility is clearly not the case with the noctuid moth preparation utilized here.

REFERENCES

Bachofer, C. S., & Wittry, S. E. Comparison of electroretinal responses to X-ray and to light. *Radiation Research,* 1962, *17,* 1–10.

Baldwin, W. F., & Sutherland, J. B. Extreme sensitivity to low-level X-rays in the eye of the cockroach *Blaberus. Radiation Research,* 1965, *24,* 513–518.

Bernhard, C. G. On the functional significance of the pigment migration in the compound eye. *Acta Physiologica Scandinavica,* 1963, *59* (Supplement 213), 22.

Bernhard, C. G., Hoglund, G., & Ottoson, D. On the relation between pigment position and light sensitivity of the compound eye in different nocturnal insects. *Journal of Insect Physiology,* 1963, *9,* 573–586.

Bernhard, C. G., & Ottoson, D. Studies on the relation between the pigment migration and the sensitivity changes during dark adaptation in diurnal and nocturnal *Lepidoptera. Journal of General Physiology,* 1960, *44,* 205–215.

Bernhard, C. G., & Ottoson, D. Quantitative studies on pigment migration and light sensitivity in the compound eye at different light intensities. *Journal of General Physiology,* 1964, *47,* 465–478.

Day, M. Pigment migration in the eyes of the moth, *Ephestia kuchniella Zeller. Biological Bulletin of the Marine Biological Laboratory (Woods Hole),* 1941, *80,* 275–291.

Elenius, V., & Sysimetsa, E. Measurement of the human electroretinographic roentgen threshold dose. *Acta Radiology,* 1957, *48,* 465–469.

Exner, S. *Die Physiologie der Facettirten Augen von Drebsen und Insecten.* Leipzig and Vienna: Deuticke, 1891.

Hoglund, G. Glow, sensitivity changes and pigment migration in the compound eye of nocturnal *Lepidoptera. Life Science,* 1963, *2,* 275–280.

Hoglund, G. Pigment migration, light screening and receptor sensitivity in the compound eye of nocturnal *Lepidopetra. Acta Physiologica Scandinavica,* 1966, *69* (Supplement 282), 11.

Jahn, T. L., & Wulff, V. J. Retinal pigment distribution in relation to a diurnal rhythm in the compound eye of *Dytiscus. Proceedings of the Society for Experimental Biology and Medicine,* 1941, *48,* 656–660.

Lipetz, L. E. *An electrophysiological study of some properties of the vertebrate retina.* Health and Biology Distribution, UCRL-2056, University of California, Radiation Laboratory, 1953.

Lipetz, L. E. The X-ray and radium phosphenes. *British Journal of Ophthalmology,* 1955, *39,* 577–598.

Newell, R. R., & Borley, W. E. Roentgen measurement of visual acuity in cataractus eyes. *Radiology,* 1941, *37,* 54–61.

Noell, W. K. X-irradiation studies on the mammalian retina. In *Response of the nervous system to ionizing radiation.* New York: Academic Press, 1962.

Pape, R., & Zakovsky, J. *Fortschritte auf dem Gebiete der Rontgenstrahlen,* 1954, *80,* 65.

Pogosyan, R. I., Trunova, N. M., & Tsypin, A. B. [On the electric reaction of the retina in the action of Co[60] gamma-radiation.] *Bulletin of Experimental Biological Medicine (USSR),* 1961, *52,* 50–53.

Post, C. T., Jr., & Goldsmith, T. H. Pigment migration and light-adaptation in the eye of the moth, *Galleria mellonella. Biological Bulletin of the Marine Biological Laboratory (Woods Hole),* 1965, *128,* 473–487.

Smith, J. C., Kimeldorf, D. J., & Hunt, E. I. Motor responses of moths to low-intensity X-ray exposure. *Science,* 1963, *140,* 805–806.

9. Visual Cells in the Pons of the Cat[1]

Mitchell Glickstein, Alan Gibson,
James Baker, Eilene La Bossiere,
George Mower, Farrel Robinson, and John Stein

Tasks that demand close coordination between eye and limb, such as a man catching a ball or a cat following a mouse, call for the combined activities of visual and motor centers in the brain. In mammals there is good evidence that both visual and motor cortex are involved in precise visual guidance of movement. How do the visual and motor cortex interact to guide the movements of the limbs? What kind of connections are there between them?

Our knowledge of the circuitry linking nerve cells in the visual and motor regions of the cerebral cortex is meager, but it is possible to trace at least three anatomic pathways by which connections might be made. One such pathway is entirely cortical: Information in the visual cortex passes through the visual association areas, which connect by a series of synaptic relays to the motor cortex. The other two routes leave the cerebral cortex and then return, one by way of the basal ganglia in the midbrain, the other by way of the cerebellum.

This latter pathway is of particular interest because a good deal is known about the internal workings of the visual cortex and the cerebellum but much less about the connections between them. We have been studying the first relay in a pathway that begins in the visual cortex and connects to the motor cortex by way of the cerebellum, a circuit that appears to be one of the important pathways for the visual guidance of movement.

Early workers thought that only the motor cortex sent fibers to the cerebellum. Snider and Stowell (1944) found evidence for a functional visual input to the cerebellum when they observed that flashes of light could evoke potentials in the vermis, the middlemost part of the cerebellar cortex. Subsequent work (Fadiga & Pupilli, 1964) has confirmed Snider's observation, and it has also revealed that in a

[1]An expanded version of this article appeared in *Scientific American* under Glickstein and Gibson, "Visual Cells in the Pons of the Brain," *235*, November 1976, 90–98. Copyright © 1976 by Scientific American, Inc. All rights reserved.

lightly anesthetized experimental animal a bright flash can evoke potentials over nearly all of the cerebellar cortex. Most of the input to the cerebellum is relayed by way of the visual cortex; another important source of inputs is from the superior colliculus.

The connections between the visual cortex and the cerebellum are part of a massive fiber system that includes output fibers from almost every region of the cerebral cortex. These outflowing cortical fibers do not go to the cerebellum directly but are relayed by way of the pons. This structure was first described accurately by the sixteenth-century Italian anatomist, Constanzo Varolia (1591), who dissected the brain from below. He thought that the great transverse fiber bundle overlying the protuberance resembled a bridge, with the brainstem flowing under it like a canal; hence, he named the region *pons*. In those mammals with a large cerebral cortex, the pons and the cerebellum are prominent; all three structures are strikingly developed in the human brain.

The pathway connecting the visual cortex to the cerebellum by way of the pons interested us for several reasons. First, since the cerebellum plays an important role in the control of movement, we felt that analysis of its visual input might reveal the nature of one of the major circuits involved in visual–motor guidance. Second, we believed that examining the connections between the visual cortex and the pons would help us clarify another problem concerning the representation of the visual world in the visual cortex. Anatomic studies had shown that fibers from cells in the lateral geniculate body project to several regions of the cat visual cortex, among them Areas 17 and 18 (Glickstein, King, Miller, & Berkley, 1967). Each of these areas appears to embody an essentially complete representation of the half-retinas.

Why are the visual fields mapped in parallel onto two different areas of the cortex? If it is because these areas have different functions, their difference might be reflected in the nature of their outputs. For example, one area might show a heavier projection of fibers to the pons. If that were the case, it would have a monosynaptic connection to the cerebellum and might therefore be specialized for the visual guidance of movement.

Our first goal, then, was to learn which are the main areas of the visual cortex that project to the pons, and where their fibers terminated in the pontine nuclei. Once we had found a visual area in the pontine nuclei we could proceed to examine the function of the cells in that region. In our initial anatomic experiments (Glickstein, Stein, & King, 1972), we made lesions in those parts of either Area 17 or Area 18 in the visual cortex that receive their input from the center of the visual field. After an appropriate time the cats were reanesthetized, sacrificed, and their brains removed, fixed, and cut into sections. Sections of the pons were then stained silver to reveal the location of degenerating fibers projecting from the visual cortex.

When the lesions were made in Area 18, a clear-cut focus of degenerating fibers appeared among a group of cells in the pontine nuclei. Lesions in the corresponding part of Area 17, however, caused only negligible degeneration in the pons, suggesting that the two cortical regions might be functionally separate. This hypothesis received support when Per Brodal (1972) found that the input to the pons from Area

17 was limited to those parts of the area that receive information from the periphery of the visual field.

There are two other visual regions in the cerebral cortex of the cat. One of them, Area 19, is continuous with Area 18; the other, the suprasylvian area, is somewhat separated from the others. All four regions of visual cortex receive direct inputs from the eyes by way of the lateral geniculate bodies (Glickstein *et al.*, 1967). When we made lesions in Area 19 and the suprasylvian area, we found that the projections from Area 19 were light, but that the suprasylvian area projected heavily into the same region of the pontine nuclei as Area 18 did. Area 18 and the suprasylvian area may thus be specialized for the visual guidance of movement, and they probably play a less important role in the visual perception of form.

These findings from degeneration studies have recently been confirmed and enlarged using the horseradish peroxidase (HRP) method.

We surgically exposed the bottom surface of the pons in cats and injected a small amount of HRP into the visual area of the pontine nuclei. By approaching the pons from below we were able to avoid the possibility that the enzyme might accidentally leak into other structures that might also receive fibers from the cortex. When the brains were later sectioned and examined unstained under the microscope, large pyramidal cells containing HRP reaction product were visible in all areas of the visual cortex except the central portion of Area 17. The labeled cells were confined to lamina V of the area of the cortex known to be a major source of outputs from the cortex to lower brain structures. These cells must therefore have been sending visual information to the pons.

Having located a set of cells in the pons that received fibers from cells in the visual cortex, we went on to see if these pontine cells could be physiologically activated by visual stimuli. We recorded the activity of single pontine cells in cats without lesions and under light anesthesia (Baker, Gibson, Glickstein, & Stein, 1976). The surface of the brain was exposed and tungsten microelectrodes were advanced into the pons. When our microelectrodes were placed in the region of the pons that receives fibers from the visual cortex, all the cells encountered responded to visual stimulation. Figure 9.1 summarizes these results.

Visually responsive cells could also be activated by electrically stimulating the visual cortex. Cells outside a certain small area in the pontine nuclei did not respond at all to the visual stimuli. These observations suggest that visual cells in the pons are located within definite regions that are exclusively visual.

In neighboring parts of the pons we encountered cells that responded to other sensory stimuli, such as clicks or tactile stimulation of the cat's fur or skin. Although we did not study the response properties of these cells in detail, they too were found in distinct clusters. All of the pontine cells we have tested so far have responded to only one form of sensory stimulation, be it visual, auditory or tactile; we have not yet found any cells that receive convergent information from more than one sense organ.

About half of the pontine visual cells we studied could be activated by a bright flash, although a flash was rarely the best stimulus. The flash response was useful,

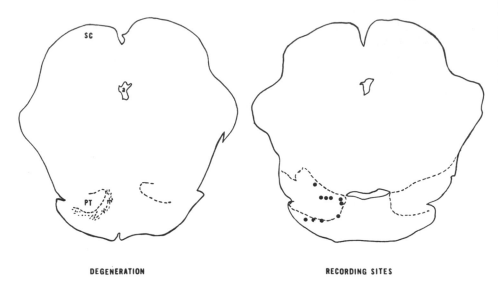

DEGENERATION   RECORDING SITES

Figure 9.1. Two tracings of frontal sections through the pons and midbrain of a cat. The stippling on the left tracing illustrates the area of degeneration that was found following a lesion of cortical Area 18. The filled circles on the right tracing show the location in which visual cells were recorded. A, Cerebral aqueduct; PT, pyramidal tract; SC, superior colliculus.

however, because it enabled us to measure precisely the latency of activation, that is, the time between the flash and the first spike. Knowing this time we could estimate the shortest pathway by which pontine cells receive their visual input. Of the 232 cells we studied, 13 were activated in 20 msec or less after a bright flash, a short latency that allowed enough time for the activation of only a few cells in the visual cortex. The circuit from the lateral geniculate body to the visual cortex to the pons thus was direct, with few synaptic relays along the way. We then proceeded to study the receptive properties of pontine visual cells. The receptive fields ranged in size from 3° by 4° up to a complete hemifield of each eye. On the average pontine receptive fields were larger than those of cells in the visual cortex. One possible way in which such large receptive fields may be achieved would be if the outputs of several cells in the visual cortex, each with a small and slightly different receptive field, converged on a single cell in the pons.

Although the visual cells in the pons receive their input from the visual cortex, their responses differ markedly from those of the cells in the cortex. Nearly all the pontine cells we tested responded maximally to a particular direction of target motion; in most cases the motion of the target in the opposite direction either failed to drive the cell or actively inhibited it. Figure 9.2 shows an example of such a receptive field. We studied the motion sensitivity of some cells in detail. The pontine cells responded to a broad range of target speeds, from a few angular degrees per second up to more than 1000° per sec, without losing their directional specificity, although there was an optimum speed for each cell. This range of speeds

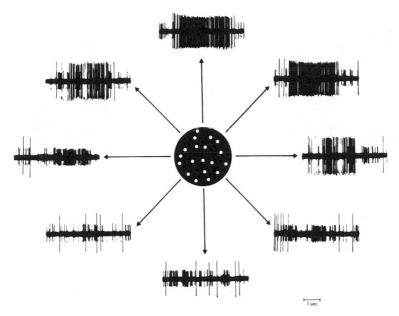

Figure 9.2.   Response of a cell to a multiple spot target moving in each of eight directions. The sharpness of directional tuning is typical of many pontine visual cells.

is considerably larger than that of cells in the visual cortex, again suggesting that several cells in the cortex, each with a different preferred speed, might converge on a single cell in the pons.

Direction and speed are the major determinants of the firing rate of visual cells in the pons, with the precise shape and orientation of the target usually being less important. However, the pontine cells do differ in their preference for different target configurations and sizes. Large receptive fields containing many spots were the most effective stimuli for activating about half of the pontine cells we studied. Figure 9.3 shows an example of a typical pontine cell receptive field. Some cells had a strong preference for such multiple-spot targets; they were not activated at all by single spots. They would fire in response either to several black spots on a white background or to several white spots on a black one, although the white spots were usually the more effective. A second group of pontine cells were preferentially driven by single moving spots. There was usually an optimum size for the spot, and large targets often failed to activate the cell at all. For most cells in the pons oriented bars and edges were no more effective stimuli than spots, and often they were less so. This behavior is in contrast to that of cells in the cortex, whose response to edges is highly specific.

The response properties of the visual cells in the pons tell us something about the kind of information that is relayed from the visual cortex to the cerebellum. The cells responding preferentially to a single moving spot could be specialized for following the rate and direction of movement of a single object, as in the case of the

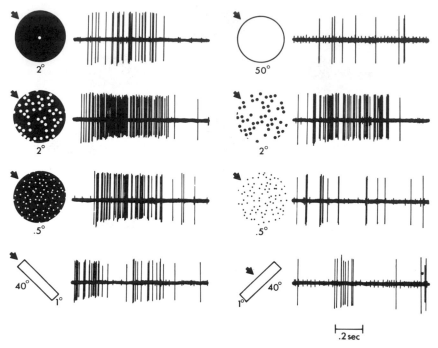

Figure 9.3. Responses of a typical pontine visual cell to spot and slit stimuli. All stimuli evoked a response. The optimal stimulus was a field of 2° diameter white spots; large spots and slits oriented orthogonally to movement were relatively ineffective.

cat, a small running animal. Those responding to the movement of large textured fields usually prefer movement down and away from the vertical meridian, and thus they could be responsible for detecting the position and direction of the ground as seen by a walking or running animal.

Since the behavior of the visual cells in the pons differed so much from the previously reported behavior of visual cells in the cortex (Hubel & Wiesel, 1962, 1965), we decided to study receptive field properties of those cortical cells projecting to the pons. Corticopontine cells were identified by antidromic invasion following electrical stimulation of their terminals in the visual area of the pons. To increase our cell catch, we simultaneously recorded with four electrodes in the cortex and switched among them with each stimulus pulse; the stimulating electrode was also an array of four electrodes placed in the visual area of the pons. To date we have recorded from 57 corticopontine cells and detected 466 antidromic potentials. The relative ease with which we could find potentials indicates that the visual area in the pons of the cat received direct inputs from broad regions of Area 18 in the cortex. In all cases we tested each cortical cell for ''collision'' by causing the cell to fire in response to a visual stimulus (such as a multispot target) and then using the elicited spike to trigger the electrical stimulator, which in turn drove an antidromic

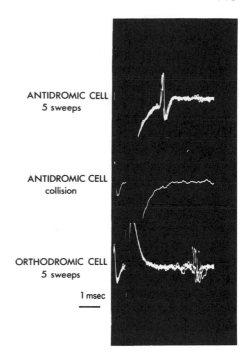

ANTIDROMIC CELL
5 sweeps

ANTIDROMIC CELL
collision

ORTHODROMIC CELL
5 sweeps

1 msec

Figure 9.4.   Top two traces: Area 18 cortical cell antidromically activated by stimulation of pontine nuclei. Bottom trace: A record of one of four orthodromically driven cells.

spike up the cell's axon. A cell which is driven antidromically will fail to be activated if its axon is stimulated shortly after a spontaneously occurring spike. Figure 9.4 shows an example of such a cell as well as the record of an orthodromically driven cell in Area 18.

A surprising finding that has resulted from the antidromic invasion experiments is that the corticopontine cells comprise a subset of cortical cells behaving more like pontine cells than other cortical cells. Much of the convergence needed to produce the large receptive fields and broad speed ranges typical of visual cells in the pons thus appears to be occurring in the cortex. One property in which corticopontine and pontine cells differ is that the corticopontine cells are more responsive to the exact orientation of line stimuli. This responsiveness to orientation, however, is largely independent of the corticopontine cell's responsiveness to the direction in which the target is moving. It may be that many cells in the cortex converge on a single cell in the pons in such a way that directional specificity is preserved even though a sharp orientation preference is lost.

In sum, movement across the retina is necessary to activate a visual cell in the pons, but such cells are not highly selective for a definite stimulus, orientation, or shape, suggesting that the analysis of visual features is done by other brain pathways. The motion of objects in the view of a stationary cat and the movement of the ground past a walking or running cat each activate a different class of cells in the pons. This information is sent to the cerebellum, which also registers the position and velocity of every muscle and joint. The cerebellum then combines these two kinds of information to control the position of the body and limbs in an actively moving animal.

REFERENCES

Baker, J., Gibson, A., Glickstein, M., & Stein, J. Visual cells in the pontine nuclei of the cat. *Journal of Physiology,* 1976, *255,* 415–433.

Brodal, P. The corticopontine projection from the visual cortex in the cat. *Brain Research,* 1972, *39,* 297–317.

Fadiga, E., & Pupilli, G. C. Teleceptive components of the cerebellar function. *Physiology Review,* 1964, *44,* 432–486.

Glickstein, M., King, R., Miller, J., & Berkley, M. Cortical projections from the dorsal lateral geniculate nucleus of cats. *Journal of Comparative Neurology,* 1967, *130,* 55–76.

Glickstein, M., Stein, J., & King, R. Visual input to the pontine nuclei. *Science,* 1972, *178,* 1110–1111.

Hubel, D., & Wiesel, T. Receptive fields, binocular interaction and functional architecture in the cat's visual cortex. *Journal of Physiology,* 1962, *160,* 106–154.

Hubel, D., & Wiesel, T. Receptive fields and functional architecture in two non-striate visual areas (18 and 19) of the cat. *Journal of Neurophysiology,* 1965, *28,* 229–289.

Snider, R. S., & Stowell, A. Receiving areas of the tactile, auditory, and visual systems in the cerebellum. *Journal of Neurophysiology,* 1944, *7,* 331–357.

Varolio, C. *De nervis opticis nonnullisque aliis, praeter communem opinionem in humano capite observatis, epistolae.* Padua: Paulum et Antonium Meiettos, Fratres, 1573.

10. Properties of Cortical Inhibition in Directionally Selective Neurons: Some Neurophysiological Parallels to the Perception of Movement[1]

Leo Ganz

I. Introduction

The illusion of motion obtained from stroboscopic sequences of stimulation is, from a phenomenological point of view, one of our strongest visual illusions. In spite of much experimental, theoretical, and applied interest devoted to it, the illusion of stroboscopic movement remains today without an adequate explanation (Kolers, 1972).

We have been analyzing the mechanism of directional selectivity in simple neurons of Area 17 of the cat, and have used as stimuli both continuous motion of edges across the neuron's receptive field as well as sequences of static stimuli, as in a stroboscopic movement paradigm. The purpose of this chapter is to show that by understanding the properties of inhibition in directionally selective neurons, an increase in our understanding of the mechanisms underlying both real and stroboscopic movement can be obtained.

II. Method

There is not sufficient space here to describe techniques in detail. The surgical preparation, microelectrode procedures, techniques of stimulation, and data analysis that we have used are described by Felder and Ganz (in preparation). In brief, the material discussed here is taken from two samples of visual cortex neurons: 70 neurons from 23 cats in which rectangularly shaped stimuli of standard intensities were presented on an oscilloscope, and 21 neurons, collected from an additional 11 cats, where moving edges varying in contrast were employed. The

[1]This work was supported by National Institute of Health Research Grant R01 EY 01241.

cats were anesthetized with short-term barbiturate anesthetic (sodium thiopental) during surgical preparation. During recording, muscle paralysis was induced using gallamine triethiodide (Flaxedil). Anesthesia was maintained with a mixture of 70% N_2O and 30% O_2. We used glass-coated platinum/iridium microelectrodes. Microelectrode penetrations into visual cortex were made at stereotaxic coordinates P2–P4 and L.5–L2 in an effort to reach a projection of the cat's area centralis in Brodmann's Area 17. In the cat, the center of the visual axis projects cortically to Brodmann's Area 17 at Horsley–Clarke stereotaxic coordinates: posterior 3 mm, lateral 2 mm (Joshua & Bishop, 1970).

III. Linearity

One experimental approach to the question of the linearity or nonlinearity of cortical inhibition we employed was to move a single edge through the neuron's receptive field, systematically varying contrast as well as velocity and direction of movement. In these experiments, mean luminance level remained constant. Results obtained from a simple unimodal neuron are illustrated in Figure 10.1. Preliminary receptive field mapping had revealed neuron T11-55 to be selective for rightward motion. Temporal response to stimulus pulses was sustained in character. It had a discrete on-excitatory discharge center of approximately .9°, with adjoining inhibitory flanks. We estimated the width of the on-center plus abutting inhibitory flanks at about 1.5°. Spontaneous activity level was very low. Figure 10.1 shows, first, that when a white leading edge moves in the preferred direction, spike rate elicited from the excitatory discharge center increases as the intensity of the moving edge increases. The curves depict log mean impulses per second during the edge's traverse plotted as a function of log intensity. The traverse was 5° in extent. Each symbol represents an average calculated from nine traverses. Looking first at the frames representing the four slowest velocities (i.e., $1.5°$–$8.5°$ sec^{-1}), one sees monotonic functions at lower contrasts. Simple cortical neurons typically operate dynamically over about a 1–2 log-unit range of intensity. T11-55 is typical in this regard.

The data points in Figure 10.1 have been fitted by eye to the function

$$R_p = aI^c/(I^c + k), \qquad (1)$$

a function derived from measurements of rod and cone receptor potentials (Boynton & Whitten, 1970; Normann & Werblin, 1974), where R_p is the response rate for movement in the preferred direction, I is the stimulus intensity, k is the stimulus intensity at which the receptor potential is half saturated, and a is a proportionality constant. All the curves in Figure 10.1 have been fitted with an exponent value of c = 1.2 and k = 10 cd m^{-2}; only a varies from curve to curve. A fairly good fit results for data obtained at different velocities with parameters c and k held constant. In other words, for motion in the preferred direction the same receptor-operating characteristic function operates at different velocities. Changing velocities, at least

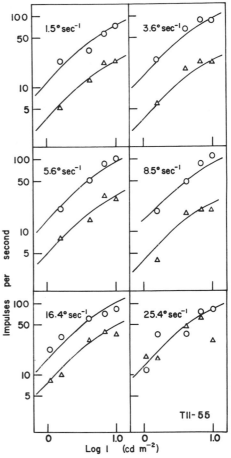

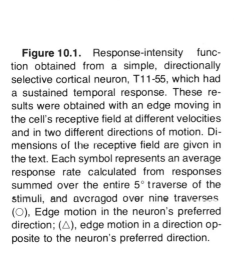

Figure 10.1. Response-intensity function obtained from a simple, directionally selective cortical neuron, T11-55, which had a sustained temporal response. These results were obtained with an edge moving in the cell's receptive field at different velocities and in two different directions of motion. Dimensions of the receptive field are given in the text. Each symbol represents an average response rate calculated from responses summed over the entire 5° traverse of the stimuli, and averaged over nine traverses (○), Edge motion in the neuron's preferred direction; (△), edge motion in a direction opposite to the neuron's preferred direction.

within the ranges employed here, only changes the multiplier a. This in turn implies an independence of intensity and velocity effects. Note further that in Figure 10.1 a fairly good fit can be obtained using the same parameter values for c and k for both motion in the preferred and in the null direction; only a changes.

In other words, Eq. (1) also gives the response rate for movement in the null direction, R_n:

$$R_n = a'I^c/(I^c + k),$$

and hence,

$$\log R_n = \log R_p - \log(a/a'). \tag{2}$$

Eq. (2) states that when plotted on log–log coordinates the response to null-direction motion is a simple downward displacement of the entire operating characteristic function.

A plausible explanation for the fact that null-direction movement yields an operating characteristic function that is simply parallel to the preferred-direction movement function, but displaced vertically downward (on log–log coordinate plots) is as follows: When the moving object travels in the preferred direction, it stimulates a family of receptors that eventually activate the excitatory part of the cortical sequence analyzer's receptive field. The same thing occurs during null-direction motion, but this step is preceded by the moving object stimulating a family of receptors that eventually activate an inhibitory cortical internuncial neuron (Felder & Ganz, in preparation). We know that this directional inhibition most probably originates intracortically (Creutzfeldt & Ito, 1968; Bishop, Coombs, & Henry, 1971). However, the power-function operating characteristic is determined by the peripheral receptors. Therefore, two power-function processes are generated at the receptors and then one of the processes is *linearly* subtracted from the other at the cortex.

Note also that the validity of Eq. (2) at numerous contrasts and velocities, postulating as it does a simple subtractive process, implies that many postsensory-transducer processes interact linearly in the visual system.

One further implication of Eq. (2) is that the absolute difference between responses to edges moving in the preferred and to those moving in the null direction is given by

$$R_\mathrm{p} - R_\mathrm{n} = (a - a') \, [I^c/(I^c + k)]. \tag{3}$$

In other words, the difference between null- and preferred-direction responding is itself a simple power function of stimulus intensity. The difference between null- and preferred-direction responding increases as edge contrast increases. If the organism uses such differences between sequence analyzer populations to determine whether motion is from one or another direction, then motion–direction resolution should improve monotonically with increases in edge contrast.

IV. Cortical Inhibition, Underlying Directional Selectivity, and the Long Decay Constant

One way in which we have estimated the temporal characteristics of cortical inhibition in directionally selective neurons is to examine the neuron's response to moving square wave gratings varying in spatial frequency, velocity, and direction of motion. For example, neuron T6-29 depicted in Figure 10.2 was a simple, directionally selective neuron with transient response properties. It responded optimally to large gratings moving quickly through its receptive field, preferably at about 25° sec^{-1}. We are able to examine the response to various combinations of velocity and spatial frequency to find the temporal rate of periodicity yielding the deepest inhibition, that is, the least responsiveness in the nonpreferred direction of motion. For example, with a .16 cycle deg^{-1} grating, the deepest inhibition is obtained at a velocity of 10° sec^{-1}. That corresponds to a repetition rate of one stripe crossing the receptive field at about every 600 msec. With a grating of .22 cycle deg^{-1}, the

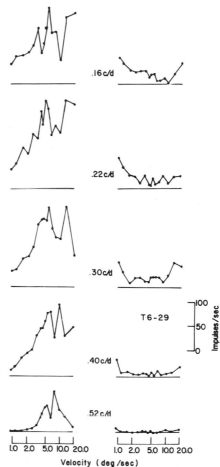

Figure 10.2. The response rate of a directionally selective simple neuron with transient response properties, T6-29, to a moving square wave grating. Left: Preferred direction of motion; right: null direction of motion. Average response rate is plotted against velocity of grating motion. Both spatial frequency and velocity have been varied parametrically. Each symbol represents responses summed over the entire 5° traverse of the grating; average response rate is computed from three traverses. Mean level of illumination: .0137 cd m⁻². Grating contrast = .95.

strongest inhibition is obtained at a repetition rate of about 900 msec, and so on. These findings invariably suggest long time constants for the decay of inhibition generated by a null-direction movement even in transient neurons. These values are long relative to the usual critical durations where Bloch's law begins to break down at peripheral loci of the vertebrate visual system (60–100 msec).

We have found these slow time constants to be the general case among *both* transient and sustained neurons. However, transient neurons invariably produce the deepest inhibition at spatial frequency–velocity combinations, suggesting relatively shorter time constants.

A second technique is to present sequences of white stationary bars, optimally oriented in the receptive field, in both the preferred and null direction. Typically, the first bar will come on and stay on. Then, after an interval, the second will come on and stay on, then the first will turn off, and finally the second will turn off. The time interval between the flashes, the stimulus–onset–asynchrony (SOA), varies

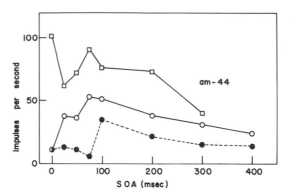

Figure 10.3. Response of a directionally selective complex neuron (am-44) with a relatively sustained temporal response to variation in asynchrony of a stroboscopic sequence. A pair of thin (.25°) stationary white rectangles is presented for a duration of 400 msec and in sequence. Stimulus–onset–asynchrony (SOA) between S_1 and S_2 is varied systematically. The response measure is the rate of action potentials at the peak of the poststimulus histogram (PSH) following S_2, that is, the S_2–PSH peak. (O), S_2–PSH peak for preferred-direction sequences; (●), S_2–PSH peak for nonpreferred-direction sequences. The squares represent sigma functions, that is, estimates of S_2–PSH peaks obtainable if S_1 and S_2 did not interact with each other in the visual system, but if their activation of am-44 were added linearly. These estimates were computed by taking the results of single-stimulus episodes, S_1 and S_2 presented alone, and adding them equally with a temporal separation to a particular SOA. This was done separately for each experimental SOA used, both for null-direction sequences and separately for preferred-direction sequences. (□), Sigma S_2–PSH peak for preferred-direction sequences.

between zero and several hundred milliseconds. Flash duration is typically 400 msec. Figure 10.3 shows the magnitude of the response (peak height in spikes per second) to the second stimulus (S_2). This was recorded from a complex directionally selective neuron with a receptive field of some 5° and a semisustained temporal response, decaying to about 300–400 msec. The open circles in Figure 10.3 depict the response to S_2 in a two-stimulus sequence presented in the preferred direction for continuous motion. The solid circles depict the response to the same S_2 when it is part of a null-direction sequence. It is obvious that S_2 yields a smaller response when it is part of a null-direction sequence. Hence, we see that complex, directionally selective neurons also show selectivity to sequences of stroboscopically presented static stimuli. Note that inhibition (as measured by the vertical distance between solid and open circles) sustains undiminished for 300 msec and lasts to 400 msec, and probably well beyond that time. Thus, cortical inhibition created by movement in the null direction is quite long-lasting. Its temporal decay, in fact, we have found to be invariably longer than the impulse response to a flash at the same receptive field location.

The square symbols in Figure 10.3 represent a prediction of what this neuron would produce as a response to S_2, as taken from data on that cell with single flashes at S_1 and separately at S_2, assuming simple additivity of the two responses. The fact that the open circles are always below the square symbols suggests that there is considerable inhibition of the S_2 response even in the preferred direction. Of course, there is even greater inhibition in the null direction.

V. Response of Transient and Sustained Neurons to Moving Edges of Diverse Velocities and Contrasts

A neuron's selectivity to direction of motion, that is, the preferred minus the null difference, seems to be affected by velocity. With neurons having *sustained* temporal properties, we noted poor direction selectivity at higher velocities. For example, in Figure 10.1, at a velocity of $25.4°$ sec^{-1}, T11-55 showed little difference between null and preferred direction in elicited response rates with moving edges of log intensities below 1.0 cd m^{-2}. When the stimulus object is moving quickly, the inhibitory process apparently does not enter in until high-contrast levels are reached and its threshold exceeded. This suggests that in a sustained response-type neuron the inhibitory process responsible for the diminution in responsiveness to null-direction motion has poor sensitivity (or long latency, or both) to fast processes. At low velocities such as $1.5°$ sec^{-1} a large preferred minus null difference is achieved even at low edge intensities.

In contrast, simple directionally selective neurons with *transient* temporal characteristics showed higher directional selectivity at higher velocities. For example, neuron T9-39 had a small, discrete receptive field with an on-excitatory discharge center of $.3$ to $.4°$. Neuron T9-39 was directionally selective, but responded optimally only to high velocities. Note in Figure 10.4 that at low velocities (e.g., $1.5°$ sec^{-1}) directional selectivity was poor though not altogether absent. Moreover, responsiveness actually dropped as the contrast of the edge increased. This suggests inhibition is generated both in the preferred and the opposite direction. As velocity increases, the intensity-response curve in the preferred direction becomes more monotonic. In other words, at higher velocities of movement in the preferred direction the transient neuron's excitatory discharge is apparently activated before inhibition has proceeded very far.

A third property of cortical inhibition responsible for directional selectivity is that in sustained neurons, inhibition has such a slow time constant that it can be eluded at high velocities of contour motion across the receptive field. This causes directional selectivity to be lost at velocities above $10-20°$ sec^{-1}. In contrast, transient neurons have a cortical inhibition that also has a fairly slow time constant, but apparently it is rapid enough to inhibit the excitatory response in the null direction within the $10-25°$ sec^{-1} range of velocities studied here. Obviously, at still higher velocities, there must be a point where even transient neurons begin to lose directional selectivity.

More generally, we infer that the velocity range within which a cortical neuron shows directional selectivity appears to be a function of the difference in temporal

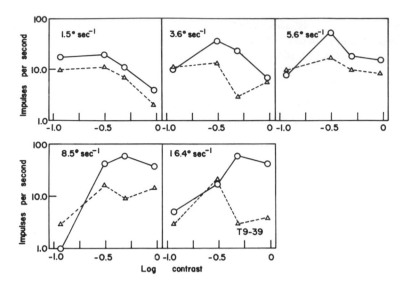

Figure 10.4. Response-intensity functions for a simple, directionally selective transient neuron T9-39, obtained with an edge moving in the cell's receptive field at different velocities and in two different directions of motion. Impulse rate is plotted against contrast on logarithmic coordinates. Contrast is defined as $(L_1 - L_d)/(L_1 + L_d)$, where L_1 and L_d are luminances of the light and dark edges, respectively. Each graph point represents an average response rate during the edge's traverse across the receptive field, calculated from nine traverses. (◯), Edge motion in the preferred direction; (△), edge motion in the nonpreferred direction. Mean luminance = 13.7 cd m⁻².

course between the excitatory impulse response of the neuron, and the inhibitory process generated when the contour crosses the inhibitory region accounting for that selectivity.

VI. Higher Threshold for Cortical Inhibition

We find that both transient and sustained neurons only show directional selectivity at higher velocities when higher contrasts are used. There seems to be a threshold for directional selectivity. Below that threshold, the neuron responds to the moving edge, but nonselectively. A fourth property is that at higher velocities the threshold for cortical inhibition is somewhat higher than the threshold for excitation.

VII. Discussion

A. Temporal Parameters of Sequence-Direction Selectivity

A consistent characteristic of visual cortex neurons is their great stability of motion–direction selectiveness. For example, the breadth of their velocity tuning for real movement is very broad (Movshon, 1975). Similarly, with stroboscopic displays, one can often stimulate in a nonpreferred-sequence direction with an asynchrony between S_1 and S_2 of 400 msec or more and still find the response to the second stimulus inhibited. If the S_2 response, coming 400 msec or more after S_1, depends on the prior position of S_1, then there must be a mechanism which, in effect, retains a short-term memory of the previous position of S_1. It will be recalled that in Barlow and Levick's (1965) model of motion–direction selectivity, a delay gate was postulated for that purpose. In cat visual cortex neurons, such a memory mechanism appears to reside in the slow buildup and decay of the inhibition generated in the inhibitory flank of the nonpreferred direction. For example, if null direction is right-to-left, the slow-decay inhibition is generated on the right side. This inhibition is measured here by the depression of the S_2–poststimulus histogram (PSH) peak. It has been found to decay over more than several hundred milliseconds in sustained neurons. The simple sequence-selective neuron acts like a gate that shuts (completely in some neurons, partially in others) and stays shut for a comparatively long period as soon as there is any activation from the nonpreferred direction.

In comparing the decay of this inhibition with the temporal impulse response for a stimulus at the same retinal position, it is repeatedly found that inhibitory decay is slower by an order of magnitude than the impulse response. What accounts for this discrepancy? It is widely believed that all direct afferent input from retinogeniculate fibers onto the visual cortex is excitatory in character. Intracellular recording studies in visual cortex have shown that electrical stimulation of lateral geniculate, optic chiasm, or optic radiations elicits excitatory postsynaptic potentials (EPSPs) and inhibitory postsynaptic potentials (IPSPs) at the cortex in which the latency of the IPSP is regularly .8 msec longer than EPSP latency for all three sites of electrical stimulation (Watanabe, Konishi, & Creutzfeldt, 1966; Toyama & Matsunami, 1968). The latency data suggest that the delay in the onset of IPSP is an intracortical phenomenon; specifically, while EPSPs can be elicited in visual cortex monosynaptically, IPSPs are always at least disynaptically elicited. If this proves to be essentially correct, it implies that the inhibition caused by movement in the visual field coming from a null-direction position must be due to the interposition of an internuncial cell (presumably a small stellate cell) between the geniculate afferent and the sequence-selective neuron. It is likely that it is the interposed internuncial which is also responsible for the slow temporal decay characterizing inhibition.

The slow temporal decay of inhibition generated by activation of the nonpreferred side of a simple neuron's receptive field has clear implications for the velocity-tuning characteristics of that neuron's directional selectivity. It is plausible to assume that a neuron's selective response to various velocities of movement is somehow related to the difference between the response to preferred- and nonpreferred-direction sequences, as given by Eq. (3). In Figure 10.3 this is represented by the vertical distance between the preferred-direction function (○) and the null-direction function (●) at each SOA value. Figure 10.3 shows that to a first approximation am-44 responds about as well differentially to stroboscopic sequence with SOA = 25 msec as with SOA = 300 msec. For the specific 1° interstimulus distance in am-44's receptive field, which was used to obtain these responses, this represents velocities ranging from $40°$ sec^{-1} to $3.3°$ sec^{-1}, or a log-unit range of velocities where approximately equal differential sensitivity is present. Thus, the velocity tuning of many neurons is inferred to be quite broad. This should be especially true for neurons with an impulse response of the sustained type (velocity tuning can also be inferred from Figures 10.1 and 10.4; it is clearly broad). It is our experience that both with real and stroboscopic movement sequences, a very broad range of velocities and SOA values is always effective (see also Movshon, 1975). The slow decay of the nonpreferred-direction inhibition gives great stability to the sequence-direction selectiveness of the neuron. As a result, however, much velocity information becomes lost.

When sustained neurons were tested with moving edges varying in velocity and in contrast, directional selectivity was shown to be lost at higher velocities. This loss in directional selectivity was primarily due to high response rates to high-velocity movement in the nonpreferred direction. The explanation is clear. Simple, directionally selective neurons in cat visual cortex have a powerful inhibitory flank on the nonpreferred side of the receptive field (Goodwin, Henry, & Bishop, 1975; Felder & Ganz, in preparation). The inhibition from that flank has a very slow time course in sustained-type neurons, slower than the time course of the excitatory discharge center. Therefore, we presume that when edge motion in the nonpreferred direction is too fast, the excitation from the excitatory discharge center is fully in progress before inhibition has developed. This occurs even though the moving edge stimulates the inhibitory flank first. In other words, as velocity in the nonpreferred direction increases, the latency difference between stimulation of the inhibitory flank and the later stimulation of the excitatory discharge center diminishes progressively. However, the impulse response from the excitatory discharge center remains considerably faster than the time course of inhibition. Therefore, as velocity increases, more excitation comes to precede inhibition, rendering the inhibition less efficacious. At these velocities, directional selectivity is lost. The same considerations apply to transient neurons, since their inhibitory time course is also slower than excitation but the loss in selectivity is shifted to a much higher velocity.

We believe that the division of neurons into two functional groups, the transient type concerned with the detection of movement and change, and the sustained type concerned with visual acuity and the detection of form (Ikeda & Wright, 1972, 1974, 1975a, 1975b) has not been correctly segmented. Our results suggest that a sustained impulse response is necessary for a selective response to slow movement. It is more probable that transient-type impulse responses participate in responses to fast change and movement, while neurons of the sustained type mediate acuity, form, and direction-selective slow-movement responses.

The fact that individual, simple, directionally selective cortical neurons lose velocity specificity leads one to wonder how this perceptual attribute is coded. Perhaps the differential activation of two different "channels," transient and sustained by fast- and slow-moving edges, respectively, provides encoded velocity information for a higher level neuron.

B. Psychophysical Parallelism

There are a number of obvious parallels between the stimulus conditions eliciting an experience of stroboscopic movement and those eliciting a selective response in simple and complex neurons.

First, it is clear that a stroboscopic sequence involving stationary pairs of stimulus pulses can elicit a highly selective response in cortical neurons. The selectiveness of the response can be strong. (It should be mentioned that we find that many neurons with large, complex receptive fields show only weak directional selectivity to sequences of strobed flashes.) The mechanism we have described here, in which selectiveness to direction of motion is created by having inhibition from visual stimulation of a nonpreferred-directed flank effectively depress the neuron's sensitivity for a prolonged period, appears designed to retain information on direction and degrade information on velocity. This combination of properties makes the mechanism selectively responsive to stroboscopic display, that is, to sequences of stationary light pulses presented within a broad range of SOAs. The selectivity mimics, to a first-order approximation, that shown to real movement, paralleling the illusion in human observers of real movement in stroboscopic movement sequences.

Second, consider the *difference* between an S_2–PSH response in the preferred and nonpreferred direction (the difference between the solid- and open-circle functions in Figure 10.3). This difference function typically rises steadily from an SOA value of zero, peaking approximately at SOA = 60–100 msec, and then steadily declining toward SOA = 200–400 msec (declining more rapidly in transient impulse-response neurons). Our measurements of this function admittedly need to be extended. But, such as they are, they are in agreement with measurements of the vividness of perceived movement to SOA sequences where the most vivid apparent movement is reported at 80 msec < SOA < 100 msec (Kahneman, 1967; Weisstein & Growney, 1969; Kolers, 1972, see especially Figures 4.4 and 4.5).

Third, velocity tuning of directional selectivity appears to be very broad in the entire population sampled here (see also Movshon, 1975). This is paralleled by the results of habituation studies in human subjects (Sekuler & Ganz, 1963; Sekuler & Pantle, 1967; Pantle & Sekuler, 1968, 1969; Breitmeyer, 1973) where velocity tuning of the inferred habituated movement-selective receptors has invariably been broad.

ACKNOWLEDGMENTS

We are grateful to R. C. Felder and to A. F. Lange for technical assistance with the experiments.

REFERENCES

Barlow, H. B., & Levick, W. R. The mechanism of directionally selective units in rabbit's retina. *Journal of Physiology,* 1965, *178,* 477–504.

Bishop, P. O., Coombs, J. S., & Henry, G. H. Interaction effects of visual contours on the discharge frequency of simple striate neurones. *Journal of Physiology,* 1971, *219,* 659–687.

Boynton, R. M., & Whitten, D. N. Visual adaptation in monkey cones: Recordings of late receptor potentials. *Science* 1970, *170,* 1423–1426.

Breitmeyer, B. G. A relationship between the detection of size, rate, orientation, and directions in the human visual system. *Vision Research,* 1973, *13,* 41–58.

Creutzfeldt, O., & Ito, M. Functional synaptic organization of primary visual cortex neurons in the cat. *Experimental Brain Research,* 1968, *6,* 324–352.

Felder, R. C., & Ganz, L. Analysis of directional selectivity in neurones of cat visual cortex. Manuscript in preparation, 1977.

Goodwin, A. W., Henry, G. H., & Bishop, P. O. Directional selectivity of simple striate cells: Properties and mechanism. *Journal of Neurophysiology,* 1975, *38,* 1500–1523.

Ikeda, H., & Wright, M. J. Receptive field organization of "sustained" and "transient" retinal ganglion cells which subserve different functional roles. *Journal of Physiology,* 1972, *222,* 769–800.

Ikeda, H., & Wright, M. J. Evidence for "sustained" and "transient" neurones in the cat's visual cortex. *Vision Research,* 1974, *14,* 133–136.

Ikeda, H., & Wright, M. J. Retinotopic distribution, visual latency and orientation tuning of "sustained" and "transient" cortical neurons in area 17 of the cat. *Experimental Brain Research,* 1975, *22,* 385–398. (a)

Ikeda, H., & Wright, M. J. Spatial and temporal properties of "sustained" and "transient" neurones in area 17 of the cat's visual cortex. *Experimental Brain Research,* 1975, *22,* 353–383. (b)

Joshua, D. E., & Bishop, P. O. Binocular single vision and depth discrimination. Receptive field disparities for central and peripheral vision and binocular interaction on peripheral single units in cat striate cortex. *Experimental Brain Research,* 1970, *10,* 289–416.

Kahneman, D. An onset-onset law for one case of apparent motion and metacontrast. *Perception & Psychophysics,* 1967, *2,* 577–584.

Kolers, P. A. *Aspects of motion perception.* Oxford: Pergamon Press, 1972.

Movshon, J. A. The velocity tuning of single units in cat striate cortex. *Journal of Physiology,* 1975, *249,* 445–468.

Normann, R. A., & Werblin, F. S. Control of retinal sensitivity. I. Light and dark adaptation of vertebrate rods and cones. *Journal of General Physiology,* 1974, *63,* 37–61.

Pantle, A., & Sekuler, R. Velocity sensitive elements in human vision: Initial psychophysical evidence. *Vision Research,* 1968, *8,* 445–450.

Pantle, A., & Sekuler, R. Contrast response of human visual mechanisms sensitive to orientation and direction of motion. *Vision Reserach,* 1969, *9,* 397–406.

Sekuler, R. W., & Ganz, L. Aftereffect of seen motion with a stabilized retinal image. *Science,* 1963, *139,* 419–420.

Sekuler, R., & Pantle, A. A model for after-effects of seen movement. *Vision Research,* 1967, *7,* 427–439.

Toyama, K., & Matsunami, K. Synaptic action of specific visual impulses upon cat's parastriate cortex. *Brain Research,* 1968, *10,* 473–476.

Watanabe, S., Konishi, M., & Creutzfeld, O. D. Postsynaptic potentials in the cat's visual cortex following electric stimulation of afferent pathways. *Experimental Brain Research, 1966, 1,* 272–283.

Weisstein, N., & Growney, R. L. Apparent movement and meta-contrast: A note on Kahneman's formulation. *Perception & Psychophysics,* 1969, *5,* 321–328.

Sensitivity and Adaptation

11. "Compression" of Retinal Responsivity: V–log I Functions and Increment Thresholds[1]

Theodore P. Williams and John G. Gale

I. Introduction

Naka and Rushton (1966a) were the first to show that retinal responses (from horizontal cells in their study) followed the hyperbolic relationship

$$V/V_{max} = I/(I + \sigma),\qquad(1)$$

where V is the amplitude of the response evoked by a flash of intensity, I, and V_{max} is the saturation response. The intensity eliciting half-maximal response is called "σ," the semisaturation constant. It appears that Eq. (1) also provides an adequate description of receptor responses (Boynton & Whitten, 1970; Dowling & Ripps, 1972; Fain & Dowling, 1973; Grabowski, Pinto, & Pak, 1972) and of PIII responses (Ernst & Kemp, 1972; Witkovsky, Dudek, & Ripps, 1975). This is interesting because no theoretical reason for this equation was given by Naka and Rushton in their original work. More recently, Hagins and Yoshikami (1975) have presented a transmitter model of receptor function and have suggested that under certain conditions this model will give rise to the hyperbolic relationship. The conditions to which they refer are those in which the transmitter is found in either of *two states,* namely, it is bound either to the disk or to the plasma membrane.

In this chapter we present a model also based on the idea that a response-producing system can exist in one of two states. In the development of the model, response generators are treated as simple "black boxes" but could be thought of as retinal volumes within which photons can be absorbed and responses produced. This kind of generalized view is sufficient for present purposes because we are only interested in the input–output behavior of those systems to which the model will be applied. The two-state nature of the model leads directly to a description of simple

[1]This work was supported in part by NSF Grant BNS74-24655, by an institutional grant from ERDA, and by NIMH Training Grant No. MH 11218.

129

"compression" adaptation, such as seen, for example, in human rod "signals" (Alpern, Rushton, & Torii, 1970). We also suggest that it is applicable to two nonneural responses of the retina, c-wave (from pigment epithelial cells), and slow PIII (from glial cells), since these responses have certain properties that characterize compression systems. In addition, the two-state model gives a simple, testable meaning to σ, the semisaturation intensity, and it leads to increment threshold functions closely resembling those reported for certain retinal responses.

II. Results and Discussion

A. The Model

We start by assuming that "generators" of the given response exist in *finite* number. When this maximum number is activated the maximum response, V_{max}, is obtained. The formalism of the model is expressed in the following way:

$$A + I \underset{k_2}{\overset{k_1}{\rightleftharpoons}} B,$$

where As are responsive generators that absorb light of intensity I and are driven to state B in which each produces a unit of response. As long as they are in state B, the generators continue to produce this response, and when B is reconverted to A (without added light), the response unit is also removed. Thus, Bs are responding generators, and their concentration is proportional to the response V. They are also considered to be unresponsive to additional photons absorbed within them.

The rate at which A is driven to B by light is proportional to k_1, which in the simplest case is the photosensitivity of the generator (i.e., volume element) expressed as generators per photon. The designation k_2 represents the rate of removal of the response, for example, by the process of rapid "neural" dark adaptation. Note that A reappears at this same rate. In other words, the model does not incorporate any *long-lived* intermediates in either the forward or reverse paths. [For an example of such an intermediate state, compare the Y-binding site of Hagins and Yoshikami (1975).] Thus, compression is built into this model: The generators must either be responding to light or be available for response to it. This is expressed as

$$A_0 = A + B. \tag{2}$$

Here, A_0 is the total number of generators, and is the quantity that is proportional to V_{max}, as mentioned earlier.

The rate equation appropriate for the production of response at intensity I is

$$dB/dt = k_1 I A - k_2 B. \tag{3}$$

We shall assume that steady state is quickly attained and that therefore $dB/dt \simeq 0$. Hence

$$k_1 I A = k_2 B, \tag{4}$$

and since $A = A_0 - B$,

$$k_1 I (A_0 - B) = k_2 B. \tag{5}$$

This gives

$$B/A_0 = I/(I + k_2/k_1). \tag{6}$$

Since B is proportional to V and A_0 to V_{max}, Eq. (6) is the same as the original Naka–Rushton Eq. (1) where k_2/k_1 is identified with σ. This ratio of rates has the units of intensity (photons $sec^{-1} \cdot$ generator^{-1}) as it should: $k_1 =$ generators per photon (the photosensitivity), $k_2 = 1$ sec^{-1}, and $k_2/k_1 =$ photons $sec^{-1} \cdot$ generator^{-1} $= I$. A simple test of Eq. (6) and therefore of this two-state model would be to measure the temperature dependence of k_2, and assuming k_1 to be independent of temperature (since photosensitivity is), to compare this with a measurement of the temperature dependence of the midpoints of V–$\log I$ functions obtained in separate experiments.

It is interesting to note that k_2/k_1 also has an appropriate intuitive meaning. If a response-producing system has a rate of recovery that is much greater than its rate of excitation, then it will be able to remain responsive even at high intensities. The effect of this would be to confer upon the system a large σ. For example, the photosensitivities of rod and cone pigments are quite similar (Weale, 1965), but their rates of rapid dark adaptation are different—cones are faster than rods. Hence, the V–$\log I$ functions should show a larger σ for cones than for rods. And this is observed (cf. Norman & Werblin, 1974).

To summarize: A two-state model of response generators gives an equation identical in form to the one originally proposed by Naka and Rushton for horizontal cell responses. The model predicts that σ is the ratio of the rate constants for recovery and excitation.

B. Increment Threshold Functions

Formulation of the response of a simple compression system in the presence of a background is accomplished as follows. Consider Figure 11.1. Here the idealized time course of responses is shown: A background of intensity I_B comes on at the arrow and remains on. The response, V_B, to it quickly reaches the steady-state level and stays there (since this is a simple compression model). If a saturating test flash were now imposed on top of this background, the maximum possible response to such a flash is $V'_{max} = (V_{max} - V_B)$. If other than saturating test flashes are given the responses to them follow the usual hyperbolic relationship, the only difference being that now this relationship must be modified to account for the unavailability of a part of V_{max}, namely V_B.

Thus

$$V_T/(V_{max} - V_B) = I_T/(I_T + \sigma). \tag{7}$$

The denominator of the left-hand side of Eq. (7) represents the redefinition of the

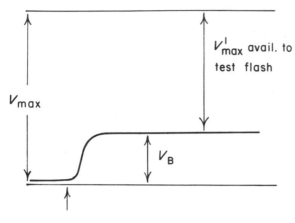

V'_{max} avail. to test flash

Figure 11.1. Idealized time course of response to background in a simple compression system. I_B comes on at arrow and a steady response, V_B, is maintained. After this time, a saturating test flash can elicit no greater response than $V'_{max} = V_{max} - V_B$. This redefines the maximum response available to any test flash in the presence of a background for a compression system.

maximum response available to the test flash. It states that test flashes are processed in a way that depends upon the response elicited by the background and in fact shows what the dependence is. This denominator is the "compression factor" and will be shown to have the same form as the one used by Alpern *et al.* (1970).

Figure 11.2 shows V–log I functions calculated from Eq. (7) for various I_Bs. These were done in the following way: A σ was picked and assumed to be constant for all conditions of adaptation (again because we are dealing only with simple compression systems). Then V_{max} was set equal to 1 and $V_B = I_B/(I_B + \sigma)$ was substituted. This fixes the denominator of the left-hand side of Eq. (7) for any given value of I_B. Finally, I_T values were picked and V_T calculated for each. The V–log I functions of Figure 11.2 are compressed and the dashed vertical line shows that the apparent σ does not change.

In order to calculate increment thresholds, Eq. (7) is rearranged as

$$I_T = \sigma V_T/(1 - V_T - V_B), \tag{8}$$

where V_{max} has been set equal to unity; thus V_T and V_B are fractions of the maximum response. Substituting $V_B = I_B/(I_B + \sigma)$, one sees that Eq. (8) becomes

$$I_T = \sigma V_T/[1 - V_T - (I_B/I_B + \sigma)]. \tag{9}$$

Eq. (9) was solved numerically by picking values of σ and V_T (the criterion response) and varying the value of I_B. Thus, I_T becomes the dependent variable just as it is experimentally. (Note: For accurate results it is necessary to carry at least as many decimal places in all the parameters as there are in V_T.) The results of such calculations are given in Figure 11.3 for two values of σ.

Several features of these curves are of interest. First, Weber lines of unit slope are evident when small criteria are chosen. An earlier equation for increment thresholds presented by others (Naka & Rushton, 1966b; Boynton & Whitten, 1970) does not give this result (for a critique of the earlier equation see the Appendix). Second, the low I_B limit on I_T is σV_T and this agrees with Alpern *et al.* (1970). Third, saturation

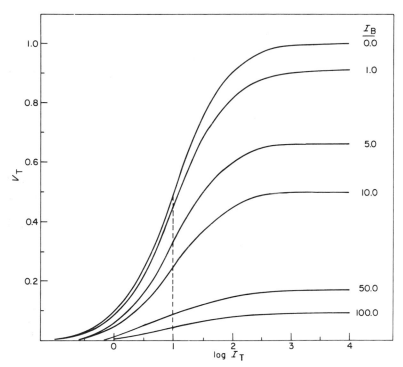

Figure 11.2. V–log$I$ functions calculated for a simple compression system in the presence of various I_Bs as shown. The value of σ used in Eq. (7) was 10 and the apparent σ of these curves stays at that value over all the I_B values used.

occurs at $I_B = \sigma/V_T$. This ratio has a simple meaning: It is the number of jnds of size V_T available to the system over an intensity range equal to σ. Fourth, of further interest in Figure 11.3 is the fact that the functions "break" at $I_B = \sigma$ and enter the linear Weber region. This implies that when a simple compression system is obeying the Weber law, it is responding in the "top-half" of its operating range. More specifically, Table 11.1 shows that strict linearity does not obtain until the background elicits at least 90% of V_{max}. Above such a background intensity, one log unit of I_T is required to reach criterion for every log unit of I_B imposed. Finally, it is clear that the curves move upward and subtend smaller ranges of I_B when the criterion is increased. This feature is of special interest because data obtained from a compression system are available for comparison. Not only have Alpern *et al.* (1970) indicated that human rod signals behave as a compression system, but they have also varied the criterion response in a systematic way. Their results are shown as symbols with error bars in Figure 11.4, and the lines drawn through these are from our Eq. (9). The fit is nearly exact. The parameter on the curves is the criterion rod signal just needed to suppress other given rod signals. Alpern *et al.* cite the criterion on the lowest curve as 10^{-4}—exactly the one we find gives the best fit in our Eq.

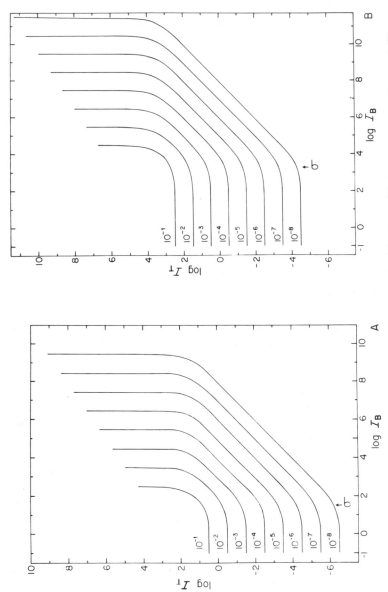

Figure 11.3. Increment threshold functions calculated from Eq. (9). (A) σ = 30 photons generator^{-1} · sec^{-1}. (B) σ = 3000. The parameter on each curve is the criterion of threshold V_T. Higher criteria move the curves upward on the I_T axis. All curves are horizontal lines at low I_B, the value of I_T being equal to $\sigma \times V_T$ (see Alpern et al., 1970). Weber relationships are obvious in some curves but only when V_T is small and only then when T_B exceeds σ. The range of backgrounds over which the linear (log–log) region extends is roughly the inverse of the criterion chosen. Saturation occurs at σ/V_T.

TABLE 11.1

Dependence of I_T on the Fraction of Maximum Response Elicited by Backgrounds[a]

$V_B V_{max}$	I_T
.001	3.0×10^{-5}
.01	3.0×10^{-5}
.10	3.3×10^{-5}
.20	3.7×10^{-5}
.50	6.0×10^{-5}
.80	1.5×10^{-4}
.90	3.0×10^{-4}
.99	3.0×10^{-3}
.999	3.0×10^{-2}
.9999	3.0×10^{-1}
.99999	3.0

[a]Calculated from Eq. (9) with $V_T = 10^{-6}$, $\sigma = 30$. Entries below the broken line reflect Weber relationship.

(9). They do not give explicit values for the criteria on the other curves, but their experimental paradigm implies it was increased by factors of 8. These values, 8 × 10^{-4} and 6.4 × 10^{-3} used in our equation, also correspond well.

Another test of our two-state model derives from the results of Witkovsky *et al.* (1975) on slow PIII of carp and from the work of Steinberg (1971) on pigment epithelial responses from cat. These responses resemble compression systems in

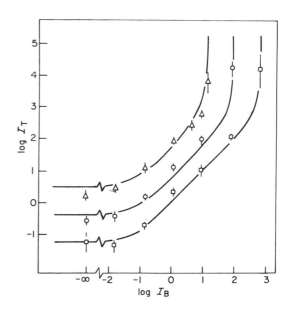

Figure 11.4. Comparison of experimental and calculated results. Symbols with error bars are from Alpern *et al.* (1970) and lines drawn through them are calculated from Eq. (9). The parameter on the curves is the criterion rod response needed to just suppress rod signals elicited with lights of various intensities. Alpern *et al.* indicate that the criterion is 10^{-4} for the bottom curve and we find it fits their data exactly when used in our Eq. (9). The criterion on the middle curve is 8 × 10^{-4} and on the top curve it is 6.4 × 10^{-3}.

some respects, especially in their saturation mechanisms. In both of these studies, increment threshold functions are presented which break and enter the Weber region at or near σ of the dark-adapted V–$\log I$ function. An attempt was made to compare our model with these published functions in more detail. Without any scaling, the agreement was good but not excellent: The model failed to duplicate the absolute thresholds of the slow PIII by .5 log unit but fit the rest of the points well. However, it reproduced the epithelial responses exactly in the low-background region but failed to predict saturation by .7 log unit. Perhaps these inadequacies arise from the fact that the responses in question are not simple compression systems. For example, both have V–$\log I$ functions which shift slightly to higher intensities as backgrounds are increased; that is, σ is not constant as it is in our model or as it is in human rod signals.

In Eq. (7) redefinition of the maximum response available to the test flash is embodied in the term $V_{\max} - V_B$. This is the compression factor of our equation. Alpern et al. (1970) in their treatment of rod signals as a compression system have used the following equation for increment threshold which also involves a compression factor:

$$N = [\Phi/(\Phi + \sigma)] \times [\Theta_D/(\Theta_D + \Theta)].$$

Here N is the amplitude of the rod signal (analogous to our V_T) which is elicited by a test flash of intensity Φ in the presence of a background whose intensity is Θ. Θ_D is the "eigengrau" or dark light (noise) and is a constant characteristic of the system. In the absence of a background the rod signal depends only upon intensity, Φ, but in the presence of a background whose intensity is Θ, there is a compression factor, $\Theta_D/(\Theta_D + \Theta)$, which reduces the effectiveness of the $\Phi/(\Phi + \sigma)$ term. On first inspection, this multiplicative compression factor bears no resemblance to our simple subtractive one, $V_{\max} - V_B$, but a closer look suggests they may well be analogous; to wit: Let $V_{\max} = 1$ and $V_B = I_B/(I_B + \sigma)$. Then our compression factor becomes

$$V_{\max} - V_B = 1 - I_B/(I_B + \sigma) = \sigma/(\sigma + I_B),$$

and upon substituting this and cross-multiplying, our Eq. (7) becomes

$$V_T = [I_T/(I_T + \sigma)] \times [\sigma/(\sigma + I_B)].$$

This now has the same form as that used by Alpern et al. since our compression factor has become a multiplicative term. But while the form of the equations is the same, it is difficult to pursue this comparison further, since it would then be necessary to identify σ with Θ_D. While both are characteristic constants of the systems, it seems unlikely that they are one and the same. Hence, the actual numerical value of our compression factor need not be the same as that of Alpern et al. (1970). This assumption seems appropriate since psychophysical and electrophysiological thresholds seldom match.

III. Appendix

Naka and Rushton (1966a) presented the following equation which they suggested was appropriate for describing responses of horizontal cells to test flashes in the presence of backgrounds:

$$(V_T + V_B)/V_{max} = (I_T + I_B)/(I_T + I_B + \sigma). \qquad (a)$$

(We have changed their symbolism but not the form of the equation.) Here, the Vs are responses (voltage changes) and Is are intensities, with subscripts T and B referring to "test" and "background," respectively. V_{max} is the maximum (i.e., saturation) response and σ is the intensity which elicits one-half of V_{max}. This equation seems to be intuitively correct since it appears to embody the actual experimental conditions; that is, it shows that test flash intensities are *added* to those of the background and that the overall response is the $sum (V_T + V_B)$. As Naka and Rushton (1966b) put it: "This is what must follow if the flash $[I_T]$ simply adds to $[I_B]$ and gives a total potential $[V_T + V_B]$ as though $[I_T + I_B]$ was [sic] a single flash [p. 598]." We shall refer to these features of the equation as the additivity properties and to the equation itself as the additive equation. At the end of this critique, we shall call attention to one of the consequences of these additive terms.

Boynton and Whitten (1970) slightly modified the additive equation by raising the intensity terms to powers less than 1. However, they retained the additivity of the terms. Important for the present critique is the fact that Boynton and Whitten present increment threshold data which have a Weber line whose slope is 1. Others who have presented data with Weber lines of unit slope have also referred to this equation (Dowling & Ripps, 1972). Thus, using it in conjunction with data whose slopes are unity implies that the equation gives rise to such slopes.

The main point of this appendix is to show that the additivity equation gives Weber functions whose slopes are, in fact, 2, not 1.

Apparently, those who have used or cited this equation have not tested it numerically. We have put numbers into it and the results are shown in Figure 11.5. To do these calculations we have proceeded as

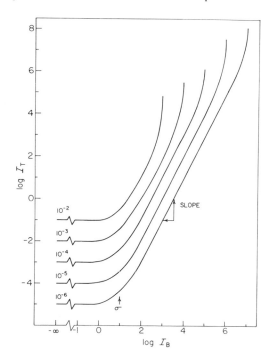

Figure 11.5. Increment threshold functions calculated from the additive equation. The equation predicts slopes of 2 but experimental results typically have slopes of unity (or less). The parameter on the curves is the criterion response, V_T/V_{max}.

follows: A fixed σ was chosen (10 photons absorbed per rod per second in Figure 11.1, but values up to 3000 have also been used with no change in the slopes of the Weber lines). A criterion response V_T/V_{max} was picked. Then an I_B was chosen and the response to it, V_B, was calculated from $V_B/V_{max} = I_B/(I_B + \sigma)$. Then σ, V_T/V_{max}, I_B, and V_B were substituted into the additive equation and I_T was calculated.

Not only does direct numerical solution of this equation give Weber lines of slope 2 but an analytical solution of the equation corroborates this result:

$$(V_B + V_T)/V_{max} = (I_B + I_T)/(I_B + I_T + \sigma), \tag{a}$$

whence

$$V_T/V_{max} = [(I_B + I_T)/(I_B + I_T + \sigma)] - [I_B/(I_B + \sigma)]. \tag{b}$$

After obtaining the LCD and collecting terms

$$V_T/V_{max} = \sigma I_T/(I_B + I_T + \sigma)(I_B + \sigma) \tag{c}$$

$$= \sigma I_T/[(I_B + \sigma)^2 + I_T(I_B + \sigma)]. \tag{d}$$

It must be recognized that the Weber fraction region (a) lies at intensities greater than σ of the dark-adapted V–$\log I$ function (cf. Dowling & Ripps, 1972; Witkovsky et al., 1975) and (b) in this region $I_T \ll I_B$. These conditions mean that $(I_B + \sigma)^2 \simeq (I_B)^2$ and $(I_B + \sigma)^2 \gg I_T(I_B + \sigma)$.

Therefore, Eq. (d) becomes

$$V_T/V_{max} = \sigma I_T/I_B^2, \tag{e}$$

whence

$$\log I_T = 2 \log I_B + \log(V_T/V_{max}) - \log \sigma. \tag{f}$$

Thus a plot of Eq. (f) with $\log I_T$ as ordinate and $\log I_B$ as abscissa will have a slope of 2 (compare Glantz, 1972).

We now make a final point regarding the additivity properties of the equation. While it is true that test and background intensities are physically added to each other, it does not follow that the response elicited will be the sum $V_T + V_B$ "as though $[I_T + I_B]$ was a single flash." If this were true, the phenomenon called "summation period" would be unknown; that is, two lights could always be added together, at any time between their onsets, and the result would be a response of fixed amplitude determined only by the relationship given in the additive equation. Obviously this is not observed. The only time it is true is when the onsets are synchronized or, at most, separated by a few milliseconds. But these are not the conditions under which increment thresholds are typically determined.

In summary, we conclude that the additive equation does not reproduce Weber lines with unit slopes. This conclusion is based on direct numerical solution as well as analytical solution of the equation.

REFERENCES

Alpern, M., Rushton, W. A. H., & Torii, S. The attenuation of rod signals by backgrounds. *Journal of Physiology*, 1970, *206*, 209–227.

Boynton, R. M., & Whitten, D. N. Visual adaptation in monkey cones: Recordings of late-receptor potentials. *Science*, 1970, *170*, 1423–1427.

Dowling, J. E., & Ripps, H. Adaptation in skate photoreceptors. *Journal of General Physiology*, 1972, *60*, 698–719.

Ernst, W., & Kemp, C. M. The effects of rhodopsin decomposition on PIII responses of isolated rat retinae. *Vision Research*, 1972, *12*, 1937–1946.

Fain, G. L., & Dowling, J. E. Intracellular recordings from single rods and cones in the mudpuppy retina. *Science*, 1973, *180*, 1178–1181.

Glantz, R. M. Visual adaptation: A case of nonlinear summation. *Vision Research,* 1972, *12,* 103–109.

Grabowski, S. R., Pinto, L. H., & Pak, W. L. Adaptation in retinal rods of axolotl: Intracellular recordings. *Science,* 1972, *176,* 1240–1245.

Hagins, W. A., & Yoshikami, S. Ionic mechanisms in excitation of photoreceptors. *Annals of the New York Academy of Sciences,* 1975, *264,* 314–325.

Naka, K., & Rushton, W. A. H. S-potentials from colour units in the retina of fish (*Cyprinidae*). *Journal of Physiology,* 1966, *185,* 536–555. (a)

Naka, K., & Rushton, W. A. H. S-potentials from luminosity units in the retina of fish (*Cyprinidae*). *Journal of Physiology,* 1966, *185,* 587–599. (b)

Normann, R. A., & Werblin, F. S. Control of retinal sensitivity. I. Light and dark adaptation of vertebrate rods and cones. *Journal of General Physiology,* 1974, *63,* 37–61.

Steinberg, R. H. Incremental responses to light recorded from pigment epithelial cells and horizontal cells of the cat retina. *Journal of Physiology,* 1971, *217,* 93–116.

Weale, R. A. Vision and fundus reflectometry: A review. *Photochemistry and Photobiology, 4,* 1965, 67–87.

Williams, T. P., & Gale, J. G. Critique of an increment threshold function. *Vision Research,* 1977, *17,* 881–882.

Witkovsky, P., Dudek, F. E., & Ripps, H. Slow PIII component of the carp electroretinogram. *Journal of General Physiology,* 1975, *65,* 119–127.

12. Psychophysical and Physiological Tests of Proposed Physiological Mechanisms of Light Adaptation[1]

Donald C. Hood

I. Introduction

The major problem of visual adaptation is usually stated in the following way: An organism must be able to detect naturally occurring contrasts (which rarely produce intensity differences of more than a factor of 100 even with shadows) over a range of naturally occurring ambient intensities that exceeds 10^8. In the last 15 years, a wealth of physiological data that bear on the mechanisms of adaptation has been collected. These data have led to a variety of proposals for the possible physiological bases of visual psychophysics. In this chapter I will summarize some of our work in which both psychophysical and physiological experiments were designed to test some physiological proposals.

II. A Psychophysical Test of Physiological Proposals: Use of the Cone Saturation Paradigm

At any moment, ambient intensity is relatively constant, and the visual system is responsive to a small range of intensities (the dynamic range) around this ambient level. Adaptation has long been thought to involve an ambient-light-induced change in the dynamic range of the visual system (cf. Craik, 1938). There is general agreement among recent physiological studies about the nature of the dynamic range. However, there is wide disagreement about how the dynamic range changes with ambient intensity.

[1]This research was supported in part by National Institutes of Health Grants EY 01877 and EY 02115.

A. Dynamic Range and the Effect of Ambient Intensity

To study a cell's dynamic range the physiologist measures its response to a range of flash intensities. Figure 12.1 shows a typical response–intensity function that relates peak amplitude of the response to intensity of a light flash. Notice that the response does not continue to grow as flash intensity is increased much beyond the value of the intensity marked I_s. This response function is described by Eq. (1), which has been shown to fit a wide variety of physiological data. In Eq. (1),

$$R(I_f) = [I_f^n/I_f^n + \sigma^n] \times R_{max}, \tag{1}$$

$R(I_f)$ refers to the amplitude of the incremental response, the response above ongoing activity, elicited by a flash of intensity I_f. R_{max} is the largest incremental response amplitude possible to any flash. The term σ is called the semisaturation constant since, when $I_f = \sigma$, $R(I_f) = .5$ or one half of its maximum, R_{max}.

There is fair agreement that the shape of the response–intensity function, at least for flashes presented in the dark, is described by Eq. (1) with n between .7 and 1.0. There is also agreement that increases in ambient-light level decrease the response R to any flash intensity I_f. This is analogous to the decrease in sensitivity measured psychophysically. What is not agreed upon is how the response amplitude decreases. We have found at least four physiological explanations in the literature, and these are presented in Figure 12.2. Each panel shows three response–intensity functions, each for a different adapting intensity, along with the equation describing how the response amplitude $R(I_f, I_A)$ depends upon the flash and adapting field intensities. Notice that in every panel the response to any given flash intensity is smaller as the adapting intensity I_A is increased. However, the dynamic range is modified differently in each of these four theoretical response–intensity functions (see the legend to Figure 12.2).

All four physiological explanations must take pigment bleaching into consideration. With increases in the steady ambient-light level I_A, the proportion p of pigment molecules present in receptors decreases. Pigment bleaching can be thought of as changing the effective intensity from I to pI. So, for example, if an ambient light bleaches half the pigment molecules, a light flash of twice the intensity will be

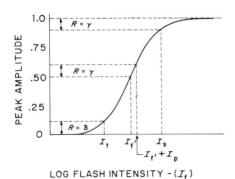

LOG FLASH INTENSITY - (I_f)

Figure 12.1. A hypothetical response–intensity function.

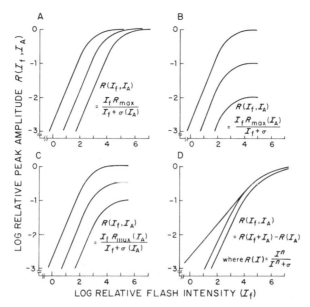

Figure 12.2. Four sets of theoretical response–intensity functions describing changes in the incremental response amplitude R as a function of the incremental flash intensity I_f and the steady adapting intensity I_A. The incremental response R is the response elicited over and above any tonic response to I_A. Each panel gives the theoretical expression and shows three response–intensity functions, plotted on log–log coordinates, for three different adapting intensities, I_A. The lowest adapting intensity is considered to be zero (darkness) and response amplitudes, $R(I_f, I_A)$, are expressed relative to the maximum, R_{max}, in the dark [i.e., for $I_A = 0$, $R_{max}(0) = R_{max} = 1$]. (A) The semisaturation constant, σ, increases with increased I_A (cf. Werblin, 1971). This shifts the response–intensity function parallel to the log I_f axis as I_A increases (see Section V, Note 1). (B) R_{max} decreases with increased I_A (cf. Alpern et al., 1970). This shifts the response–intensity function parallel to the log R_{max} axis. (C) Both σ and R_{max} change with I_A (cf. Kleinschmidt & Dowling, 1975) and the response–intensity functions shift down and to the right on log-log coordinates. (D) This theoretical expression does not have a parameter that is free to vary with I_A. The incremental response to the flash is assumed to be the difference between the response to the flash plus the adapting field $R(I_f + I_A)$ and the response to the adapting field alone $R(I_A)$, both determined by the same response–intensity function (cf. Boynton & Whitten, 1970).

required to produce the same number of quantal absorptions as before bleaching. In order to take bleaching into consideration, I in Figure 12.2 can be replaced by J where $J_x = pI_x$ (see Section V, Note 1). When we refer to the theoretical response–intensity functions in the following, J will be used. For I_A below about 3 log td, I and J are approximately equal.

B. Psychophysical Tests

Our purpose is to form psychophysically testable models based on the theoretical response–intensity functions in Figure 12.2 and to determine which of these models best accounts for human psychophysical performance. We will attempt to show that traditional increment threshold data by themselves cannot be used to choose among the alternative models. However, these models can be tested by examining their ability to predict these data and a new psychophysical measure, saturation.

To form psychophysically testable models of human cone system adaptation based on physiological proposals requires us to make two classes of assumptions. One class (physiological) makes the physiological model explicit. A second class (psychophysiological) makes explicit the connection between the behavior and the physiological model. We will make the physiological assumption that the human visual system responds according to one of the response–intensity functions in Figure 12.2. For now we are making no specific assumptions about the locus in the visual system at which cells respond as shown in Figure 12.2. The locus may be the receptors; it may be further upstream, or perhaps no single cell type is responsible. The form of response function may be determined by events at several levels. For our psychophysiological assumption, let us assume that threshold intensity I_t is the intensity of a light flash that produces an incremental response of a criterion size $R(I_t, I_A) = \delta$ (see Figure 12.1). This says that regardless of adapting field intensity, physiological responses of the same size are equally detectable psychophysically.

With these assumptions, there are four models, each consisting of the assumptions plus one of the sets of theoretical response–intensity functions. We can ask how well these four models handle human cone increment threshold data. We know that the threshold intensity I_t of a flash varies with I_A. (Over a wide range of values of I_A, I_t increases in proportion to the increases in I_A—Weber's law.) All four models predict these changes in threshold. In fact, three of the models fit the data perfectly. This should not be surprising from either the appearance of the response functions or the theoretical expressions. For Models A and B, the functions $\sigma(J_A)$ and $R_{max}(J_A)$ can be chosen to fit the threshold data. Model C with two such functions can easily describe these data. Only Model D does not have a parameter that is free to vary with I_A, but the human threshold data can be fit reasonably well if σ is large and n in Eq. (1) is less than 1 (see Boynton & Whitten, 1970).

1. SATURATION INTENSITY AND THE MODELS

Since all the models discussed can easily handle one empirical measure, namely, threshold, a second psychophysical measure is needed. Notice that if one covers the upper portion of the curves in Figure 12.2, the lower parts near threshold look similar for the four models. We need another point on the response–intensity function such as the point labeled I_s in Figure 12.1. The flash intensity I_s, which will be called saturation intensity, is the intensity that brings the response to within a constant, γ, of the peak response just as I_t raised the response to δ above zero. The psychophysiological assumption is similar to the one previously stated. In particular, assume that the saturating intensity I_s is the intensity of the flash that produces an incremental response within a constant value of the maximum response, that is, $R(I_s, I_A) = R_{max}(I_t, I_A) - \gamma$. Figure 12.3 shows predictions of I_s as a function of I_A according to models A, B, and D; the parameters in Models A and B are chosen

Figure 12.3. Predicted changes in the log of the saturating intensity I_s with, changes in adapting intensity I_A are shown for models based on the theoretical response–intensity functions of Figures 12.2A, B, and D. Curve P (bleaching curve) shows the way log-relative I_s would have to change to maintain a constant quantal catch (see Section V, Note 1). For Models A and B, the predicted changes in I_s are generated by choosing $\sigma(I_A)$ for A and $R_{max}(I_A)$ for B to fit threshold I_t data which fall on the Weber line of a slope of 1. For Model D the predicted I_s changes can be derived without any consideration of threshold data. Model C predictions are not shown since they are not uniquely determined from threshold data. Since both σ and R_{max} change in Model C the predictions must fall between curves A and B. For more details see Note 2 (Section V) and the Appendix of Hood et al. (1978). The data points are from an experiment by Hood et al. (1978)—see text for details.

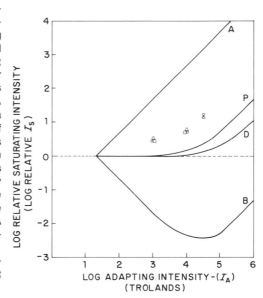

based on threshold data (see Section V, Note 2, and the legend to Figure 12.3). Notice that for this saturation measure, unlike the threshold measure, the models make very different predictions.

We have used the cone saturation paradigm introduced by Alpern, Rushton, and Torii (1970) to obtain a psychophysical estimate of the intensity I_s (see also Geisler, 1978a; King-Smith & Webb, 1974; Shevell, 1977).[2] Figure 12.4A illustrates our experimental conditions; Figure 12.4B presents the data obtained with this paradigm and two values of I_A. Notice that the probe threshold intensity first increases in proportion to I_f for a range of flashed light intensity but then rapidly and dramatically increases for further increases in flash intensity. Saturation intensity I_s is defined as the asymptotic intensity of I_f that would produce an infinite rise in the probe threshold intensity.

The empirical measure of I_s can be related to the theoretical point on the response–intensity function. Figure 12.1 shows the response elicited by three values of flash intensity: one at threshold intensity I_t; one at saturating intensity I_s; and one at an intermediate intensity I_f'. The difference between saturating intensity I_s and lower values of I_f is that light (the probe) added to I_s cannot be detected. When the flash is at intensity I_f' a probe of I_p can be found which, when added with I_f', produces a response increment of γ. However, for a flash intensity of I_s, no value of

---

[2]This paradigm can be found in Alpern et al.'s Figure 6 and is not to be confused with their contrast flash technique.

I_p will produce this criterion increment because a near maximum response has been reached.

The data points in Figure 12.3 show how the psychophysical measure of I_s changes with I_A (Hood, Ilves, Maurer, Wandell, & Buckingham, 1978). Saturation intensity I_s increases as the steady adapting intensity increases. Our I_s data can be used to reject Models A, B, and D. The predictions of Models A, B, and D shown in Figure 12.3 clearly do not conform to these data. However, Model C can be fit to them.

C. The Model and Recent Physiology

The model that fits our data is based on the response–intensity function in Figure 12.2C and the assumption that σ and R_{max} vary as power functions of J_A. In particular,

$$R(J_f, J_A) = \{J_f/[J_f + \sigma(J_A)]\} \times R_{max}(J_A) \tag{3}$$

where

$$\sigma(J_A) = k_1 J_A^m; \qquad R_{max}(J_A) = k_2 J_A^{-r}; \qquad m + r = 1.0. \tag{4}$$

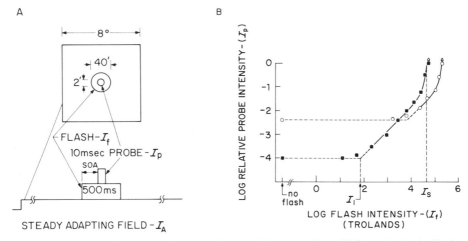

Figure 12.4. (A) Cone saturation paradigm used in our studies. (B) Data obtained with the paradigm in (A), and SOA of 250 msec, and a steady adapting field of 1.3 (■) or 4 (○) log trolands. The smooth curve is a template that we have found fits a variety of cone saturation data from different observers and conditions. This curve changes smoothly from a slope of 1 to an infinite slope over a range of I_f of .5 log unit. The saturating intensity I_s is defined as the asymptotic value of I_f determined from template fit to the data. "No flash" marks the condition in which the probe is presented on the steady adapting field without any flash present. [Modified from Hood et al. (1978).]

The incremental response amplitude, R, to flashes of J_f on adapting fields of J_A is dependent upon σ and R_{max}, both of which change as power functions of J_A (see Section V, Note 3). (Remember $J = pI$ and is a measure of relative quanta absorbed.) Figure 12.5 shows how the model consisting of Eqs. (3) and (4) and the psychophysiological assumptions previously stated fit our threshold (I_t) and saturation (I_S) data.

Kleinschmidt and Dowling (1975) introduced Eq. (3) and showed that it fit their intracellular recordings from gecko receptors. They found that σ and R_{max} varied as power functions of I_A with exponents of .83 and $-.17$, respectively. P. A. Hock and D. C. Hood (unpublished) found Eq. (3) also fit aspartate-isolated receptor data from frog cones if the exponents in Eq. (4) were .79 and $-.21$. Our psychophysical data just stated are well fit by Eq. (3) if σ and R_{max} are power functions with exponents of .63 and $-.37$. All three studies agree that σ is changing much more rapidly than R_{max}.

There are a number of other physiological studies that are at least in qualitative agreement with Eq. (3) (Dowling & Ripps, 1971, 1972; Normann & Werblin, 1974; Werblin, 1974; G. S. Easland & G. S. Wasserman, personal communication). More physiological data are needed to assess the general applicability of Eqs. (3) and (4); at least Eq. (4) will need modifying to deal with low adaptation intensities (see Section V, Note 3). It is particularly important that future physiological studies use a full range of flash intensities and at least two adapting field intensities if Eqs. (3) and (4) are to be distinguished from alternative formulations.

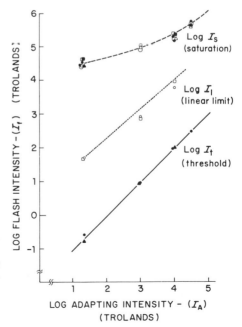

Figure 12.5. Three psychophysical measures of flash intensity (see Figures 12.1 and 12.4). The lower data points show the threshold intensity I_t of the flash needed for detection by two observers. The solid line through these points has a slope of 1. The upper data points show the intensity I_s of the flash at saturation. The data are for three observers (denoted by symbol shape) and different area-duration probe conditions (denoted by open and closed symbols) (see Hood et al., 1978). The middle data points (from Hood & Finkelstein, unpublished) show the intensity I_1 of the flash that marks the breakdown of linearity for two observers (see Section V, Note 4). The curves through each set of points are the theoretical functions.

D. Psychophysical Extensions of the Model

There are at least two criticisms that must be considered before our psychophysical model can be taken seriously. First, the model's fit to the data may depend upon the particular parameters of the probe (see Figure 12.4A). Second, the model has two functions of adapting field intensity, σ and R_{max}, and there are only two data points, I_t and I_s, to be fit at each adapting field intensity.

The area, duration, and time of onset (SOA) of the probe do not seem to affect the model's fit. We found that changing the area or duration of the probe does not affect the value of I_s (Hood et al., 1978). Shortening the SOA (Buckingham, Hood, & Ilves, 1977) decreases the value of I_s for any I_A. However, the relative change in I_s with I_A is preserved and the same model fits the data.

Even though the number of functions in the model equals the number of data points to be fit at each I_A we would have rejected the model if the functions $\sigma(I_A)$ and $R_{max}(I_A)$ had been unreasonable. They are not; in fact, to fit the data we assumed, consistent with recent physiology, that they were power functions. Of course, our faith in the model will be determined by its ability to predict new data. Two recent findings have encouraged us. First, using the same values for σ and R_{max}, we (Hood & Finkelstein, unpublished) have had reasonable success in predicting a third aspect of our data, the change with I_A of the intensity of the flash which marks the end of the horizontal portion of the cone saturation function [see I_1 in Figures 12.4 and 12.5 and Note 4 (Section V)]. Second, we (Hood & Finkelstein, 1978) found that our magnitude estimation data for the brightness of the flash deviated from Stevens' law in ways that were predictable from Eq. (3). To conclude, the model consisting of the response–intensity functions of Eqs. (3) and (4) and the previously stated psychophysiological assumptions fits a variety of data. It will require further specification and additional psychophysical tests (see Section V, Note 5).

III. A Physiological Test of a Physiological Proposal: Comparison of Receptor and Ganglion Cell Activity

The response–intensity functions in Figure 12.2, especially C and D, are based on physiological recordings from receptors. However, in the psychophysical work previously discussed we made no assumption about the locus of these functions in the human visual system. Our approach is common in the study of the physiological bases of behavior; namely, the physiological literature is used as a source of suggestions about possible physiological mechanisms. These suggestions are then formalized into testable models. Once formalized the physiological explanations can be tested behaviorally (psychophysically) and physiologically. The work previously discussed is one example of a psychophysical test of models of human vision based upon physiological proposals. We will now consider a physiological test.

Our physiological recordings from frog receptors are part of a literature showing that functions can be obtained for receptors that are qualitatively similar to the psychophysical functions obtained from humans. The increment threshold functions, intensity–time functions, and dark-adaptation functions for frog rods and cones all bear a striking resemblance to corresponding human psychophysical data (Hood & Mansfield, 1972; Hood & Hock, 1973, 1975; Hood, Hock, & Grover, 1973; Hood & Grover, 1974). For example, Figure 12.6 contains increment threshold functions for frog receptors. Notice that receptor type and flash exposure duration affect these functions in a manner similar to the way they affect human psychophysical functions.

Of course this correspondence between frog receptor and human behavioral data

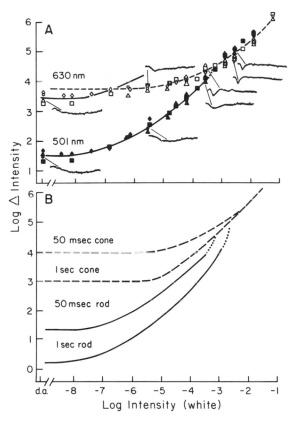

Figure 12.6. Increment threshold functions for frog receptors. The incremental intensity of the test light needed for a threshold response is plotted as a function of the adapting field intensity. Threshold is defined as a peak response amplitude of 10 μV. (A) Data and sample records of threshold responses (10 μV) for test flashes of 50 msec and either 501- or 630-nm light. The solid curve is the rod increment threshold function drawn through the 630- and 501-nm data points; the dashed curve is the cone function drawn through the 630-nm data points. (B) Increment threshold curves for the 502 rod and 580 cone and two test flash durations. These curves were obtained using procedures analogous to those of Stiles (1959). [Modified from Hood & Hock (1975).]

does not mean that the receptors are the physiological locus for all, or even most, of the sensitivity changes seen in human psychophysical functions. However, we can use the frog to test a general model of vertebrate vision that places sensitivity changes with adaptation at the receptors. Consider a simple physiological proposal in which receptors are said to be the locus of all sensitivity changes in the visual system during light and dark adaptation. A physiological test of this proposal could consist of a comparison of receptor activity to the activity of cells further upstream in the visual system. We have recorded from frog ganglion cells under the same conditions used in receptor experiments to test such a simple explanation.

Before examining the data from one ganglion cell experiment we must consider what is meant by the proposal that receptor activity is the locus for sensitivity changes seen at the ganglion cell. This physiological proposal cannot be tested unless assumptions are added to make the proposal explicit. To say that the receptors are the locus for all sensitivity loss is to assume what we have called the "linear-connection" model (see Hock & Hood, 1978). The basic assumption of this model states that ganglion cell activity elicited by quantal absorptions in one receptor type, for example, the frog's 580 cone,[3] is linearly related to the activity of this receptor type. One simple linear assumption is that peak ganglion cell response (measured as peak spike frequency) is linearly related to peak amplitude of the receptor potential. This assumption is usually implicit in experiments that compare activity at different levels of the nervous system. When threshold experiments are performed (see the following), the peak ganglion cell response is defined as one spike and the peak receptor response is defined as a criterion peak amplitude (e.g., 10 μV).

In Figure 12.7, increment threshold functions are presented for cone receptor (smooth curve) and cone-driven ganglion cell responses (data points). If the linear-connection model holds, then the receptor curve should fit the data points with only a vertical displacement (see the legend to Figure 12.7). The smooth receptor curve does not fit the ganglion cell data. Before we examine in detail this misfit to the data, we shall consider two possible results. First, if the receptors and ganglion cells lost the same amount of sensitivity as the adapting field was increased in intensity and thus the receptor curve fit the ganglion cell data, then we would conclude that we have evidence for a linear-connection model. Such was the case for most of the increment threshold curves recorded from rod-driven ganglion cells (Fusco & Hood, unpublished; see Gordon & Hood, 1976, Figure 13). Second, if the receptor curves exhibited a smaller range of sensitivity changes than was seen for the ganglion cells, we would then conclude that sensitivity changes take place beyond the receptors. Such was the case for the dark adaptation functions for rod-driven ganglion cells (Fusco & Hood, unpublished; see Gordon & Hood, 1976, Figure 15B) and skate ganglion cells (Green, Dowling, Ripps, & Siegel, 1975). Neither of these "simple"

---

[3]The frog has four types of receptors: 580 cone, 502 cone, 502 rod, and 432 rod. The numbers refer to the wavelength of light that is maximally absorbed [see Gordon and Hood (1976, pp. 29–33) for a summary].

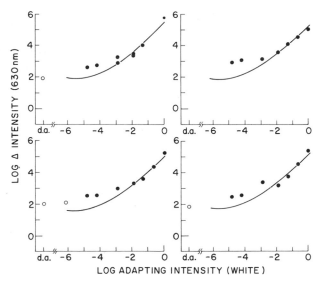

Figure 12.7. Cone increment threshold curves for four ganglion cells. The test flash was a 50-msec, 630-nm light presented upon a steady "white" adaptation light. The open data points denote thresholds that are probably rod-influenced while the closed points are probably 580-cone controlled [see Hock and Hood (1978) for details]. The solid curve is the cone function (see Figure 12.6B) positioned vertically to fit the upper points. For any ganglion cell threshold intensity, the receptor response to that intensity is within the linear range of the receptor's response-intensity function. As long as the receptor response stays within its linear range, changing the receptor response criterion (to compare the receptor curve at any given ganglion cell threshold intensity) will simply shift the entire increment threshold function vertically, without changing its shape. For the linear-connection model to fit these data the cone curve must fit the data when only vertically shifted. The curves are adjusted for best fit at the upper (cone controlled) part of the data. However, no vertical positioning of the cone curve brings the ganglion cell data and receptor curve into agreement. [Modified from Hock & Hood (1978).]

cases holds for the cone light adaptation data in Figure 12.7. In Figure 12.7 the receptors exhibit a larger range of sensitivity changes than do the ganglion cells; surprisingly, it appears that receptors lose more sensitivity than ganglion cells as the adapting field is increased in intensity. There are at least two reasonable explanations for this finding. First, the ganglion cell threshold response may not be triggered by the peak receptor amplitude. Since the waveform of the cone receptor response changes with the intensity of the adapting field, different measures of the response give differently shaped increment threshold functions. In fact, there are alternative threshold response criteria for which the receptor shows a smaller range of sensitivity changes and the fit to the ganglion cell data is better, although still not good (Hock & Hood, 1978). Second, other receptor types influence the ganglion cell's sensitivity even though the response to the test light has an action spectrum consistent with the 580 cones. By using a Stiles-type technique, Hock (1978) has shown that at least some of the ganglion cells violate Stiles' independence assumption. In particular, at low adapting intensities the response (or sensitivity) of ganglion cells to the 580-cone input is decreased by activity of other, probably 430 rods, receptor types.

The cone system data in Figure 12.7 are presented here, rather than some of our data previously mentioned which fit the simpler cases, because they illustrate two general problems that must be considered when comparing activity of one level of the nervous system to another. Such problems can be easily ignored when one or the other of the simpler cases holds. First, the higher order cell may not be responding to the same aspect of the lower order cell's response that we as experimenters are examining. And, second, other cells may be influencing the higher order cell's response to the lower order cell's input, and this influence may be complex and difficult to detect without sophisticated techniques such as the Stiles procedure.

To summarize, under some conditions receptor activity can be simply related to ganglion cell activity and perhaps to human psychophysics. Under other conditions postreceptor factors influence sensitivity, and tests of explicit models such as the linear-connection model are designed to allow specification of these influences. The data presented in Figure 12.7 illustrate some general problems that must be confronted when activity of two levels in the nervous system is compared.

IV. Concluding Remarks

In this chapter I have tried to show how physiological suggestions can be formalized and tested both psychophysically and physiologically. I would like to think, however, that the experiments we have done can stand without a particular theory. The cone saturation paradigm, for example, can be related to a wide range of classic psychophysical paradigms. Thus it is of interest to compare data from this paradigm to data from other paradigms. (For example, flashed fields are more effective in decreasing areal summation and less effective in decreasing temporal summation than are steady fields.) Such comparisons among data are potentially important in understanding the visual system as well as providing data to be handled by future theories.

V. Notes

1. The proportion, p, of the molecules in the unbleached state is given by

$$p(I_A) = C/(I_A + C), \tag{a}$$

where $C = 4.3$ log td for the middle- and long-wave human cone pigments (cf. Rushton & Henry, 1968). Since pigment density is relatively low, the effective intensity, J, is equal to $p(I_A)I$.

An increase in σ with I_A (as in Figure 12.2A) or a decrease in p are both equivalent to decreasing the intensity, I_f, of the flash. To derive this we replace I with pI and rewrite Eq. (1) as

$$R(I_f) = \{(pI/\sigma)/[(pI/\sigma) + 1]\} \times R_{max}.$$

Changing either p or σ will shift the response–intensity function parallel on the log I_f axis since log $pI/\sigma = \log I + \log p - \log \sigma$.

Models in which σ does not change with I_A need pigment bleaching to decrease I at high I_A values and keep the system from saturating to steady lights (cf. Alpern *et al.*, 1970; Boynton & Whitten, 1970; Mansfield, 1976). These models must have values of σ that are relatively large. In fact, σ must be close to or greater than C in Eq. (a).

2. In Model A σ changes and the response functions in Figure 12.2A stay the same shape and merely shift parallel along the $\log I_f$ axis. This model predicts that I_s and threshold must change in the same way, and therefore the predicted change in I_s is a line of slope 1. For this model, bleaching is not really necessary. Although pigment bleaching does occur, it shifts the response functions in the same way as increases in σ (see Note 1).

For Model B, if $R_{max}(J_A)$ is chosen to fit the threshold data, then this model predicts that I_s would decrease with increases in I_A, along a line of slope -1. The only mechanism in this model that protects the cones from saturating with intense steady lights is bleaching. Bleaching in this case is vital; bleaching shifts the response functions. Therefore, for this model, the reduction in response amplitude due to the decrease in $R_{max}(I_A)$ decreases I_s, but bleaching increases I_s. The result is the curve in Figure 12.3 labeled B.

In Model D, the maximum response to the combination of the flash and a steady adapting field is always 1 [i.e.; $R_{max}(J_f + J_A) = 1$]: Therefore, as I_A increases, I_s [the value of I_f for which $R(J_f + J_A) = R_{max} - \gamma - 1 - \gamma$] must decrease. As in Model B, pigment bleaching is vital—only through the decrease in effective intensity with bleaching does the cone system stay responsive at high I_A. I_s increases with increased I_A due to pigment bleaching. The theoretical curve falls below the pigment bleaching curve since these two factors trade off. Since the combined intensity of J_s and J_A, which produces saturation, is constant, once J_s is determined for one value of J_A (for $I_A = 1.3$ log td in Figure 12.3) it can be predicted for all other values of J_A.

3. The value of $m + r$ must equal 1 to fit the threshold data in Figure 12.5 that fall along the Weber line. By substituting Eq. (4) into Eq. (3) and making use of the fact that at threshold $J_t \ll \sigma$ and $R(J_t, J_A) = \delta$, it can be shown that $J_t = \delta k J_A^{m+r}$. Consequently, $m + r$ must equal 1 if J_t is to increase in proportion to J_A. However, the power functions of Eq. (4) must be replaced by the functions

$$\sigma(J_A) = [(\Theta + J_A)/\Theta]^m \quad \text{and} \quad R_{max}(J_A) = [\Theta/(\Theta + J_A)]^r$$

with $m + r = 1$ for the model to handle J_A values below the Weber line. Further, if the response–intensity functions are fit by Eq. (1), with $n \neq 1$, then

$$R_{max}(J_A) = [\Theta/(\Theta + J_A)]^{nr} \quad \text{and} \quad m + nr = 1$$

[see the Appendix in Hood *et al.* (1978)].

4. To obtain a third point on the response–intensity function, we considered the intensity at which the function deviates from linearity. The response–intensity function of Eq. (1) is linear for $I \ll \sigma$ if n equals 1. If the response function were linear and a constant response difference were required for detection, then the cone saturation function of Figure 12.4B would be a horizontal line. Therefore, I_1, the limit of the linear range, is defined empirically as that value of I_f for which a horizontal line no longer fits the data (see Figure 12.4). In Figure 12.5, empirical values of I_1 are shown for two observers and an SOA of 250 msec. The data for one observer ($\square$) have been shifted up by .2 log unit for comparison.

We can define I_1 theoretically as the value of I_f that satisfies the following expression:

$$[J_1/\sigma(J_A)] \times R_{max}(J_A) - \{J_1/[J_1 + \sigma(J_A)]\} \times R_{max}(J_A) = \epsilon. \tag{b}$$

If ϵ is estimated for one value of J_A, then the complete theoretical curve expressing J_1 as a function of J_A can be determined. The value of ϵ was determined for each observer using the I_1 data for an I_A of 1.3 log td and the values of σ and R_{max} determined from previous experiments. The dotted line in Figure 12.5 is this curve expressed in terms of I_1 and I_A. The fit here is not great, but both data and theory show that log J_1 increases linearly with log J_A with a slope of less than 1. The 0-msec SOA data (not shown) fit the theoretical curve better.

5. In its present form, the model does not predict the shape of the cone saturation functions in Figure 12.4B. If one assumes that $\delta = \gamma$ (in Figure 12.1) and, in fact, that to detect I_p on any I_f that $R(I_p)$ must

equal δ [i.e., $R(I_p + I_f) - R(I_f) = R(I_p) = \delta$], then the complete cone saturation curve in Figure 12.4 can be derived. If $R(I)$ is given by Eq. (1) with $n = 1$, then the slope of this theoretical cone saturation curve equals 2 (see Williams and Gale, Chapter 11, this volume). This is in clear contradiction to the slope of approximately 1 in Figure 12.4. Before concluding that the model cannot be extended to predict the entire curve, at least three aspects of the above extension must be examined: the value of n, the constancy of δ, and the experimental paradigm of Figure 12.4A. It can be shown (Buckingham, unpublished) that the slope of the theoretical function decreases as n decreases; for example for $n = .3$ the function has a slope of approximately 1 over a range of more than 3 log units. Second, there is no a priori reason to expect δ to remain constant with increased I_f. If δ depended upon I_f and, in fact, decreased with I_f, then a slope less than 2 would result. Since synaptic release by the receptors decreases with increases in intensity (cf. Schacher, Holtzman, & Hood, 1974, 1976), it is not unreasonable to think that δ might decrease with increased I_f. Finally, changing the paradigm of Figure 12.4A such that SOA = 0 actually produces results that can be fit by the above extension of the model for at least the lower range of I_f values (Geisler, 1978b; Hood & Finkelstein, 1978).

ACKNOWLEDGMENTS

I thank Norma Graham for her helpful comments and Gene Buckingham, Anne Campbell, Marcie Finkelstein, and Peggy Hock for their considerable help on versions of this manuscript and for numerous enjoyable discussions. I also thank Elijah Schachter for the use of his room without which this chapter may not have been written.

REFERENCES

Alpern, M., Rushton, W. A. H., & Torii, S. Signals from cones. *Journal of Physiology,* 1970, *207,* 463–475.

Boynton, R. M., & Whitten, D. N. Visual adaptation in monkey cones: Recordings of late receptor potentials. *Science,* 1970, *170,* 1423–1426.

Buckingham, E., Hood, D. C., & Ilves, T. Tests of models of the dynamic range: Parametric studies of cone saturation. *Investigative Ophthalmology and Visual Science,* 1977, suppl., p. 28.

Craik, K. J. W. The effect of adaptation on differential brightness discrimination. *Journal of Physiology,* 1938, *92,* 406–421.

Dowling, J. E., & Ripps, H. S-potentials in the skate retina: Intracellular recordings during light and dark adaptation. *Journal of General Physiology,* 1971, *58,* 163–189.

Dowling, J. E., & Ripps, H. Adaptation in skate photoreceptors. *Journal of General Physiology,* 1972, *60,* 698–719.

Geisler, W. S. Adaptation, afterimages and cone saturation. *Vision Research,* 1978, *18* (in press). (a)

Geisler, W. S. Rod saturation and the short-term rod afterimage. *Investigative Ophthalmology and Visual Science,* 1978, suppl., 153. (b)

Gordon, J., & Hood, D. C. Anatomy and physiology of the frog retina. In K. Fite (ed.), *The amphibian visual system: A multidisciplinary approach.* New York: Academic Press, 1976.

Green, D. G., Dowling, J. E., Ripps, H., & Siegel, I. M. Retinal mechanisms of visual adaptation in the skate. *Journal of General Physiology,* 1975, *65,* 483–502.

Hock, P. A. Rod–cone interactions and light adaptation in the frog retina. *Investigative Ophthalmology and Visual Science,* 1978, suppl., p. 110.

Hock, P., & Hood, D. C. Light adaptation of the frog's cone system: A comparison of receptor and ganglion cell increment threshold functions. *Vision Research,* 1978, *18* (in press).

Hood, D. C., & Finkelstein, M. Brightness estimates and cone saturation. *Investigative Ophthalmology and Visual Science*, 1978, suppl., p. 155.

Hood, D. C., & Grover, B. G. Temporal summation of light energy by a vertebrate visual receptor. *Science*, 1974, *184*, 1003–1005.

Hood, D. C., & Hock, P. A. Recovery of cone receptor activity in the frog's isolated retina. *Vision Research*, 1973, *13*, 1943–1951.

Hood, D. C., & Hock, P. A. Light adaptation of the receptors: Increment threshold functions for the frog's rods and cones. *Vision Research*, 1975, *15*, 545–553.

Hood, D. C., Hock, P. A., & Grover, B. G. Dark adaptation of the frog's rods. *Vision Research*, 1973, *13*, 1953–1963.

Hood, D. C., Ilves, T., Maurer, E., Wandell, B., & Buckingham, E. Human cone saturation as a function of ambient intensity: A test of models of shifts in the dynamic range. *Vision Research*, 1978, *18* (in press).

Hood, D. C., & Mansfield, A. F. The isolated receptor potential of the frog isolated retina: Action spectra before and after extensive bleaching. *Vision Research*, 1972, *12*, 2109–2119.

King-Smith, P. E., & Webb, J. R. The use of photopic saturation in determining the fundamental spectral sensitivity curves. *Vision Research*, 1974, *14*, 421–429.

Kleinschmidt, J., & Dowling, J. E. Intracellular recordings from gecko photoreceptors during light and dark adaptation. *Journal of General Physiology*, 1975, *66*, 617–648.

Mansfield, R. J. W. Visual adaptations: Retinal transduction, brightness, and sensitivity. *Vision Research*, 1976, *16*, 679–690.

Normann, R. A., & Werblin, F. S. Control of retinal sensitivity. I. Light and dark adaptation of vertebrate rods and cones. *Journal of General Physiology*, 1974, *63*, 37–61.

Rushton, W. A. H., & Henry, G. A. Bleaching and regeneration of cone pigments in man. *Vision Research*, 1968, *8*, 617–632.

Schacher, S. M., Holtzman, E., & Hood, D. C. Uptake of horseradish peroxidase by frog photoreceptor synapses in the dark and the light. *Nature*, 1974, *249*, 261–263.

Schacher, S. M., Holtzman, E., & Hood, D. C. Synaptic activity of frog retinal photoreceptors: A peroxidase uptake study. *Journal of Cell Biology*, 1976, *70*, 178–192.

Shevell, S. K. Saturation in human cones. *Vision Research*, 1977, *17*, 427–434.

Stiles, W. S. Color vision: The approach through increment-threshold sensitivity. *Proceedings of the National Academy of Sciences*, 1959, *45*, 110–114.

Werblin, F. S. Adaptation in a vertebrate retina: Intracellular recording in Necturus. *Journal of Neurophysiology*, 1971, *34*, 228–241.

Werblin, F. S. Control of retinal sensitivity. II. Lateral interactions at the outer plexiform layer. *Journal of General Physiology*, 1974, *63*, 62–87.

13. Discriminability and Ratio Scaling

Eric G. Heinemann

I. Introduction

Direct ratio estimation methods are used in attempts to determine the function relating the physical magnitude of a stimulus I to the magnitude of the sensation produced by I, $S(I)$. The most frequently used of such methods are *magnitude estimation* and *pair estimation*. In experiments with magnitude estimation the subject is presented with many values of I and is instructed to assign to each I a number proportional to the magnitude of the sensation produced by I. In experiments with pair estimation the subject is presented with pairs of stimulus values, I_s and I_v. For each of several values of I_s the experimenter determines a value I_v for which the subject is willing to say that the ratio of the sensations produced by I_s and I_v is equal to some specified value, for example, that I_s is twice as bright as I_v (multiplication) or half as bright as I_v (fractionation).

Stevens (1957) has summarized the results of a large number of experiments which show that for many prothetic continua the subjects assign approximately equal number ratios to equal stimulus ratios, so that the average magnitude estimate M is approximately a power function of I:

$$M = M_0 I^B, \tag{1}$$

where the value of the exponent B depends primarily on the nature of the stimulus continuum. If it is assumed that the number ratios that the subjects assign accurately reflect ratios of sensation magnitudes then it follows that sensation magnitude S is also a power of function of I:

$$S = S_0 I^B. \tag{2}$$

Further support for the psychophysical law given by Eq. (2) can be derived from

157

the results of cross-modality matching experiments in which subjects are required to equate the sensations of two different sense modalities. These results show that the intensity I_2 that must be presented to modality 2 in order to match intensity I_1 of modality 1 is approximately a power function of I_1, with an exponent equal to the ratio of the exponents obtained by direct ratio estimation for the two modalities (Stevens, Mack, & Stevens, 1960; Stevens, 1966).

Though the agreement between results obtained by direct ratio estimation and cross-modality matching is consistent with the assumption that the number ratios that the subject assigns during direct estimation accurately reflects ratios of sensation magnitudes, a full justification of that assumption must deal with the difficult question of how a subject could possibly learn the rules of correspondence between number names and sensation magnitudes. Since the community that teaches word usage has no access to the subject's sensations it clearly cannot teach him by the usual method of giving examples and correcting mistakes. This chapter examines this problem and advances a possible account of how subjects learn number names and apply them in direct estimation experiments. Several experiments that bear on this account will be presented.

The question raised in the previous paragraph was discussed several years ago by Krantz (1972a). Krantz suggests that subjects are taught to assign number names to *physical quantities* on a special continuum, such as line length. I shall call this special continuum the *training continuum*. When dealing with physical quantities the community can, of course, give examples and correct the subject's usage when it is wrong. Krantz assumes that having been trained to use number names correctly for stimuli from the training continuum, the subject will be able to apply number names consistently to stimuli from other continua. The problem now is to state the rules that specify how number names are transferred from the training continuum to other continua. Krantz discusses two possible theories of transfer which he calls *mapping theory* and *relation theory*. In discussing these theories the symbols I_i' and I_i will be used to represent a pair of stimulus values from continuum i, the training continuum, and I_j' and I_j will be used to represent a pair of stimulus values from another continuum, j.

According to mapping theory, if the subject is required to specify the ratio of the sensation magnitudes produced by I_j' and I_j, he matches the sensation produced by I_j' to the memory of a sensation produced by an I_i' (e.g., a particular line length), and he matches the sensation produced by I_j to the memory of a second training stimulus value, I_i. He then computes the ratio I_i'/I_i and speaks the "ratio name" that he has learned to apply to I_i'/I_i.

Relation theory eliminates the mental arithmetic required to get the ratio. It assumes that the subject does not associate number names with single training stimuli but instead associates ratio names with the relation between the sensations produced by pairs of training stimuli. When required to state the ratio of the sensations produced by I_j' and I_j, the subject matches the relation of the sensations produced by these stimuli to a relation of the sensations produced by stimuli I_i' and I_i, and then speaks the ratio name for I_i'/I_i. Krantz shows that these theories can account for the consistency of the results obtained by direct estimation and cross-modality matching methods.

Another possible account of the transfer process will now be presented. This account has two interesting general features: It does not use the concept of sensation magnitude, and it relates results obtained in scaling experiments to discriminability.[1]

Suppose that during training to estimate stimulus magnitudes the subject has been taught to assign the number M_0 to an arbitrary reference stimulus I_i. Then the number M that a well-trained subject will assign to any stimulus I_i' on the training continuum will be

$$M = M_0 \ (I_i'/I_i). \tag{3}$$

Now let us assume that Weber's law is true for the training continuum. Then the number of just-noticeable-differences (jnds) from I_i' to I_i, to be called n_i, is given by

$$n_i = [\log(I_i'/I_i)]/[\log(1 + W_i)], \tag{4}$$

where W_i is the Weber fraction for continuum i (see Woodworth, 1938, p. 436). From Eqs. (3) and (4) it follows that

$$\log(M/M_0) = \log(I_i'/I_i) = n_i \log(1 + W_i). \tag{5}$$

In words, the logarithm of the ratio that the subject assigns to any pair of stimuli, I_i', I_i, is proportional to the number of jnds from I_i' to I_i. Let us assume that this is the relation the subject learns. Let us assume further that when required to estimate the ratio of sensations produced by stimuli I_j' and I_j from continuum j, the subject follows exactly the procedure he has learned, that is, that he counts the number of jnds from I_j' to I_j, multiplies this number by the constant he has learned to use, namely, $\log(1 + W_i)$, and so on.[2] It will then be true that on continuum j

$$\log(M/M_0) = n_j \log(1 + W_i), \tag{6}$$

where n_j, the number of jnds from I_j' to I_j, is equal to n_i.

Rewriting Eq. (4) for continuum j shows that

$$n_j = [\log(I_j'/I_j)]/[\log(1 + W_j)], \tag{7}$$

where W_j is the Weber fraction for continuum j.

Substituting the right-hand part of Eq. (7) for n_j in Eq. (6) gives

$$\log(M/M_0) = [\log(1 + W_i) \log(I_j'/I_j)]/\log(1 + W_j). \tag{8}$$

Equation (8) implies that

$$M = M_0 \ (I_j'/I_j)^{[\log(1 + W_i)]/[\log(1 + W_j)]}. \tag{9}$$

---

[1]The formal development presented here is an extension of that presented by Auerbach (1973) in his analysis of cross-modality matching.

[2]If, as in magnitude estimation, the subject is to speak number names rather than ratio names, a number M_0, called the "modulus," must be assigned to I_j either by the experimenter or by the subject.

Equation (9) has the same form as Eq. (1), where $B = [\log(1 + W_i)]/[\log(1 + W_j)]$, and I_j is the stimulus unit. This account then is consistent with the form of the magnitude estimation function.

In experiments with the pair estimation procedure the experimenter assigns a constant value to the ratio M/M_0. The subject is presented with various stimulus magnitudes I and is required to search for a second stimulus magnitude I' such that I and I' form a pair to which he is willing to assign the number ratio M/M_0. Empirical results obtained with this procedure are consistent with those predicted by Eq. (8).

An analysis of cross-modality matching that is entirely consistent with the account just given has been presented by Auerbach (1973). Auerbach assumes that if a subject equates stimuli I_i and I_j of modalities i and j, then he will also equate stimuli of magnitudes I_i' and I_j' whenever I_i' is n_i jnds from I_i, and I_j' is n_j jnds from I_j. He shows that it follows from these assumptions that the exponent obtained in cross-modality matching of stimuli from continua i and j is equal to the ratio of the exponents determined by magnitude estimation for these continua.

The arguments presented show that it is possible to account for the major results of experiments on magnitude estimation, pair estimation, and cross-modality matching by assuming that the subjects' behavior is governed by the discriminability of the stimuli presented in these experiments. As will be brought out in Section III, this interpretation is compatible with several interpretations based on the concept of sensation magnitude. The major advantage of the present interpretation is that it relates scales obtained by direct estimation to quantities that are more easily measured than sensations.

The basic assumption that transfer of ratio names from a training continuum to other continua is based on discriminability can be tested empirically. Some experiments that bear on this matter will now be described.

II. Experiments

The general plan was to train subjects to make an arbitrary verbal response (analogous to a ratio name) to a ratio of two stimulus magnitudes chosen from a portion of a training continuum for which Weber's law holds, and then to examine the manner in which the learned name is transferred to (a) stimuli chosen from a portion of the training continuum on which the Weber fraction is not constant, and (b) stimuli from another sense modality.

The subjects in these experiments were four women, 19 to 22 years of age. The stimuli used in training were weights suspended from small metal rings that the subjects lifted with the index finger of the right hand. During training two such rings rested on the top of a small table. The strings by which the weights were suspended passed through small holes in the table so that the subjects could not see the suspended objects. On each trial the subjects lifted the two weights in succession. They were told that each pair of weights had the name "A," "B," or "C," and that their task was to learn the names of the various pairs. After each correct response the subjects were immediately given a small monetary reward.

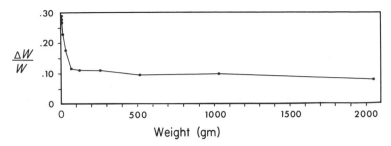

Figure 13.1. The Weber fraction as a function of base weight. Means of four subjects.

The weights presented in training were four ''standard'' weights, W_s, ranging from 1088 to 1792 gm, each paired on different trials with one of six ''comparison'' weights, W_c. The comparison weights were so chosen that the ratio W_s/W_c varied from 1.4 to 2.8. The 24 pairs of weights were presented in random order. The names the experimenter defined as correct were ''A'' for $W_s/W_c \geqslant 2.33$, ''B'' for $W_s/W_c = 2$, and ''C'' for $W_s/W_c \leqslant 1.6$. The transfer tests were done after the subjects' performances ceased to improve with further training.

During the first transfer test the subjects were presented with standard weights ranging from 2 to 160 gm. For each standard they were required to form a pair they were willing to call ''B'' by selecting a second weight (heavier than the standard) from a large array of comparison weights.

Difference thresholds for weight were also obtained for each subject in a separate experiment that used the same basic apparatus and method of lifting. These experiments used the method of limits with two response categories.

Figure 13.1 shows the mean relative difference thresholds for weight. These data agree well with a summary of results of other experiments that is presented by Woodworth (1938, p. 433). It should be noted that the Weber fraction is approximately constant over the range of stimuli used in training, but that it increases with decreasing weight over the range of stimuli presented during the transfer test.

Figure 13.2 shows the ratios of the weights in each pair that the subjects called ''B'' during the transfer test (solid line). Let us consider now the relation between

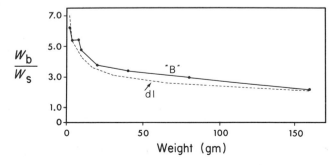

Figure 13.2. W_b/W_s is the weight ratio that was called "B." The solid line represents mean results obtained for four subjects in the transfer test. The dashed line, labeled dl, represents ratios predicted on the basis of the data shown in Figure 13.1.

the results in Figures 13.1 and 13.2. Equation (4) shows that if the Weber fraction is constant, the number of jnds from I' to I depends only on the ratio I'/I. Thus the weights in each pair the subjects were taught to call "B" were separated by the same number of jnds, namely, about 8 according to the data in Figure 13.1. If the subjects' assignment of the name "B" is indeed governed by discriminability, then the weights that were called "B" during the transfer test should also be separated by 8 jnds. The ratios of weights that are in fact separated by 8 jnds, according to the data in Figure 13.1, are shown by a dashed line in Figure 13.2.[3] The agreement between the predicted and obtained performance during the transfer test is reasonably good.

In the second transfer test the subjects were presented with paired patches of light that differed in luminance, and were required to choose pairs of luminances that had the relation they had been taught to call "B." More specifically, the stimuli were evenly illuminated disks subtending 1.5° of visual angle, and were viewed foveally. The two disks were exposed in cyclical alternation for 1 sec each, with a dark interval of 6 sec between successive exposures. The luminance of one of the disks, I, was fixed by the experimenter; the luminance of the other disk, I_b, was adjusted by the subject by turning a circular neutral density wedge. The subjects were instructed to adjust I_b until the pair (I,I_b) formed the best possible instance of "B."

For each subject luminance difference thresholds were also determined in a separate experiment done by the method of limits with two response categories. The conditions under which difference thresholds were measured differed from those of the transfer experiment only in that the experimenter adjusted I_b and the subject was required to tell whether I_b appeared brighter or dimmer than I.

Each experiment was done in two versions. In the first version the disks appeared against a totally dark background. Four continuously exposed, dim, red points of light that surrounded the disks were used to guide fixation. In the second version the disks were surrounded by a continuously exposed annular field, subtending 8° of visual angle and separated from the disks by a dark area approximately 4 sec in width. The luminance of the surround was constant at 20 mL.

The results of the difference threshold experiments are shown in Figure 13.3. Those obtained under the surround condition are similar to results obtained under roughly similar conditions by Heinemann (1961). The results obtained under the no-surround condition are somewhat unusual in that they do not show the increase in the Weber fraction often found as I is decreased to levels approaching the photopic threshold. However, most experiments in which Weber's law has been found to fail at low photopic levels have been done by methods that require the subject to detect a small luminance that is added to a continuously exposed adapting field. The results obtained in the present experiment agree well with results obtained by Cornsweet and Pinsker (1965) with a procedure which required the subject to compare the brightness of two simultaneously exposed patches of light.

The results of the transfer tests are shown in Figure 13.4 by solid lines. The

[3]The method used to count jnds is that described by Luce and Edwards (1958).

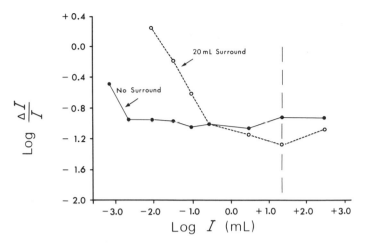

Figure 13.3. The logarithm of the Weber fraction as a function of log luminance. Means of four subjects.

dashed lines in Figure 13.4 represent predicted values derived from the difference threshold measurements on the assumption that all pairs of luminance values, I and I_b, that the subject called ''B'' during the transfer tests were separated from each other by 14 jnds. The agreement in the form of the obtained and predicted ''B functions'' is reasonably good. The discrepancy in the actual number of jnds that separate pairs of lights that are called ''B'' and pairs of weights that are called ''B'' (14 versus 8) may be the result of procedural problems that will be discussed briefly in Section III.

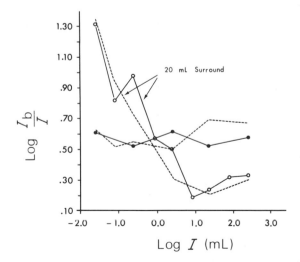

Figure 13.4. The solid lines represent the log luminance ratios that were called ''B'' during the transfer tests. The dashed lines represent values of this ratio predicted on the basis of the data shown in Figure 13.3. Means of four subjects.

After all the experiments were completed the four subjects were interviewed in an attempt to determine whether they had realized that the name "B" was equivalent to the ratio name "two." All the subjects spontaneously referred to "B" as a "distance" between two stimuli and seemed to take it as new information when the experimenter finally explained that during training "B" represented a ratio of two weights.

III. Discussion

It seems clear that results of direct estimation and cross-modality matching procedures can be accounted for on the basis of transfer of learned concepts that is mediated by stimulus discriminability, without introducing the concept of sensation. However, a complete account of results of ratio scaling procedures should include a theory of discrimination, and virtually all theories of discrimination find it necessary to refer to internal states induced by stimuli. For example, in Thurstone's theory and the closely related theory of signal detection, internal states induced by repeated presentations of a specific stimulus are represented by a normally distributed random variable. One can choose to identify this random variable with sensation magnitude. Then the mean of the distribution that corresponds to each stimulus represents the mean sensation evoked by that stimulus, and one can consider how the results of direct estimation procedures are related to mean sensations. The relations that follow from a number of different assumptions have been discussed in detail by Krantz (1972b).

If it is assumed that the sensations evoked by different stimuli used in a discrimination experiment are statistically independent, and that the distributions corresponding to different stimuli differ in the value of the mean but have a common standard deviation, then it follows that equally discriminable stimuli correspond to equal differences in (mean) sensations. Provided Weber's law holds, Fechner's logarithmic law of sensation would then be correct. With this interpretation the theory of transfer that has been presented is a form of *relation theory*. Specifically, it would be true that subjects trained with, say, line lengths are taught to apply ratio names to sensation differences.

Other assumptions lead to different psychophysical laws and to different forms of relation theory. Of particular interest is the assumption that the correlation between the sensations evoked by repeated presentations of pairs of stimuli is a function of discriminability. Krantz (1972b) has shown that in this case sensation follows a power law. Since the power law implies that equal stimulus ratios give rise to equal sensation ratios, it follows that subjects trained with line lengths would be taught to apply ratio names to sensation ratios. The possibilities considered in this and the previous paragraph together with the outcome of the present experiments illustrate the importance of discrimination theory for the interpretation of scales obtained by direct estimation methods.

Returning to the principal argument presented here, we should point out that measurements obtained in experiments on discrimination and direct estimation can be expected to be related to each other in the manner specified only if the two kinds of experiments are done under comparable conditions. To illustrate what is meant: Most measurements of luminance discrimination are made by methods that enable the subject to respond to transients produced by sudden changes in stimulus level, or to the appearance of a contour in a previously uniform field. There is no reason to think that the discriminability measured in such experiments is related in any simple way to the discriminability of stimuli that are presented one at a time, with relatively long intervals between exposures, as in a typical direct estimation experiment. For the purposes under consideration an appropriate method of determining discriminability would seem to be one that requires the subject to judge the brightness of successively presented stimuli.

There are still other complexities to be considered. The psychophysical method used to measure discrimination (e.g., the method of limits; or constant stimuli) appears to have no strong effect on the form of the Weber function, but it does affect the absolute values of the Weber fractions. The latter may also be affected, within each method, by the range of stimuli presented during the experiment. In spite of the successes of modern discrimination theories such as the theory of signal detection, methods of extracting a pure discriminability measure from the results obtained by different psychophysical procedures have not yet been perfected (one of the main stumbling blocks is the effect of stimulus range). Finally, the size of jnds may be affected by subtle factors that are under the control of the subject. For example, evenly illuminated fields tend to appear brightest at the edges and darkest in the center (cf. Davidson, 1968). When assessing the brightness of such fields, subjects may base their judgments on an arbitrarily chosen feature, such as the brightness of the center, or of the edges, or perhaps some average of the two. Measures of discriminability may well depend somewhat on which feature the subject responds to.

Given this state of affairs it is difficult to find a rational basis for comparing jnds obtained for different sense modalities, and therefore the finding that the number of jnds that separated pairs of weights that the subjects called "B" differed from the number of jnds that separated lights they called "B" is not really surprising.

REFERENCES

Auerbach, C. A note on cross-modality matching. *Quarterly Journal of Experimental Psychology,* 1973, *25,* 492–495.

Cornsweet, T. N., & Pinsker, H. N. Luminance discrimination of brief flashes under various conditions of adaptation. *Journal of Physiology,* 1965, *176,* 294–310.

Davidson, M. L. Perturbation approach to spatial brightness interaction in human vision. *Journal of the Optical Society of America,* 1968, *58,* 1300–1309.

Heinemann, E. G. The relation of apparent brightness to the threshold for differences in luminance. *Journal of Experimental Psychology,* 1961, *61,* 389–399.

Krantz, D. H. A theory of magnitude estimation and cross-modality matching. *Journal of Mathematical Psychology,* 1972, *9,* 168–199. (a)

Krantz, D. H. Visual scaling. In D. Jameson & L. M. Hurvich, (Eds.), *Handbook of sensory physiology* (Vol. VII/4): *Visual psychophysics*. New York: Springer-Verlag, 1972. (b)

Luce, R. D., & Edwards, W. The derivation of subjective scales from just noticeable differences. *Psychological Review*, 1958, *65*, 222–237.

Stevens, J. C., Mack, J. D., & Stevens, S. S. Growth of sensation on seven continua as measured by force of handgrip. *Journal of Experimental Psychology*, 1960, *59*, 60–67.

Stevens, S. S. On the psychophysical law. *Psychological Review*, 1957, *64*, 153–181.

Stevens, S. S. Matching functions between loudness and ten other continua. *Perception & Psychophysics*, 1966, *1*, 5–8.

Woodworth, R. S. *Experimental psychology*. New York: Holt, 1938.

14. Suppressive Interactions between Fused Patterns[1]

Walter Makous and R. Kevin Sanders

I. Introduction

One of the defining properties of binocular rivalry is that a pattern presented to one eye cannot always be seen; that is, it is periodically suppressed. An old idea is that the singleness of vision during fusion is due to a suppression of one or the other retinal image by the same process or processes similar to those of binocular rivalry (Porta, 1593; Du Tour, 1760; Verhoeff, 1935; Asher, 1953; Kaufman, 1964; Hochberg, 1964a, 1964b; Levelt, 1965). Others disagree with this interpretation (Werner, 1937; Sperling, 1970; Nelson, 1975).

The visibility of a dim, monocularly presented test flash fluctuates in synchrony with the visibility of the pattern presented to the same eye during rivalry (Bouman, 1955; Fox & Check, 1966b, 1968, 1972; Wales & Fox, 1970; Collyer & Bevan, 1970). Thus, the detectability of the test flash can be used as an objective index of suppression. The limited use of this technique to test for suppression during fusion, however, has yielded unclear results (Fox & Check, 1966a; Fox & McIntyre, 1967).

The purpose of our observations was to use the visibility of a test flash to monitor the suppression associated with binocular rivalry while successively increasing the similarity of the binocular stimuli by discrete steps until they were able to be fused, ultimately ending with presentation of identical stimuli to both eyes. The question we asked was, where in the transition from rivalry to fusion does the suppression cease? The answer we obtained was that it never does: Even the fusion of identical stimuli is associated with suppression, just as occurs during rivalry.

[1]This research was supported by National Institutes of Health Grant EY 00788.

II. General Methods

A. *Observers*

The authors were the observers. Both have normal, 20–20 vision, although WM required correction by clinically prescribed lenses, which were mounted on the optical apparatus.

B. *Stimuli*

The four pairs of stimuli used in the various experiments are illustrated in Figure 14.1. Each eye viewed a grating through a 1° aperture, surrounded by a grating seen through a 2° annulus. Each grating was either horizontal or vertical. The gratings were square waves of 5 cycles per degree; thus, the stripes were 6' wide. The white stripes were 2.6 log td, when not attenuated [measured by the technique described by Westheimer (1966)]. The observer fixated the top of a thin, circular line that separated the two gratings. The point of fixation is indicated in Figure 14.1 by an "X," although the X was not actually part of the stimulus. The test flash was 2.6 log td when not attenuated; 100 msec in duration; 2' in diameter; and 6' below the point of fixation, in the center of a black stripe. All stimuli were in Maxwellian view. The 1-mm exit apertures of the optical system were positioned within each pupil so as to produce the sharpest images of the stimuli. The observer's head was steadied by a bite bar with his dental impression that made contact with all of his teeth. The bite bar was mounted on a three-dimensional manipulator by means of an Aloris quick-change tool, and the optical apparatus for the right eye was mounted on a laterally adjustable table, so that the apparatus could be readjusted for a change of observer quickly and reproducibly between sessions.

C. *Procedure*

The observer adapted to the stimuli a minimum of 3 min before beginning a session. In the first three experiments, sessions alternated randomly between those in which the gratings in the two eyes were of equal troland value and those in which the troland values of the grating in one eye were attenuated (1.2 log unit in the left eye of KS and 2.0 log units in the right eye of WM). As these manipulations of troland values were intended to control the relative dominance of the two eyes, dominance was monitored by beginning and ending each session with a 3-min period during which the cumulative amount of time each eye was dominant and the total number of alternations of dominance were recorded. According to these observations, the two eyes of each observer were approximately equally dominant during half of the sessions, and one of the eyes was dominant about 60% of the time during the other half of the sessions. (The right eye of KS was dominant 51 ± 1% of the time when the pattern was attenuated, and 60 ± 3% when neither pattern was attenuated; the right eye of WM was dominant 52 ± 1% of the time when neither

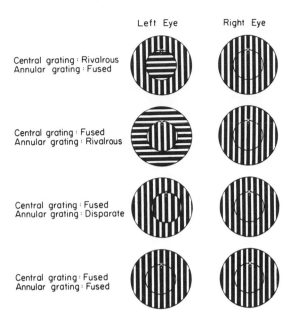

Left Eye   Right Eye

Central grating : Rivalrous
Annular grating : Fused

Central grating : Fused
Annular grating : Rivalrous

Central grating : Fused
Annular grating : Disparate

Central grating : Fused
Annular grating : Fused

Figure 14.1.   Patterns of stimulation presented to the left and right eyes. The top pair of stimuli were used for Experiments 1 and 4; the second pair, for Experiment 2; the third pair for Experiment 3; and the last pair for Experiments 4 and 5.

pattern was attenuated, and $60 \pm 1\%$ of the time when the troland value of the left eye was attenuated.)

The observer triggered the test flash when he was ready (except in Experiment 5). On any given trial, there was equal probability that the test flash would be presented to the left eye, to the right eye, or not at all. The observer reported whether or not he saw a test flash, and he was told whether or not one was presented. The attenuation of the flash followed a double-random staircase, but the data so obtained were used to construct frequency-of-seeing curves.

III. Experiment 1

A. Procedure

The steadily viewed stimuli are shown in the top row of Figure 14.1. Note that the pair of annuli are identical; they promote the appropriate convergence, they would be expected to fuse, and they were described by the observers as being fused. The gratings in the center, however, are crossed; hence, they are rivalrous. The test flash fell within this region of rivalry.

Each session was divided into double-alternating blocks of six trials. During a given block of trials the observer presented the test flash only when a particular eye appeared to be dominant. Dominance was judged according to which pattern was visible in the vicinity of the fixation point.

Thus, thresholds were measured under two conditions of dominance, in both eyes of two observers, under two conditions of relative illumination of the two eyes. Therefore, 16 frequency-of-seeing curves were generated with 336 observations per curve.

B. Results

Figure 14.2A shows an example of the results of this experiment. Notice that the probability of detecting the test flash is greater when the eye to which it is presented is dominant. Although this figure shows the result of only one of the eight pairs of curves resulting from this experiment, the results were the same for all eight conditions represented.

C. Discussion

These results merely show that, by means of the frequency-of-seeing curves obtained under our particular conditions, we can replicate the previously cited findings on the suppressive effects of rivalry on test flashes.

IV. Experiment 2

A. Procedure

The stimuli are shown in the second row of Figure 14.1. In this experiment the gratings in the annuli are crossed and therefore rivalrous, while the gratings in the centers are identical and reported as being fused. Thus, the test stimulus in this experiment falls within a fused region, although rivalry in nearby regions can be used as an index of any changes of dominance between the two eyes. Except for this difference in the stimuli, Experiment 2 is similar to Experiment 1.

B. Results

Figure 14.2B shows an example of the results of this experiment. Here the detectability of a test stimulus presented within a fused region of a pattern varies with the phase of dominance within a nearby region of rivalry. Again, the results of all eight conditions of this experiment were the same as those exemplified here.

C. Discussion

These results clearly show a fluctuation of sensitivity inside a fused region, a fluctuation that is directly analogous to what is observed during binocular rivalry.

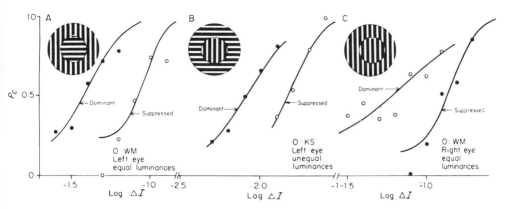

Figure 14.2. Examples of frequency-of-seeing curves from Experiments 1 (A), 2 (B), and 3 (C). The ordinate, P_c, is probability of detection. The abscissa, log ΔI, is intensity of the test flash, relative to 2.6 log td. The insets show the patterns presented to the left eye. (The right eye had vertical gratings in all three cases.) The filled circles represent conditions where the stimulus was triggered when the left eye was dominant; open circles, when the right eye was dominant. The lines are cumulative normal curves that minimize residual variance; that is, they are least-square fits achieved by an iterative computer program that takes into account the number of observations per point. Points with four or fewer observations were omitted from the figure although they were included in the fit.

Perhaps, however, this can somehow be attributed to the nearby region of rivalry by reference, for example, to such things as spread of suppression (Kaufman, 1963).

V. Experiment 3

A. Procedure

The stimuli are shown in the third row of Figure 14.1. The gratings in the central region of the patterns presented to the two eyes are identical and thus they can be fused. The gratings in the annular region are of the same spatial frequency and orientation, and they also can be fused. However, the gratings in the center and annulus of the pattern presented to the left eye are 180° out of phase with respect to one another. Thus, this stimulus is a stereogram wherein the center appears closer than the annulus. The test flash, as always, appears within the central region. This experiment is similar to the previous two in all respects except for the steadily viewed stimulus.

B. Results

The stereogram is fused, in the sense that the two patterns fuse into a single pattern with the impression of the appropriate difference of depth. However, when the pattern is fixated steadily, under the stable conditions that are possible on a bite bar, the appearance of the pattern fluctuates between that visible to the left eye and that visible to the right eye; that is, the singleness of vision persists, and the perception of depth persists, but the appearance of the grating suddenly changes as though the observer had abruptly shifted his point of view from one directly in front of the pattern to one slightly to the side, or vice versa. As in the previous experiments, for purposes of stimulus presentation a given eye was considered dominant when the pattern presented to that eye was visible in the vicinity of the test stimulus.

Figure 14.2C shows an example of the results: The observer is more likely to see a test flash in a given eye when he sees the background pattern viewed by that eye. These results were obtained in all eight conditions of this experiment.

C. Discussion

Thus, even fused stereograms produce an alternation of sensitivity analogous to the alternation of dominance and suppression seen during rivalry, and the results of the preceding experiment appear not to be due to the nearby rivalry. However, it is possible that the fluctuations of sensitivity, such as were observed here, occur only when the two eyes view rather different stimuli, whether singleness of vision results or not. Perhaps as the patterns in the two eyes approach exact correspondence, the suppression associated with rivalry decreases or disappears, and both eyes are freed of suppression.

VI. Experiment 4

A. Procedure

In order to test the foregoing idea, we presented identical patterns to the two eyes, as shown in the bottom row of Figure 14.1. However, owing to the obvious difficulty of observing any rivalry between identical patterns, the observer was not asked to present the stimuli during any particular phase of dominance. Instead, the observer presented the test flash whenever he was ready.

The rationale is as follows. If fluctuations of dominance were occurring, and if the test flash were presented as described, then at some times it would fall on a suppressed retina and at other times on a dominant retina. The probability of detecting the test flash on a large number of trials must be somewhere between the probabilities obtaining under these two conditions. If, however, each of the eyes is liberated from any suppressive effect of the other eye, then the probability of seeing should be stable, at the unsuppressed value corresponding to a dominant retina.

Thus, sessions of the kind of trial just described were randomly alternated with sessions in which the steadily viewed stimuli were equally luminous patterns of Experiment 1, and the procedures were those of Experiment 1. Thus, in the case of the rivalrous stimuli, the observer was careful to present the test flash during prescribed phases of dominance. In this experiment trials of particular phases of dominance were run in blocks of 10. Twenty sessions of 160 trials were run with KS and 12 such sessions were run with WM.

B. Results

Figures 14.3 and 14.4 show the results. In three of the four eyes, the probability of detecting the test flash during fusion is not as great as it is while the eye is free of suppression (dominant) during rivalry. Control observations have shown that any difference in sensitivity to test flashes presented against horizontal as opposed to vertical gratings in the left eye is too small to be detected in this experiment.

C. Discussion

One would expect these results if the eyes, while viewing these identical gratings, were alternately dominating and being suppressed. In any case, the reduced sensitivity during fusion is difficult to reconcile with the idea that both eyes are continually at their most sensitive during fusion.

However, this experiment has a defect. The observer's task is more difficult when he can present the test flash only during a particular phase of rivalry than when he can present it at any time, as during the fused condition of this experiment. Owing to this difference of difficulty, the difference of sensitivity between the two conditions may be greater than it appears in this experiment. Therefore, we designed the next experiment to avoid this defect.

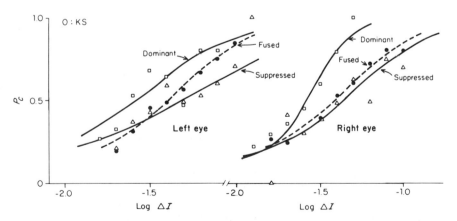

Figure 14.3. Frequency-of-seeing curves from Experiment 4, left and right eyes of KS. Squares and triangles represent data obtained when the test flash was triggered when the test eye was dominant and suppressed, respectively, and when the steadily presented patterns were the top pair in Figure 14.1. The circles represent data obtained when the steadily presented patterns were the bottom pair in Figure 14.1. Otherwise this figure is similar to Figure 14.2.

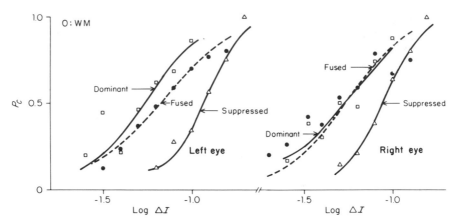

Figure 14.4. Frequency-of-seeing curves from Experiment 4, left and right eyes of WM. See Figure 14.3 for explanation.

VII. Experiment 5

A. Procedure

In this experiment the observers viewed the same two pairs of stimuli as in the previous experiment. The experimenter instead of the observer presented the test flash in both the fused and rivalrous conditions. Thus, as the experimenter could not know which eye was dominant at any given time, presentation of the test flash was independent of the phase of dominance in both fused and rivalrous conditions; further, the observer's task did not differ according to which pair of stimuli he viewed.

The pairs of patterns were presented in four blocks of 52 trials each, in an ABBA sequence. Observer KS participated in 7 such sessions and WM in 4.

B. Results

The results, in Figures 14.5 and 14.6, show that in this experiment no release from suppression is detectable during fusion. The filled circles represent the detectability of the test flash against a fused pattern, and the open circles show the analogous detectabilities when the test flash is presented against the rivalrous gratings.

Statistical evaluation of these results shows that if there was any less suppression in the fused than in the rivalrous condition for either eye of KS or for the right eye of WM, it occurred on fewer than 2% of the trials. The left eye of WM was more sensitive during rivalry than during fusion.

WM responded "yes" significantly more often on blank trials during the fused condition than during the rivalrous condition. This corresponds to a bias in favor of

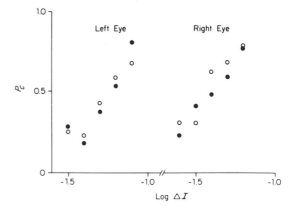

Figure 14.5. Frequency-of-seeing curves from Experiment 5, left and right eyes of KS. Open circles represent data obtained when the top pair of stimuli shown in Figure 14.1 was used; filled circles, when the bottom pair of stimuli was used. Ordinate and abscissa as in Figure 14.2.

the fused condition. In an effort to present the results in a way that is as free as possible from the effects of such bias, we have shown them in Figure 14.6 in terms of d', the parameter that reflects sensitivity in signal-detectability theory. This was the only condition in the experiments reported here in which the false positives in two conditions being compared differed sufficiently to affect the interpretation.

C. Discussion

If the eyes alternate in dominance regardless of the similarity of the patterns presented to opposite eyes, then the probability of detecting the test flash should be the same whether the alternation can be seen, as in rivalry, or not, as in the binocular viewing of identical patterns. However, if fusion involves a release from suppression, then the probability of detecting the test flash should be greater during fusion than it is during rivalry.

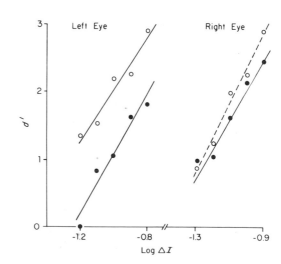

Figure 14.6. Sensitivity (d') of WM to varying test flash intensities in Experiment 5. Abscissa as in Figure 14.2, and symbols as in Figure 14.5. Curves are lines fit by least squares.

These results are clearly difficult to reconcile with the idea that rivalrous stimuli cause significantly more suppression than fused stimuli. The greater sensitivity of the left eye of WM during rivalry than during fusion is puzzling, but it offers no obvious refuge for the idea that fusion involves less suppression than rivalry.

VIII. Other Results

A. Sources of Variance

The first three experiments were identical except for the pattern imaged in the left eye. Thus, any difference in the detectability of the test flash in the right eye must be due to the influence of the stimulus to the other eye. Analysis of variance performed on the means of the 12 frequency-of-seeing curves obtained for the right eye in these three experiments revealed that 66% of the variance is due to the conditions of dominance at the time that the test flash was presented.

The pattern of the stimulus presented to the left eye accounted for 24% of the variance of the thresholds in the right eye. Post hoc analysis of this effect revealed that is was entirely due to an elevation of the thresholds measured against stereo-scopic backgrounds (Experiment 3). Any attempt to interpret this result, however, must take into account the fact that although the two observers did the experiments in different sequences, no effort was made to randomize or to counterbalance the sequence of experiments.

No detectable influence on thresholds in the right eye could be attributed to (a) any of the interactions, or (b) the relative troland values in the two eyes or the relative dominance of the two eyes, which was controlled by these troland values. All told, these effects accounted for only 10% of the variance.

B. Dominance

The relative dominance of the two eyes did not differ reliably among Experiments 1–3. The rate at which dominance alternated also did not differ reliably between observers or between Experiments 1 and 2. However, in Experiment 3, during which the observers viewed a fused stereogram, the rate of alternation was only 14 ± 2 reversals per minute, half the rate of alternation in the other two experiments (31 ± 1 reversals per minute). This is in agreement with the finding of Kaufman (1963) and with Ogle and Wakefield's suggestion (1967) that stereoscopic detail tends to stabilize binocular rivalry.

C. Phenomenological Observations

The foregoing experiments deal with rivalry and fusion of contours. Both rivalry and fusion of colors also can be observed. Hence we experimented with varying combinations of color and contour rivalry to determine whether or not they are linked. For example, suppose that a hortizontal green and black grating is presented to one eye, and an equally luminous vertical grating that is red and black is presented to the other eye. We observed that the color of the grating fluctuates with the orientation of the contours, but the reds and greens are not as saturated as they are when the same color is presented to both eyes or when only one eye is stimulated. However, if both gratings are vertical, stable color mixing is possible.

IX. General Discussion

The results of these experiments suggest that presence of a contour on one retina tends to suppress stimuli presented to corresponding regions of the contralateral retina, whether that stimulus is an orthogonal contour, a congruent contour, or a test flash.

Test flashes were used to monitor suppression of a given eye partly in order to avoid the subjectivity of phenomenology, but the technique does have the drawback that it is not very sensitive to the suppression it is used to measure. This is because presenting a stimulus as a flash greatly increases its capacity to be seen. A steadily presented stimulus that is, for example, a hundred times above threshold can be completely suppressed during binocular rivalry, but if the same stimulus is presented as a flash, it need only be two or three times threshold in order to be seen (cf. Wales & Fox, 1970). Thus, although the detectability of the test flash serves to monitor changes of dominance and suppression, the magnitude of these changes is only a weak reflection of the magnitude of the suppression being monitored. For this reason, we have not emphasized the magnitudes of the effects we have observed. Nevertheless, these observations do not support the idea that the magnitude of the suppression is smaller during fusion than during rivalry.

A variable that is of the utmost importance here and in all experiments on binocular fusion, and yet often overlooked, is fixational disparity. For example, fixational disparities can cause a test flash delivered to the nondominant eye to appear off-center with respect to the grating visible at the time (i.e., that presented to the other eye). The parameters of the stimuli are critical in this respect. For example, in Experiment 3, we have found that increasing the size of the annulus tends to shift fixation from correspondence between the gratings in the center toward correspondence between those in the annuli. This can cause either or both gratings to appear to shift phase slightly as dominance shifts.

The evidence from these observers is strong, but a larger number of observers would be necessary to be certain of the general applicability of these findings. The conclusions of Fox and McIntyre (1967) support the present results, but Fox and Check (1966a) failed to find evidence of suppression during fusion. A possible explanation of these negative findings is that Fox and Check attempted to monitor the suppression within their fused area by observing rivalry in a distinctly different field that was separated from the fused field by 1° 20′ at the closest. It is well known that different eyes can dominate in different parts of the visual field at the same time. Possibly a low correlation between dominance in their two fields contributed to their negative findings.

These results permit the statement that the process of suppression closes a channel of information that would otherwise allow information on the presence or absence of a test flash to be observed in the response. Other kinds of information in suppressed images presumably are also blocked somewhere in transmission. Possibly visual direction of suppressed contours is one kind. Nevertheless, at least three kinds of information in images that are suppressed from some response systems can be observed in other classes of response. As others have pointed out (e.g., Kaufman, 1964), reports based on stereopsis require information from a contour in each eye, whether one is suppressed or not. Further, contours in the suppressed eye control its position. Finally, if the color of the image between suppressed contours affects the reported color of corresponding regions in the other eye, then information on color is getting into the response even though information on the contours is not.

X. Summary

We have used the detectability of a test flash to monitor the sensitivity of both eyes against varying patterns of binocular rivalry and fusion. Experiment 1 established that the test flash can be used to monitor suppression; Experiment 2 showed a suppression within a region of identical fused contours in synchrony with rivalry in a nearby region; Experiment 3 showed an alternating suppression within a completely fused stereogram; and Experiments 4 and 5 showed suppression during fusion of identical patterns containing no patently rivalrous contours. No differences between the suppression of rivalry and the suppression of fusion could be detected. These results suggest that binocular rivalry and the singleness of vision during fusion may be due to the same processes.

REFERENCES

Asher, H. Suppression theory of binocular vision. *British Journal of Ophthalmology*, 1953, *37*, 37–49.
Bouman, M. A. On foveal and peripheral interaction in binocular vision. *Optica Acta*, 1955, *1*, 177–183.
Collyer, G., & Bevan, W. Objective measurement of dominance control in binocular rivalry. *Perception & Psychophysics*, 1970, *8*, 437–438.
Du Tour, E. F. Discussion d'une question d'optique. *Mémoirs de Mathématique et Physique d'Académie Royale Science (Paris)*, 1760, *3*, 514–530.
Fox, R., & Check, R. Binocular fusion: A test of the suppression theory. *Perception & Psychophysics*, 1966, *1*, 331–334. (a)
Fox, R., & Check, R. Forced-choice form recognition during binocular rivalry. *Psychonomic Science*, 1966, *6*, 471–472. (b)
Fox, R., & Check, R. Detection of motion during binocular rivalry suppression. *Journal of Experimental Psychology*, 1968, *78*, 388–395.
Fox, R., & Check, R. Independence between binocular rivalry suppression, duration, and magnitude of suppression. *Journal of Experimental Psychology*, 1972, *93*, 283–289.

Fox, R., & McIntyre, C. Suppression during binocular fusion of complex targets. *Psychonomic Science,* 1967, *8,* 143–144.

Hochberg, J. Contralateral suppressive fields of binocular combination. *Psychonomic Science,* 1964, *1,* 157–158. (a)

Hochberg, J. A theory of the binocular cyclopean field: On the possibility of simulated stereopsis. *Perceptual and Motor Skills,* 1964, *19,* 685. (b)

Kaufman, L. On the spread of suppression and binocular rivalry. *Vision Research,* 1963, *3,* 401–415.

Kaufman, L. Suppression and fusion in viewing complex stereograms. *American Journal of Psychology,* 1964, *77,* 193–205.

Levelt, W. J. M. *On binocular rivalry,* Mouton: The Hague, 1965.

Nelson, J. I. Globality and stereoscopic fusion in binocular vision. *Journal of Theoretical Biology,* 1975, *49,* 1–88.

Ogle, K. N., & Wakefield, J. Stereoscopic depth and binocular rivalry. *Vision Research,* 1967, *7,* 89–98.

Porta, J. B. *De refractione. Optices parte: Libri nouem.* Ex Officia Horatii Saluiani. Naples: Jacabum Carlinum & Antonium Pacem, 1593.

Sperling, G. Binocular vision: A physical and a neural theory. *American Journal of Psychology,* 1970, *83,* 461–534.

Verhoeff, F. H. New theory of binocular vision. *Archives of Ophthalmology,* 1935, *12,* 151–175.

Wales, R., & Fox, R. Increment detection thresholds during binocular rivalry suppression. *Perception & Psychophysics,* 1970, *8,* 90–94.

Werner, H. Dynamics of binocular depth perception. *Psychological Monographs,* 1937, *49,* 1–127.

Westheimer, G. The Maxwellian view. *Vision Research,* 1966, *6,* 669–682.

15. The Influence of Color on Binocular Rivalry

Mark Hollins and Eleanor H. L. Leung

I. Introduction

Opinions differ as to the nature of binocular rivalry, a phenomenon in which targets presented to corresponding regions of the two retinas are seen in alternation, rather than simultaneously. According to one view (Panum, 1858/1940; Ogle, 1950), rivalry is the opposite of fusion, and is to be expected only when the targets are appreciably different from one another. A contrasting theory (Verhoeff, 1935) states that rivalry occurs at all times, even when the targets presented to the two eyes are the same.

Evidence against Verhoeff's position has been reported by Leung (1976). She showed that when identical targets are presented to the two eyes, the binocular impression will, under certain conditions, be brighter than that resulting from either target presented alone. This finding is incompatible with the notion that only one of the targets is actually being seen at any given time.

If fusion occurs when the targets are identical, and rivalry occurs when they are very different, how discrepant would the stimuli presented to the two eyes have to be before fusion would give way to rivalry? Perhaps if the difference between the targets were gradually increased, it would be possible to see evidence of increasingly vigorous binocular rivalry. This is the possibility which we explore in the present set of experiments.

Our plan was to present a pair of targets that were equivalent in their ability to dominate one another (so that each would be dominant for half of an extended period of time), and somehow to measure the strength of the suppressive force they exerted on one another; then to replace one of them with a target that was different in color but equal to the first in dominating ability, and again measure the intensity of the rivalry occurring, and so on.

The first step was to choose a set of targets differing in color but all capable of

181

dominating, for 50% of the time, a constant grating presented to the other eye: It was necessary to know, for example, whether highly saturated colors are dominant over others of equal brightness. We therefore determined an action spectrum of binocular rivalry, using the traditional procedure (Breese, 1899) of having the subject indicate which of two rivaling targets was dominant.

It sometimes happens during rivalry that both targets, or portions of them, are visible simultaneously; at other times, however, one target completely suppresses the other. In the course of our initial experiments, we became convinced that this distinction, to which Breese's method is insensitive, is an important one for understanding the relation between color and binocular rivalry. We therefore decided to make our measurements of the strength of rivalry in a way that would take this distinction into account. For this purpose we adopted (with modifications) a procedure introduced by Wade (1974), who had subjects indicate throughout rivalry not just which target was the more visible, but whether the left eye's target alone, the right one's alone, or a composite of the two targets was seen. We have called this procedure the *method of exclusive visibility,* because it calls on subjects to record the amount of time during which one target is visible to the exclusion of the other. Our use of the method rests on the assumption that rivalry can be considered stronger or more vigorous when the targets alternate crisply than when they blend together into a composite.

Wade (1974) used this method to assess rivalry between gratings, the orientation of one of which he varied; this manipulation had no significant effect. Later, however, Wade (1975) showed that orthogonal gratings form a composite less often if one is red and one green than if they are both red or both green.

We undertook the present experiments to determine whether the strength of rivalry increases in any lawful way with the difference in color between the targets presented to the two eyes, and to what component(s) of color difference it is related. We also hoped that studying the influence of color on binocular rivalry would provide some insight into the nature of the rivalry mechanism itself.

II. Apparatus and Subjects

The experiments were run on a Maxwellian view optical system consisting of four channels: one for the background and one for the test target in each eye. The system is the one used by Leung (1976), with modifications. Achromatic lenses and front surface mirrors were used to bring light from a pair of quartz–halogen lamps, run on 6.6 A dc, to the subject's eyes. Light from one of the sources passed through heat-absorbing glass and a daylight filter before dividing at a beamsplitter to provide the two background fields. Identical field stops, produced photographically on glass, defined the 8° diameter circular backgrounds. Each had a 5′ diameter black dot at its center. Throughout these experiments, both backgrounds were present and were seen fused; the dot served as a fixation point. The backgrounds were adjusted with neutral density filters to a retinal illuminance of 1.25 log trolands, measured according to the method described by Westheimer (1966) with an S.E.I. meter and a Macbeth reflection plate.

Two beams of light from the second lamp provided the test targets. Each passed through a circular 1° field stop with a photographically produced square-wave grating attached to it. The grating for the right eye was vertical, the one for the left eye, horizontal. Except for orientation, these gratings were identical, with a spatial frequency of 6 cycles deg^{-1}. Each target was concentric with the background on which it was superimposed, the fixation point being located in the gap between two bright bars of the grating.

The beam for the right test target passed through a Bausch and Lomb high-intensity monochromator; its spectral properties were further controlled at wavelengths shorter than 500 nm and longer than 580 nm with Wratten gelatin filters.

The test beam for the left eye came out of the lamp house from the side, bypassing the monochromator; it passed through narrow band interference filters, in conjunction with blocking filters to provide light of either 455 or 651 nm. For the final experiments in the study, the spectral composition of this channel was controlled with Wratten filters. A heat-absorbing filter was always present.

The subject's head was held in place with a bite bar and forehead rests. Each beam passed through a 2-mm artificial pupil located just before the eye and was brought to a filament image less than 2 mm in diameter in the subject's pupil plane. Because of the eye's chromatic aberration, the target stop for the left eye was moved in depth to the position of best focus every time the color of this beam was changed; these movements did not affect the visual angle subtended by the target, since the Maxwellian lens was located one focal length from the subject's pupil plane. An achromatizing lens was used in front of the right eye.

An inconel wedge, which could be adjusted by the subject, was located at a filament image in each test beam. These wedges were calibrated in the system using a United Detector Technology radiometer. Calibrated inconel filters were also used. Daco electromagnetic shutters, located at filament images and operated by Hunter timers, controlled target presentation.

In different conditions of the experiment, the subject held in a push button whenever the prescribed phase of rivalry occurred; these periods of time were cumulated within a trial on a Hunter Klockounter.

The authors served as the subjects. EHL is 29 and MH 31 years of age. Both have normal color vision as determined with American Optical pseudoisochromatic plates and the Farnsworth–Munsell 100 hue test. Field stops were positioned so that the test targets and backgrounds were seen clearly despite the subjects' slight myopia.

III. Action Spectrum Experiment

In order to learn whether some colors are more dominant than others, we wanted to determine the action spectrum of binocular rivalry. It is known that as the luminance of one of a pair of rivaling stimuli is increased, it comes to dominate the other member of the pair for a larger and larger fraction of the time (Kaplan & Metlay, 1964). It therefore seemed reasonable that by varying the luminance of one of a pair of colored gratings, we could find some luminance at which it and the constant grating would be equal in their ability to dominate one another. Our question was how the color of the variable grating would influence these measurements.

We carried out the experiment in the following way. The left eye's grating was held constant in wavelength (455 nm) and luminance (1 log unit above threshold), but both the wavelength and luminance of the right eye's grating were systematically varied. At each wavelength, this grating was first presented at a luminance .4 log unit above threshold, and then increased in .3 log-unit steps on subsequent trials until a value 1.6 log units above threshold, or the maximum output of the system, was reached.

The standard and variable gratings came on simultaneously at the beginning of each 100-sec trial. During the trial, the subject indicated by depressing a push button those periods of time during which the variable grating was dominant over the standard. Both gratings went off at the end of the trial, and the subject viewed the background alone for the 100-sec interval that followed.

A complete luminance series was obtained for one wavelength at a time, the wavelengths being ordered randomly; when a series of measurements had been made at each wavelength, the experiment was repeated using a new random order. In all, four series were run at each wavelength.

The lowest luminance we used always caused the variable grating to dominate the standard for less than 50 sec, the highest luminance always produced a value above 50 sec, and the amount of dominance increased systematically in between, never falling below 50 sec after it had risen above that level. We were therefore able to calculate the (log) luminance value that would have produced 50 sec of variable grating dominance by interpolating between the two points that bracketed this criterion.

The results are shown in Figure 15.1, where each upright triangle represents the average of the four values obtained at each wavelength. It can be seen that for both subjects, the function peaks in the midspectral region.

How do these measurements compare with the photopic luminous efficiency functions for these same observers? The answer to this question is reflected by the filled circles, which represent threshold measurements made on the same apparatus as a preliminary to the action spectrum experiment. For these threshold determinations, the standard grating was blocked off and the variable grating flashed for 100 msec once per second. (As usual, the background was present in both eyes.) The subject was instructed to adjust the luminance of the variable grating until the flashing target could just be seen, not necessarily resolved as a grating.

The threshold measurements have been slid down the ordinate to facilitate comparison with the action spectrum of rivalry. It is clear that the two functions are very

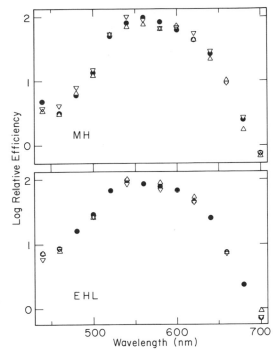

Figure 15.1. Action spectrum of binocular rivalry. The ordinate plots as a function of wavelength the effectiveness of a vertical grating presented to the right eye in dominating a horizontal grating presented to the left eye, which had a wavelength of either 455 nm (upright triangles) or 651 nm (inverted triangles). The circles represent threshold measurements and have been slid down the ordinate for comparison with the triangles. Each point is the mean of four determinations.

similar. This result suggests that the ability of the variable grating to dominate the standard depends, at least in this situation, on brightness rather than on hue, saturation, or some combination of these factors. However, before we could conclude that this rule was a general one, independent of the colors involved, it was necessary to determine whether the action spectrum of rivalry was the same for different standard gratings. To settle this question we changed the wavelength of the left eye's grating to 651 nm and repeated the experiment; these measurements are shown by the inverted triangles in Figure 15.1. The two sets of triangles are in close agreement, lending support to the idea that when a subject indicates which of two gratings is the more dominant during rivalry, it is brightness, independent of hue and saturation, that determines the results.

In the course of these experiments, however, we had noticed that the colors of the gratings did have a conspicuous effect on the appearance of rivalry, an effect to which our psychophysical procedure was insensitive. We had observed that with certain pairs of wavelengths, the two gratings were simultaneously visible for long periods of time, with first one and then the other being seen slightly more strongly; with other wavelength combinations, however, there was more of a tendency for one or the other of the gratings to disappear entirely for a few seconds, then reappear and completely replace the other in awareness. We undertook additional experiments to study these periods of "exclusive visibility."

IV. Exclusive Visibility Experiment

We had the subjects indicate, by pushing the button, those periods of time during which only the right eye's grating was visible. The two gratings were always equal in luminance: 1 log unit above threshold for MH, and .7 log unit above threshold for EHL, who found exclusive visibility easier to judge at the lower level because of the slower course of rivalry.

As before, trials lasted 100 sec and were separated by intervals of the same length. During one series, the left eye's grating was kept at 455 nm, while the wavelength of the right eye's grating was varied between 440 and 700 nm. Wavelengths were presented in random order, with the restriction that each had to be used once before any could be used a second time, and so on; this was continued until five trials had been run at each wavelength.

The results are shown by the filled circles in Figure 15.2, where the number of seconds out of 100 for which the right eye's grating was visible alone is plotted as a function of its wavelength. For both subjects, the amount of exclusive visibility is small when the variable grating (like the standard) is blue, but rises as the difference in color between the two gratings increases. The measurements level off in the red region of the spectrum, which is to be expected in view of the fact that chromaticity does not change much at these long wavelengths. To determine whether the color of the right eye's grating also influenced exclusive visibility with the left eye, we obtained at three wavelengths additional measurements in which subjects depressed the push button when the constant grating was seen alone. These results (filled

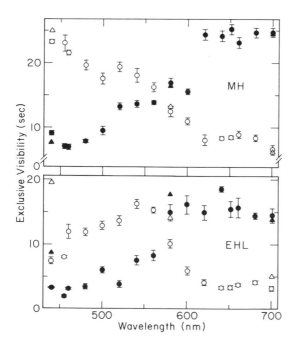

Figure 15.2. Seconds of exclusive visibility for either a vertical grating presented to the right eye (circles) or a horizontal grating presented to the left (triangles) are plotted as a function of the wavelength of the former. The wavelength of the left eye's grating was held constant at either 455 nm (filled symbols) or 651 nm (open symbols). Each point is the mean of five determinations. Error bars for the circles plot one standard error above and below the mean.

triangles) parallel the earlier measurements, although in the case of EHL exclusive visibility tended to be somewhat greater for the left eye than for the right. These data indicate that the amount of exclusive visibility is smallest when rivaling targets are the same color.

To determine the generality of this finding, we changed the wavelength of the left eye's grating to 651 nm and repeated the experiment (open symbols). Once again, the targets rivaled more vigorously when they differed in color than when they were the same color.

There is, however, a clear difference between the data for the two subjects at short wavelengths. We do not yet have an explanation for this difference, but have begun to look for one by asking what aspect(s) of color difference between the gratings is important in rivalry. The measurements to be discussed now represent a first step in this investigation.

V. Is the Binocular Rivalry Mechanism Tritanopic?

The data reported are puzzling because for neither subject is exclusive visibility related in any close way to differences in perceived color (e.g., Hurvich & Jameson, 1956). For example, the data for MH show that more exclusive visibility occurred when a red grating was paired with a blue or a violet one than when it was paired with green; this was the opposite of what we had expected. To gain some insight into this problem, we plotted the data for this subject in another way (open symbols in Figure 15.3): Each wavelength of the variable grating was represented by a point, its position along the ordinate representing the amount of (right eye) exclusive visibility when paired with 455 nm, its position along the abscissa representing exclusive visibility when paired with 651 nm. The resulting plot defined what might be called a "spectrum locus in binocular rivalry space," and was fit reasonably well

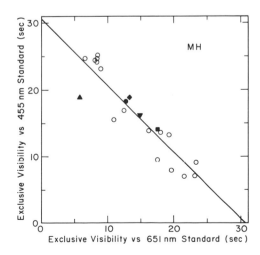

Figure 15.3. The amount of exclusive visibility of 16 spectral lights (open symbols) and 5 nonspectral lights (filled symbols) when each was paired with a 455-nm grating is plotted as a function of the amount of exclusive visibility when each was paired with a 651-nm grating. All measurements are for subject MH: The open symbols represent the same measurements shown for this subject in Figure 15.2. The nonspectral lights were Illuminant A (●), and tungsten light filtered through Wratten filters 34 (▲), 38A (▼), 65 (■), and 78 (◆). The position of each point along each axis is the mean result of five 100-sec trials.

by a straight line with a slope of -1. This suggested to us that, from the point of view of the binocular rivalry mechanism, the test stimulus might be varying in only one dimension.

One way in which this could occur would be if only two of the three classes of cones made a contribution to binocular rivalry. To test this notion, we studied rivalry in subject MH when nonspectral colors were used for the left eye's grating. Four of these colors were produced with Wratten filters 34, 38A, 65, and 78, and a fifth (considered to be Illuminant A) by removing all filters but the heat-absorbing glass from the tungsten beam. The positions of these stimuli on the CIE chromaticity diagram are shown in Figure 15.4. In each case, the subject recorded exclusive visibility of the nonspectral light when the wavelength of the right eye's grating was 455 nm (on some trials) or 651 nm (on others). In this way the position of each of the five nonspectral colors in binocular rivalry space could be determined (filled symbols in Figure 15.3). All lay reasonably close to the spectrum locus, as would be predicted by the idea that the binocular rivalry mechanism is dichromatic.

Which two classes of cones contribute to rivalry? Clearly, it must be the middle- and long-wave-sensitive cones that do so, since the rivalry mechanism distinguishes very well among wavelengths in the 540- to 600-nm range, where short-wave-sensitive cones absorb negligibly. Therefore, if the rivalry mechanism is dichromatic, it must be the signals from blue-sensitive cones that make no contribution. As a test of this idea we recorded, in the case of MH, exclusive visibility of the same five nonspectral colors when each was paired with that wavelength (shown in Figure 15.4) with which it would be confused by a tritanope. For no pair did the amount of exclusive visibility average more than 8 sec. The results were comparable to those obtained earlier when the same wavelength (either 455 or 651 nm) was presented to both eyes. In other words, when confronted with pairs of colors that a tritanope would confuse, the binocular rivalry mechanism behaves as if they were indistinguishable.

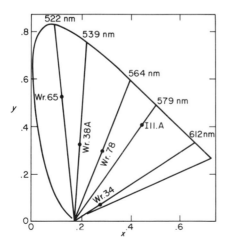

Figure 15.4. The positions in the CIE chromaticity diagram of the nonspectral lights used in the experiments are shown by the filled circles. Lines drawn through them intersect the spectrum locus at the tritanopic confusion wavelength of each. The copunctal point for tritanopia is assumed to lie at $x = .171, y = 0$ (Wyszecki & Stiles, 1967).

We take these findings as support for the notion that blue-sensitive cones do not contribute to binocular rivalry under the conditions of our experiment. This is not really surprising, however. Since contours play an important role in rivalry (Panum, 1858/1940; Breese, 1899), and since the acuity of the blue-sensitive system is low (Stiles, 1949; Brindley, 1954; Green, 1968), it is to be expected that rivalry between fine gratings will be influenced little, if at all, by these cones. However, it is not likely that even the use of coarse square-wave gratings would reveal much input from blue-sensitive cones to the rivalry mechanism, since Tansley and Boynton (1976), in a study influencing the design of the experiments reported here, showed that when subjects judge the distinctness of a single edge, they are not influenced by information from blue-sensitive cones.

Whether low-frequency sine-wave gratings would rival in a way that took account of signals from blue-sensitive cones is a question remaining to be investigated.

VI. Summary and Conclusions

These experiments show that the color of orthogonal gratings presented to the two eyes has a strong effect on binocular rivalry. When the targets are the same color the tendency for both to be seen at once is greater than when they differ in color, as Wade (1975) found using red and green gratings. If the premise is accepted that a target is more strongly suppressed when it disappears completely than when it remains visible, it follows that binocular rivalry involves more vigorous suppression when the two rivaling targets differ in color.

We found some evidence that the binocular rivalry mechanism is tritanopic, although this needs to be tested more extensively.

As shown in the action spectrum experiment, the influence of color on the strength of rivalry is obscured when subjects are asked only to indicate which of two targets is more visible at a given time; here it is brightness, rather than hue or saturation, that appears to determine the results.

Some work suggests that binocular rivalry is a selective phenomenon resulting from antagonistic interactions within specific information-processing channels in the visual system (Kaufman, 1964; Julesz, 1971; Julesz & Miller, 1975). Our results are difficult to interpret in these terms, for we find that changing one stimulus property of a target—its color—influences the amount of time for which the target, or another with which it is rivaling, will disappear in its entirety. We have never seen a grating remain visible but lose its color; nor have we seen any other dissociation of stimulus properties during rivalry, except that gratings sometimes grow dimmer during periods of partial suppression.

These observations suggest to us that rivalry is a unitary phenomenon, varying in intensity, certainly, and subject to many influences, but acting to suppress simultaneously a range of types of visual signals. This is similar to the view advanced by Fox and Check (1966, 1968) and Blake and Fox (1974), although we have no evidence to confirm their additional conclusion that the suppressive force is exerted equally on different classes of visual signals.

ACKNOWLEDGMENTS

The authors are indebted to Professor Riggs for loaning us much of the equipment with which the experiments were done. Additional support was provided by USPHS Grant EY-01391. Thanks are also due to Professor Robert B. Lawson for making the translation of Panum's manuscript available to us.

REFERENCES

Blake, R., & Fox, R. Binocular rivalry suppression: Insensitive to spatial frequency and orientation change. *Vision Research*, 1974, *14*, 687–692.

Breese, B. B. On inhibition. *Psychological Review Monograph Supplements*, 1899, *3*(1, Whole No. 11).

Brindley, G. S. The summation areas of human colour-receptive mechanisms at increment threshold. *Journal of Physiology*, 1954, *124*, 400–408.

Fox, R., & Check, R. Forced-choice form recognition during binocular rivalry. *Psychonomic Science*, 1966, *6*, 471–472.

Fox, R., & Check, R. Detection of motion during binocular rivalry suppression. *Journal of Experimental Psychology*, 1968, *78*, 388–395.

Green, D. G. The contrast sensitivity of the colour mechanisms of the human eye. *Journal of Physiology*, 1968, *196*, 415–429.

Hurvich, L. M., & Jameson, D. Some quantitative aspects of an opponent-colors theory. IV. A psychological color specification system. *Journal of the Optical Society of America*, 1956, *46*, 416–421.

Julesz, B. *Foundations of cyclopean perception*. Chicago: University of Chicago Press, 1971.

Julesz, B., & Miller, J. E. Independent spatial-frequency-tuned channels in binocular fusion and rivalry. *Perception*, 1975, *4*, 125–143.

Kaplan, I. T., & Metlay, W. Light intensity and binocular rivalry. *Journal of Experimental Psychology*, 1964, *67*, 22–26.

Kaufman, L. On the nature of binocular disparity. *American Journal of Psychology*, 1964, *77*, 393–402.

Leung, E. H. L. Monocular and binocular brightness of monochromatic lights. (Doctoral dissertation, Brown University, 1976). *Dissertation Abstracts International*, 1977, *38*, 394B. (University Microfilms No. 77-14, 155.)

Ogle, K. N. *Researches in binocular vision*. Philadelphia: Saunders, 1950.

Panum, P. L. [*Physiological investigations concerning vision with two eyes*] (C. Hübscher, trans.). Unpublished manuscript. Hanover, New Hampshire, Dartmouth Eye Institute, 1940. [Originally published, Kiel: Schwering's Bookstore, 1858.]

Stiles, W. S. Increment thresholds & the mechanisms of colour vision. *Documenta Ophthalmologica*, 1949, *3*, 138–163.

Tansley, B. W., & Boynton, R. M. A line, not a space, represents visual distinctness of borders formed by different colors. *Science*, 1976, *191*, 954–957.

Verhoeff, F. H. A new theory of binocular vision. *Archives of Ophthalmology*, 1935, *13*, 151–175.

Wade, N. J. The effect of orientation in binocular contour rivalry of real images and afterimages. *Perception & Psychophysics*, 1974, *15*, 227–232.

Wade, N. J. Monocular and binocular rivalry between contours. *Perception*, 1975, *4*, 85–95.

Westheimer, G. The Maxwellian view. *Vision Research*, 1966, *6*, 669–682.

Wyszecki, G., & Stiles, W. S. *Color science: Concepts and methods, quantitative data and formulas*. New York: Wiley, 1967.

Color Vision

16. Ten Years of Research with the Minimally Distinct Border[1]

Robert M. Boynton

I. Color Scaling

When P. Kaiser joined me at Rochester about 10 years ago, I had become interested in the scaling of color. My objective was to find a method whereby any two colors, whether closely similar or very different, could be compared so that the amount of that color difference could be meaningfully specified. In addition (in accord with a philosophy of research that I had learned at Brown University), I wanted to obtain results that would not only be psychologically meaningful, but also physiologically so. The existing methods that had produced results to which some physiological models had been applied [mainly those of MacAdam (1942), which produced his famous ellipses] were suitable only for measuring very small color differences, namely, just-discriminable ones. It is not at all clear whether or how one can legitimately add just noticeable differences (jnds) in order to specify differences between colors that differ a lot. Existing methods for gauging large color differences, like those of Ekman (1954), Indow and Uchizono (1960), or Burnham, Onley, and Witzel (1970), in effect require the subject to make gross psychological judgments of ill-defined global percepts. This may be adequate for some purposes, but probably not if one's goal is ultimately to understand the data in physiological terms.

II. Development of the Minimally Distinct Border Method

Kaiser and I tried several procedures that involved flicker, masking, adaptation, and induction. There seemed to be insurmountable problems with all of them.

[1]Support of this research by Research Grants EY-00187 and EY-01541 from the National Eye Institute, U.S. Public Health Service, is gratefully acknowledged. Some of this work was previously reviewed (Boynton, 1973).

193

Eventually we decided to try what seemed to be a very direct method, one where the two fields to be compared were placed side by side, yet which differed from conventional heterochromatic photometry. The logic of the approach was as follows. If two such fields are of the same spectral distribution, and each one fills half a bipartite field, then at equal brightness and luminance the field must become uniform, with no division at the center. This must be so because, if the optics are correct, there is no physical inhomogeneity anywhere within such a circular field; its two halves are merely supplied by separate optical channels. But if the two fields differ in chromaticity, then the perceived difference between them should never disappear, no matter how their relative intensities are set. At some setting the apparent difference between them should be minimized.

One aspect of the difference that remains is color per se, for example, the observation that the field might appear as saturated red on one side and desaturated yellow on the other. But the magnitude of such a color difference is difficult to gauge, and therefore it was not the *color* of the fields to which we directed our attention. Instead, we concentrated on the *border* between them which, it seemed, ought to remain visible at all relative luminances. We hoped that the strength of this residual contour could provide the index of color difference that we sought.

All new experiments present many difficulties, and this one was no exception. The worst problem we had was getting the positions of the fields just right. Our criterion was that there should be no visible artifact when fields of equal spectral distribution were set for equal brightness. Because we were unable to achieve this criterion in Maxwellian view, we abandoned that method and projected the beams of our various channels onto a diffusing surface. By placing razor blades at conjugate foci of the various beams, we could move the half-fields around and create the condition of perfect juxtaposition. By doing this we sacrificed intensity and had to settle for luminances of the order of 20 td. As a result, because the light was too dim, we could not examine wavelengths shorter than 470 nm. Although we did not think at the time that this was a very important limitation, it turned out to be critical.

Another problem was to take care of the chromatic aberration of the eye which caused blue fields to appear fuzzy and not to align properly with other fields. We solved this problem by having an achromatizing lens built in the Institute of Optics shop, according to a prescription that had been published by Bedford and Wyszecki (1957). Our first work with the minimally distinct border (MDB) was published in *Science* in July of 1968 (Boynton & Kaiser, 1968).

III. "Saturation" as Revealed by the Minimally Distinct Border

Working with spectral colors over the range of wavelengths available, we compared each of these with a reference white. The first step in the experiment was to adjust the spectral field to produce an MDB with the white. The second step was to gauge how distinct that border was. For example, 570 nm formed an indistinct

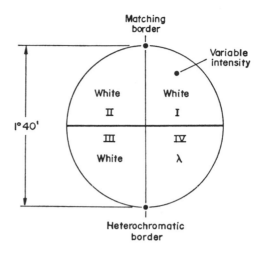

Figure 16.1. Four-part field used for determining the equivalent achromatic contrast for a minimally distinct border formed by juxtaposing a monochromatic field (IV) and a white one. The luminance (*L*) of Field I at the upper right is varied to form an upper border equally as distinct as the lower one. Contrast is defined as $(L_{max} - L_{min})/(L_{max} + L_{min})$ for the upper field pair. [From Kaiser, Herzberg, & Boynton (1971).]

border—just about at threshold for the small fields and low luminances that we were using—whereas the spectral "extremes" yielded borders with white that were very distinct indeed. Our first method for measuring border distinctness at MDB (Kaiser, Herzberg, & Boynton, 1971) was to set up a white field just above the border to be assessed (see Figure 16.1). After the MDB had been set below, a setting was made of the upper-right field above in order to produce an achromatic contrast yielding an upper border equally as distinct as the lower one (the chromatic border that had been formed by the monochromatic stimulus with white). Typical results are shown in Figure 16.2, where equivalent achromatic contrast is plotted as a function of the wavelength of the spectral color that had been juxtaposed with white.

The striking similarity between this function and saturation discrimination functions already in the literature was immediately noticed. Almost by definition, it seemed, the more saturated a color, the more it should differ from white. Apparently we had a handle on the problem that we had initially set out to solve.

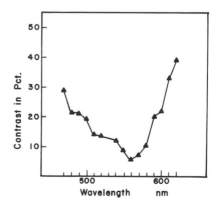

Figure 16.2. Equivalent achromatic contrast as a function of wavelength for monochromatic lights paired with white. [From Boynton (1973).]

IV. Additivity Tests and Spectral Sensitivity

So far, I have been concerned mainly with how distinct borders are when they are minimally distinct. As I indicated, this is only the second part of our experiment. What makes borders minimally distinct in the first place? To examine this, we tested to see what relative radiances were required to produce an MDB. G. Wagner, a German exchange fellow, helped me with this work. Kaiser and I had already done some additivity tests (Boynton & Kaiser, 1968) and, so far as we could tell, the MDB criterion yielded nearly perfect additivity. As an example of such a test, imagine a red field that is set to produce an MDB with white, and then a green field similarly adjusted. If the red and green fields are added together by optical superposition and then reduced by half (e.g., by inserting a 50%-transmittance neutral filter into the beam that supplies that side of the field), the mixture will still form an MDB with the white. Brightness is another story since in such a test the mixture field looks much dimmer than the white. This phenomenon has been observed by many investigators, and the general rule is that whenever there is a cancellation of hue, there is also a partial cancellation of brightness. But there is no cancellation at all for whatever it is that is responsible for the MDB.

Wagner did more additivity experiments and then extended work begun by Kaiser (1971) by doing careful measurements of spectral sensitivity (Wagner & Boynton, 1972). Figure 16.3 shows the results of some of the additivity tests, while Figure 16.4 shows spectral sensitivity as obtained by MDB and compared with Judd's corrected luminosity curve. We found that MDB and flicker photometry yield essentially equivalent results. Since the specification of equal luminance depends mainly upon the outcome of flicker photometry, it seems safe to suggest that the MDB setting is a valid method of luminance equation for an individual subject. For

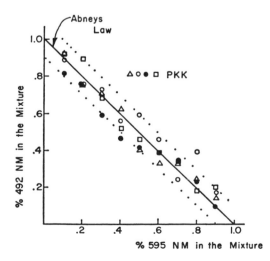

Figure 16.3. Additivity test. Percentage of relative luminance at 492 nm, in a mixture field, as a function of the percentage of relative luminance at 595 nm, with 100% (1.0) being based on minimum-border comparisons with a reference white when each component is used alone. The straight line is the predicted outcome if the additivity law obtains. Dotted lines indicate ±10%; the different symbols indicate data collected in separate sessions. [From Boynton & Kaiser (1968). Copyright 1968 by the American Association for the Advancement of Science.]

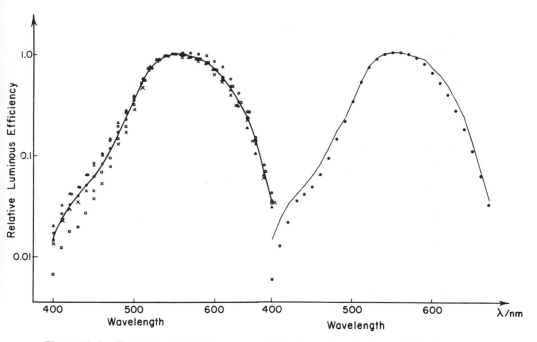

Figure 16.4. The points at the left represent data for four subjects, where relative luminance efficiency was obtained by minimum-border settings of monochromatic lights with white. The solid curve is the average curve for the four observers; it is reproduced at the right where the points represent Judd's modified V_λ function. [From Wagner & Boynton (1972).]

the remainder of this discussion, in using the expression *equal luminance,* I will refer to two fields that are equated by the MDB procedure.[2]

V. Theoretical Developments

By this time (1972), we were also involved in some heavy theorizing. Our idea was that there were five elements in the brain (RGBYW). They were presumed to exist as "interlaced mosaics" and they received their inputs from fairly restricted regions of the retina and visual field. Borders were assumed to form whenever the numbers of turned-on elements of the same kind differed for the two brain fields that received the projections from the juxtaposed fields of the visual world. The theory stated that MDB always occurred when the numbers of W (achromatic) elements

---

[2]It seems probable that brightness is signaled mostly by the achromatic channels that are concerned with luminance, but with an additional component attributable to the opponent color channels. This suggestion is made specifically by Boynton (1960, p. 943) and has been discussed extensively by S. Lee Guth and his colleagues. For example, Guth and Lodge (1973) incorporate this kind of thinking into an explicit model used to account for threshold data.

active in the two brain fields were equated. A simple formulation led to a method to calculate the equivalent achromatic contrast that can be sustained by any remaining differential activity of the four kinds of chromatic elements (RGBY) associated with the two parts of the field (Kaiser *et al.,* 1971).

VI. Equally Saturated, Psychologically Unique Fields

It was this kind of thinking that led T. Greenspon and me to do a study of "equally saturated, psychologically unique fields [Boynton & Greenspon, 1972]." A psychologically unique field, we thought, would have this property of uniqueness because of its ability to turn on only one of the four types of chromatic elements. At equal saturation, the four psychologically unique hues would then each stimulate the same number of elements. Because color space seems to be representable in two dimensions at constant luminance, we expected our results to show that the opponent hues, such as red and green, would produce borders $\sqrt{2}$ times as strong as adjacent ones, such as red and yellow. This would be so if the vectors representing the level of activity of brain elements of a particular type were related to one another so as to produce the requisite two-dimensional array of colors.

VII. Borders That Melt

The experiment just described produced very strange results, as shown in Figure 16.5. Two of the adjacent hue pairs, RB and GY, produced borders of about the

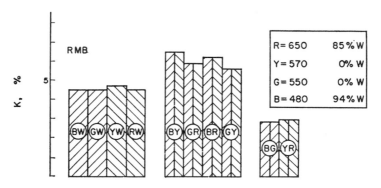

Figure 16.5. Equivalent achromatic contrast for equally saturated, psychologically unique red, yellow, green, and blue fields. Monochromatic lights were mixed with percentage of white (luminance units) as shown in the inset; when these were paired in turn with white, they produced equivalent borders at MDB, as shown by the four bars at the left. When the chromatic stimuli were paired with each other, the six possible pairs divided into two groups, four of which formed relatively distinct borders (middle set of bars), whereas the remaining two pairs tended to melt and produce very low equivalent contrasts (bars at the right). [From Boynton & Greenspon (1972).]

same strength as the opposite pairs. This was all wrong. Even worse, and much more mysterious, was the finding that the other two adjacent pairs, RY and BG, hardly produced any borders at all. One-half of the field seemed to "melt" into the other.

We had not seen these melting borders before, although our earlier comparisons of white with 570 nm had come very close to this phenomenon. But with small fields and dark surrounds, 570 nm looked very much like white, so the fact that a very poor border is sustained between them hardly seemed surprising. In these new observations, where colors were very different, the melting of the border at their junction was unexpected.

An important point here is that we defined "equal saturation" in terms of the MDB criterion. For example, for this author as observer, unique yellow at 570 nm produced an equivalent achromatic contrast of about 4.5% when juxtaposed with our reference white. To produce this same contrast with unique red, spectral red at 650 nm had to be mixed with more than five times as much white (in luminance units) in order to sufficiently desaturate it. At the time, this seemed to be an excellent operational basis for scaling saturation, which otherwise is a notoriously difficult sensory quality to judge. Moreover, in terms of the brain-element model that was guiding our work, it made specific sense to do it this way.

The melting border is difficult to describe. Liebmann had observed it long before; Koffka and Harrower worked on the problem and Koffka (1935) described the Leibmann effect in his textbook. He talks of "poor articulation," where different regions in space, though they obviously have different colors, nevertheless blend together at their junction so that there is no clear visible contour.

We had also been pursuing another approach toward achieving a two-dimensional arrangement of our colors. Boynton and Wagner (1972) reported the first of these studies; F. Ward, then a graduate student, subsequently worked with me as we extended our work in this area (Ward & Boynton, 1974).

VIII. Multidimensional Scaling of MDB Data

Psychological color diagrams and chromaticity diagrams both require a two-dimensional plane for the representation of color. Each, however, suffers from fundamental limitations. Psychological diagrams are of limited value because they have been arrived at by rather informal and qualitative procedures. If a person is given a large collection of colored chips of equal lightness and is asked to arrange them in some meaningful way, a likely outcome will be that white will be placed at the center and the most saturated colors will be positioned toward the outside, with hues arranged in their spectral order and purples completing the ring. Colors will retain their dominant hue, but with less saturation, as they are placed along a line connecting the most saturated color and white. Chromaticity diagrams suffer from the fact that the experimental operation upon which they are based (color matching) requires no judgment about color other than that of equality. The CIE diagram represents small color differences very unequally, and no linear transformation of it seems capable of representing MacAdam's ellipses as circles of the same size. Our method permitted the comparison of any two hues at equal luminance. It was our hope and expectation that the distinctness of the border that remained at equal luminance would correlate with, and indeed could be used as an index of the amount of color difference. From this, a comparison of many colors with one another would lead to distinctness values between all possible pairs of pairs that would be representable in a two-dimensional plane diagram.

In the first of these studies, Ward and I used 15 monochromatic stimuli plus white. The many permutations and combinations of these were examined in a randomized design, and the two half-matrices collapsed to give 120 experimental conditions. For each pair we had a measure of the equivalent achromatic contrast at MDB. To analyze the results we used a powerful multidimensional scaling procedure that had been previously developed by R. Shepard (1963) and J. B. Kruskal (1964). For a two-dimensional analysis a computer program attempts to arrange the stimuli of the experiment (16, in our case) in such a way that there is a good correlation—hopefully an optimal one—between distances between points in the diagram and the original estimates of the amount of difference between the stimuli.

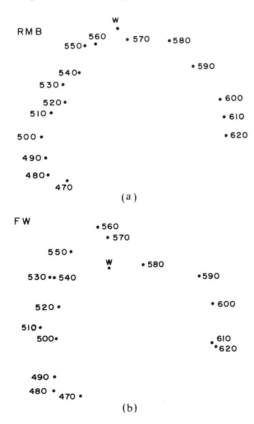

Figure 16.6. Fifteen monochromatic stimuli, plus white, were juxtaposed in all possible combinations and equivalent achromatic contrasts were determined at MDB. The distances on these diagrams correlate very well with the experimental values. [From Ward & Boynton (1974).]

In our case, equivalent achromatic contrast was the experimental measure. For the most part, the procedure seemed to work very well; our stimuli arranged themselves as we had expected along a horseshoe-shaped curve, as shown in Figure 16.6. There was one problem, however. The point representing our white stimulus did not plot where we had expected it to. For one subject, it fell just inside the spectral locus, near the yellow region of the spectrum, which was not too bad. But for the other subject, it fell slightly *outside* the spectral locus, and that made no sense to us at all. Ward and I also experimented with the use of distinctness ratings instead of distinctness matching. This gave very similar results and has been used to good advantage in subsequent experiments.

IX. Scaling of Nonspectral Colors

The next step was to fill in the center of the space by doing an experiment that utilized many nonspectral colors. B. Tansley, my last graduate student at Rochester, played a key role in this. He modified a colorimeter to provide fields by a mixture of filter primaries, using essentially the principle of the Riggs colorimeter. A light beam passing through each of three filters could be altered in its chromaticity by varying the spatial position of a slide in which the three filters were juxtaposed. Tansley followed me to San Diego where we soon did an experiment in which we compared 36 nonspectral colors in all possible combinations—and that is a lot of combinations (630).

The outcome of this experiment (Tansley & Boynton, 1976) startled us. The proper arrangement of points representing these stimuli turned out to be linear. There was no filling-in of the diagram. Each spectral point also represented many nonspectral colors. Figure 16.7 shows how these points arranged themselves in a two-dimensional configuration.

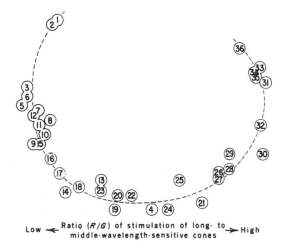

Figure 16.7. Thirty-six nonspectral stimuli were juxtaposed in all possible combinations and equivalent contrasts were determined at MDB. Distances between points on this diagram correlate .98 with experimental border distinctness ratings. The nonspectral stimuli did not plot, as expected, inside the curve defined by spectral stimuli. [From Tansley & Boynton (1976). Copyright 1976 by the American Association for the Advancement of Science.]

Low ← Ratio (*R/G*) of stimulation of long- to → High
middle-wavelength-sensitive cones

X. Insight: Tritanopic Purity

Insight came suddenly when Tansley was playing around with clusters of points that plotted nearly at the same place along one of our lines. What did these points have in common? When he plotted them on a chromaticity diagram they tended to fall along tritanopic confusion lines. A more direct experiment was devised, and we were able to confirm that any two stimuli falling along such a line fail to form a contour when juxtaposed at equal luminance, and that if any member of the set of stimuli that fall along such a line is substituted for any other member of that set, it will behave the same way in the MDB experiment (Figure 16.8).

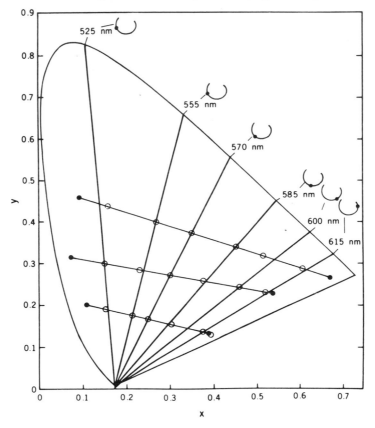

Figure 16.8. Monochromatic lights of the six wavelengths shown were matched with mixtures of three pairs of stimuli (shown as filled circles) under the subject's control. The subject adjusted the ratio of these primaries at constant luminance until an MDB was formed between the mixture and the monochromatic stimulus beside it. In most such cases the border disappeared entirely. The chromaticities of the mixture points are shown by the open circles. The experiment confirms that the border-forming properties of a nonspectral stimulus are equivalent to a monochromatic light whose wavelength can be determined by drawing a straight line from its intersection with the locus of spectral colors. [From Tansley & Boynton (1976). Copyright 1976 by the American Association for the Advancement of Science.]

When two stimuli fall along a tritan confusion line, this means that, although they stimulate the blue-sensitive cones differentially, they stimulate the red- and green-sensitive cones to exactly the same extent at constant luminance. In the spring of 1976 we were joined by a Norwegian physicist, A. Valberg, who went back through most of the data that we had previously collected. Tansley and Valberg (1977) developed the concept of "tranopic purity," this being a modification of a system of color specification that Valberg (1974) had already proposed. In common with many other models, his three-channel system featured a luminance quantity and two opponent-color vectors. His index of purity (saturation) was ordinarily obtained by comparing the activities of both red–green and yellow–blue opponent quantities, which he called "chromatic moments," to the luminance value. For the tritanope, lacking the blue cones, only the red–green discrimination remains. At constant luminance, only the ratio of red to green activity matters for determining saturation. If constant luminance implies, for different colors, that there is an equality of activity summed across red- and green-sensitive cones, then the distinctness of a border can be predicted simply by calculating the relative amount of red- (or green-) sensitive cone stimulation provided by any two fields being compared.

The key idea here is that we were right in our earlier suspicion that borders at MDB could reveal something about the relative saturation of the two fields being compared—but it is a very special kind of saturation, one that ignores the contributions of the blue-sensitive cones.

This concept led to the prediction of something that had not yet been observed, or observable. There are pairs of monochromatic lights, straddling 460 nm, which fall along tritanopic confusion lines. Therefore, it was predicted that such pairs should form melting borders with each other, and that either member of such a pair should behave in the same way when compared with some other color. By this time, with the help of D. MacLeod and M. Hayhoe, we had achieved a satisfactory MDB in Maxwellian view and, by using a high-intensity monochromator, Tansley and Valberg were able to explore these very short wavelengths which had never been available to us before. As Figure 16.9 shows, the prediction was confirmed (Valberg & Tansley, 1976).

Our new insight also led to another prediction. If the luminance channels are fed only by red- and green-sensitive cones, and if MDB equates luminance for both fields, then all borders should melt for dichromats. For the protanope, for example, if only the green-sensitive class of cones remains, the equation of luminance by MDB should cause an equal effectiveness for the two stimuli for this class of cones. The blue-sensitive cones will, in general, be differentially activated, but blue cones do not count for MDB. With the help of another graduate student, R. Glushko, Tansley (1976) tested this hypothesis and found it to be supported. By using monochromatic lights, the action spectrum of the remaining class of photoreceptors could be determined for protanopes and deuteranopes, and these values agreed well with estimates in the literature made by other methods.

One such method is the use of moderately high-frequency flicker, which the channels serving the blue-sensitive cones cannot follow well. The MDB method

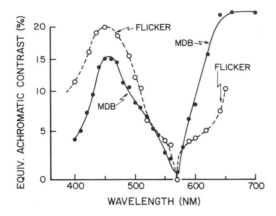

Figure 16.9. Equivalent achromatic contrasts determined by two methods. The solid curve drawn through the filled circles is for MDB [from Tansley (1976)]; the dotted curve drawn through the open circles is from research by Boynton and Kaiser (1978), where the wavelengths shown on the abscissa were alternated with 580 nm at relative luminances that produced minimum flicker.

mimics this procedure, and this is the explanation for the similarity of the results that the two methods produce.

XI. Reinterpretation of Flicker Work

As I mentioned at the outset, one of the methods that Kaiser and I tried had utilized flicker. The results for one of those experiments is also shown in Figure 16.9. Note the peak of the curve at 460 nm and that stimuli exist on each side of this wavelength that are equivalent in their ability to sustain the perception of flicker when paired with a long-wave standard. We had been able to do the flicker experiment in Maxwellian view, and it was for this reason that the shorter wavelengths were still available to us. We did not understand this complex result at all, and we were also bothered by certain pairs of lights that did not flicker well with each other. It turns out, of course, that these are pairs that are equivalent, or nearly so, for tritanopes. It seems that the melting border therefore has its counterpart in the temporal domain (Boynton & Kaiser, 1977).

XII. On the Physiological Basis of MDB

If human beings were all possessed of the vision of tritanopes, based only on two classes of cones with long-wave peak spectral sensitivity, then I would judge that the original aim of using MDB to scale color differences could have been accomplished. The physiological basis for the result is clearly evident in center-surround receptive field organization of a sort first observed by Wiesel and Hubel (1966). One of my former students, C. Ingling, together with a student of his, B. Drum, published a report demonstrating how this probably works (Ingling & Drum, 1973). Wiesel and Hubel found some units with red on-centers, others with green off-surrounds. They also found the counterparts of these, namely, units with green on-centers and others with red off-surrounds. But they found no double opponent units, for example, ones with both red on-centers and green off-surrounds. De-Valois (1973), Gouras (1974), and others have also emphasized that the role of the red–green opponent units in the formation of contour may be at least as important as their role in the mediation of hue perception.

The blue-sensitive cones, however, seem to be free of any serious spatial or temporal responsibilities in vision. This probably relates to their small numbers, especially in the central retina. Chromatic perception along the yellow–blue dimension seems to fill in and to be constrained by contours that are defined by the activity of the other two types of cone receptors. My current research is directed toward the study of discriminations that depend exclusively upon such blue-cone differences. As we now know, the MDB method is useless for these discriminations. Indeed, we find that the apparent difference between two such fields is somewhat enhanced if they are slightly separated since, if they are not, the fields tend to melt together and to become confused (Boynton, Hayhoe, & Mac-Leod, 1977).

XIII. Original Melting Borders Reinterpreted

I would like to conclude by pointing out the basis for the melting borders that Greenspon and I first observed. The saturation equivalence that we deliberately produced in that experiment, since it was based upon MDB, was precisely that component of saturation mediated only by red- and green-sensitive cones. We desaturated our hues so that the strength of the border that each provided, when compared with white, was made equal. Two of the stimuli (red and yellow) consequently produced the same activation of red- and green-sensitive cones—in other words, they fell along tritanopic confusion lines. Calculations confirm this observation. The other two stimuli (green and blue) fit the same description, but for a different ratio of red and green activation.

XIV. Summary

To summarize: One of the two major dimensions of color difference, based upon the ratio of red-to-green cone stimulation, is well characterized by the strength of the border that is maintained, at equal luminance, when any two stimuli are carefully juxtaposed. For central vision, the blue-sensitive cones have no role to play. Our failure to understand this led to theorizing that was unproductive except for the further experiments that were engendered by the effort. An extensive body of data resulted. All of these diverse results can now be accounted for simply by calculating the difference in tritanopic purity between the half-fields that were used. The other major dimension of color difference, which is dependent upon the relative activation of the blue-sensitive cones, must be dealt with by other methods.

REFERENCES

Bedford, R. E., & Wyszecki, G. Axial chromatic aberration of the human eye. *Journal of the Optical Society of America,* 1957, *47,* 564.

Boynton, R. M. Theory of color vision. *Journal of the Optical Society of America,* 1960, *50,* 929–944.

Boynton, R. M. Implications of the minimally distinct border. *Journal of the Optical Society of America,* 1973, *63,* 1037–1043.

Boynton, R. M., & Greenspon, T. S. The distinctness of borders formed between equally saturated, psychologically unique fields. *Vision Research,* 1972, *12,* 495–507.

Boynton, R. M., Hayhoe, M. M., & MacLeod, D. I. A. The gap effect: Chromatic and achromatic visual discrimination as affected by field separation. *Optic Acta,* 1977, *24,* 159–177.

Boynton, R. M., & Kaiser, P. K. Vision: The additivity law made to work for heterochromatic photometry with bipartite fields. *Science,* 1968, *161,* 366–368.

Boynton, R. M., & Kaiser, P. K. Temporal analog of the minimally distinct border. *Vision Research,* 1978, *18,* 111–113.

Boynton, R. M., & Wagner, H. G. Color differences assessed by the minimally-distinct border method. In J. J. Vos, L. F. C. Friele, & P. L. Walraven (Eds.), *Color metrics.* Soesterberg: International Color Association (AIC), 1972.

Burnham, R. W., Onley, J. W., & Witzel, R. F. Exploratory investigation of perceptual color scaling. *Journal of the Optical Society of America,* 1970, *60,* 1410–1420.

DeValois, R. L. Central mechanisms of color vision. In R. Jung (Ed.), *Handbook of sensory physiology* (Vol. 7). New York: Springer-Verlag, 1973.

Ekman, G. Dimensions of color vision. *Journal of Psychology,* 1954, *38,* 467–474.

Gouras, P. Opponent-colour cells in different layers of foveal striate cortex. *Journal of Physiology,* 1974, *238,* 583–602.

Guth, S. L., & Lodge, H. R. Heterochromatic additivity, foveal spectral sensitivity, and a new color model. *Vision Research,* 1973, *13,* 450–462.

Indow, T., & Uchizono, T. Multidimensional mapping of Munsell colors varying in hue and chroma. *Journal of Experimental Psychology,* 1960, *59,* 321–329.

Ingling, C. R., & Drum, B. A. Retinal receptive fields: Correlations between psychophysics and electrophysiology. *Vision Research,* 1973, *13,* 1151–1163.

Kaiser, P. K. Minimally distinct border as a preferred psychophysical criterion in visual heterochromatic photometry. *Journal of the Optical Society of America,* 1971, *61,* 966–971.

Kaiser, P. K., Herzberg, P. A., & Boynton, R. M. Chromatic border distinctness and its relation to saturation. *Vision Research,* 1971, *11,* 953–968.

Koffka, K. *Principles of Gestalt psychology.* New York: Harcourt Brace, 1935.

Kruskal, J. B. Multidimensional scaling: A numerical method. *Psychometrika,* 1964, *29,* 115–129.

MacAdam, D. L. Visual sensitivities to color differences in daylight. *Journal of the Optical Society of America,* 1942, *32,* 247–274.

Shepard, R. N. The analysis of proximities: Multidimensional scaling with an unknown distance function. *Psychometrika,* 1963, *27,* 125–139; 219–246.

Tansley, B. W. Psychophysical studies of the contribution of chromatic mechanisms to the visual perception of borders. Doctoral dissertation, University of Rochester, 1976.

Tansley, B. W., & Boynton, R. M. A line, not a space, represents visual distinctness of borders formed by different colors. *Science,* 1976, *191,* 954–957.

Tansley, B. W., & Valberg, A. Chromatic border distinctness: Not an index of trichromatic hue or saturation differences. *Journal of the Optical Society of America,* 1977, *67,* 1330–1335.

Valberg, A. Color induction: Dependence on luminance, purity, and dominant or complementary wavelength of inducing stimuli. *Journal of the Optical Society of America,* 1974, *64,* 1531–1540.

Wagner, G., & Boynton, R. M. Comparison of four methods of heterochromatic photometry. *Journal of the Optical Society of America,* 1972, *62,* 1508–1515.

Ward, F., & Boynton, R. M. Scaling of large chromatic differences. *Vision Research,* 1974, *14,* 943–949.

Wiesel, T. N., & Hubel, D. H. Spatial and chromatic interactions in the lateral geniculate body of the rhesus monkey. *Journal of Neurophysiology,* 1966, *29,* 1115–1156.

17. Increment Thresholds: Sensitization Produced by Hue Differences[1]

C. E. Sternheim, C. F. Stromeyer III, and L. Spillmann

I. Introduction

Stiles (1939, 1953, pp. 65–103) developed the two-color threshold technique to study the basic mechanisms of color vision. Enoch (1972, pp. 537–567) has recently summarized the assumptions underlying this technique and the properties of the derived mechanisms or π functions. Enoch (1972) concludes, "... the π functions most probably represent a relatively stable, early, reproducible stage in the biological processing of color vision 'data' [p. 564]." Although variation of the color of the small test spot and larger adapting field is inherent to the technique, the observer usually pays little attention to color appearance.[2] Rather, the observer looks for any change in the center of the field as the spot is flashed and intensity is adjusted to a threshold level. Detection may be based, at least, upon differences in brightness or hue between the test spot and adapting field, but it is difficult under these conditions to identify which cues are operating.[3]

In the present experiments spatial gratings or flickering lights were superposed as test increments upon one or more chromatic adapting fields. Hue differences domi-

[1]This work was supported by the German Research Council (SFB 70, Teilprojekt A_6), and partially supported by National Institutes of Health Grant 1 Ro1 EY01808-01 awarded to R. E. Kronauer and C. F. Stromeyer III. C. F. Stromeyer III thanks the Alexander von Humboldt Foundation, and C. E. Sternheim gratefully acknowledges the Alexander von Humboldt Foundation and the National Institutes of Health (EY00539-05) for their support during a sabbatical leave in Freiburg.

[2]In an experiment, King-Smith (1975) distinguished between simple detection and detection of hue and found that the spectral sensitivity function often differed for the two tasks. And this difference was strongly affected by overall field intensity and the size and duration of the test spot.

[3]Hurvich (1963) has argued that in the increment threshold situation, "... difference judgments are involved that depend on the surround-test wavelength combinations used and the basis on which the difference judgment rests may be brightness, saturation, or hue, or complex combinations of all three [p. 200]."

209

nated at low spatial or temporal frequencies while brightness differences prevailed at high frequencies. Adding light to the background sometimes increased hue differences in low-frequency patterns and made these patterns more visible. The degree of sensitization obtained with red patterns was greater than that obtained with green patterns. We also found differences in the shape of the field sensitivity functions that were generated when the red test gratings were varied in spatial frequency.

Stiles (1939, 1953) originally assumed that independent π mechanisms obey displacement rules that determine the position of a standard threshold versus radiance curve (tvr) depending upon the wavelengths of the test field (λ) and background field (μ). The notion of independence was questioned after interactions between mechanisms were revealed in experiments with mixtures of lights in test or background fields (Boynton, Das, & Gardiner, 1966; Boynton & Das, 1966; Boynton, Ikeda, & Stiles, 1964; Ikeda, Uetsuki, & Stiles, 1970). Our data also reveal interactions between mechanisms. The tvr curves obtained with red test patterns of low spatial frequency differed from the standard shape in that they first descended before ascending. This sensitization effect, produced by hue differences, suggests that opponent interactions are involved in the detection process.

II. Method

A. *Apparatus*

Laser-generated red and green gratings were presented on homogeneous colored fields. A diagram of the optical apparatus is shown at the top of Figure 17.1 above a spatial profile of the stimulus. A neon–helium laser (632.8 nm) and argon laser (514.5 nm) were used to produce vertical sine-wave gratings. [The helium–cadmium (441.5 nm) laser and mirror M_5 were not used in the present experiments.] Mirrors M_3 and M_4 direct light from the argon laser into a Mach–Zehnder interferometer (Françon, 1966) consisting of mirrors M_1 and M_2 and beamsplitters BS_4 and BS_5. By removing mirror M_4, light from the neon–helium laser is allowed to pass in its place. The interferometer splits the laser beam so that two beams enter the eye at different angles (controlled by micrometer adjustments of M_1). The eyepiece forms two small source images near the nodal point of the eye that produce by interference a sine-wave grating on the retina. Spatial frequency is controlled by micrometer adjustments of M_1. The contrast of such a grating is essentially unaffected by the focus of the eye or by diffraction at the pupil.

The other sources, S_1 and S_2 (quartz iodine bulbs) and S_3 (regular tungsten bulb), formed images between the laser source images near the nodal point of the eye. Interference filters were used to control the spectral nature of the adapting fields provided by these channels. A common field stop (FS) in the eyepiece determined the visual angle of all fields, usually 4°. Neutral density filters and wedges were

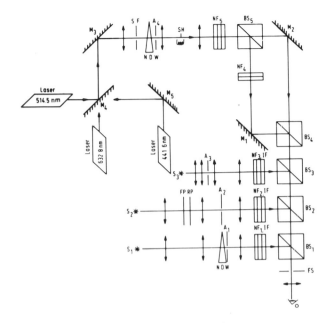

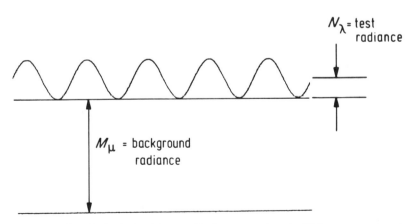

Figure 17.1. Top: Optical stimulator used in these experiments. Flicker was produced, when required, by placing a fixed and rotating polarizer in the channel supplied by source S_1. Bottom: Spatial profile of test grating superposed upon a single adapting field. [From Stromeyer, Kranda, & Sternheim (1978).]

used to attentuate the beams. The optical apparatus and calibration procedures are described in more detail elsewhere (Stromeyer, Kranda, & Sternheim, 1978).

This apparatus, with the addition of another channel, was also used to provide a red or green unity-modulated flickering light superposed upon fields of various colors. (The lasers were not used in these experiments.) Sinusoidal flicker was produced with a fixed and rotating polarizer in the channel containing source S_1. Interference filters and neutral density filters controlled the wavelength and radiance, respectively.

B. Procedure

Two of the authors who have normal vision served as observers in these experiments. The results of CES are presented here. The results of CFS agreed with those shown in all important aspects.

The observer was usually required to adjust the test radiance until the test pattern was just visible, after having become fully adapted to the background field. When thresholds were high, the test pattern itself might be expected to contribute significantly to the adaptation level. However, the estimated size of this effect was typically negligible (Stromeyer *et al.*, 1978, Appendix).

The field sensitivity of π_4 and π_5 was determined by first having the observer adjust the appropriate test pattern to threshold in the presence of one or more primary adapting fields. The wavelengths of these fields were chosen in an attempt to depress selectively the sensitivity of mechanisms other than that under study. Following the initial determination, the test pattern was made clearly visible by setting it to a multiple of the threshold value. Another background was then added and the observer adjusted its radiance to again reduce the test pattern to threshold. The wavelength of this background was varied through the spectrum from red to violet and back to red, or vice versa. For each wavelength the observer adapted to the field for a considerable time, and then made careful adjustments while avoiding large changes. Six settings were made, three going from one spectral end to the other and three upon return.

III. Results

A. Facilitation Effect Obtained with Spatial Gratings

A test grating generated with the 632.8-nm laser was presented on a primary field ($\mu_1 = 615$ nm) of approximately 5000 td. Threshold was measured, and then a secondary field ($\mu_2 = 565$ nm) was added. Threshold was again determined following adaptation to the mixed field. Data points in Figure 17.2 are based upon 10 determinations, 5 obtained when the level of μ_2 added to μ_1 was increased in successive steps and 5 obtained when the level of μ_2 was decreased in succesive steps. As can be seen the threshold of a 1 cd deg^{-1} grating is lowest at intermediate

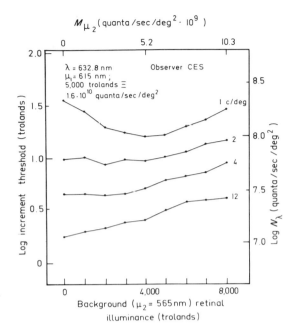

Figure 17.2. Threshold versus radiance curves for 632.8-nm test grating at different spatial frequencies. Field μ_2 (565 nm) is added to a fixed amount of field μ_1 (615 nm). Top curve is in actual position; lower curves are displaced downward by successive .3 log-unit intervals.

levels of μ_2. The slope of the thresholds versus radiance curves (tvr) thus dips at 1 cd deg^{-1}; at 2 and 4 cd deg^{-1} the tvr curves are shallow compared to that obtained at 12 cd deg^{-1}.

The color of the background changed from yellow–red through yellow to yellow–green as more μ_2 was added. A low spatial-frequency grating was seen on the yellow (mixed) field as an alternation of red and "muddy" green stripes. A high spatial-frequency grating was seen as an alternation of bright and dark red stripes.

The facilitation effect obtained at 1 cd deg^{-1} was confirmed for observer CFS using a signal detection procedure. The d' value for a fixed test level was significantly higher for a mixed field, μ_1 (5000 td) + μ_2 (5000 td), than for a single μ_1 (5000 td) by itself.

The results of a similar experiment using the 514.5 test grating are shown in Figure 17.3. In this case μ_1 (529 nm) appeared green. As more μ_2 (620 nm) was added the mixed field looked yellow and then reddish yellow. Hue differences between striations were much less noticeable with the green gratings. A facilitation effect at 1 cd deg^{-1} was not observed; however, the threshold was not significantly elevated as more μ_2 was added. As before, the slope of the tvr curve increased slightly as spatial frequency increased.

B. Facilitation Effect Obtained with Sinusoidal Flicker

A slowly flickering red light ($\lambda = 620$ nm) was more visible on a mixed field that looked yellow (μ_1, 615 nm, + μ_2, 548 nm) than upon a single component of that

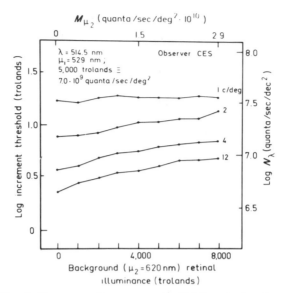

Figure 17.3. Threshold versus radiance curves for 514.5-nm test grating at different spatial frequencies. Field μ_2 (620 nm) is added to a fixed amount of field μ_1 (529 nm). Top curve is in actual position; lower curves are displaced downward by successive .3 log-unit intervals.

field (μ_1) that looked red. Thresholds were lower on the mixed field when flicker was below 4 Hz (Figure 17.4, left). Strong hue shifts were seen at these low frequencies. At higher frequencies hue shifts were absent and adding μ_2 slightly raised the threshold.

The facilitation effect for a slowly flickering green light was smaller in degree than for red light (Figure 17.4, right) and occurred only at frequencies below 2 Hz. This difference was even more marked for observer CFS (not shown here). Adding μ_2 to μ_1 slightly raised the threshold for high-frequency green flicker for both observers.

C. Field Sensitivity Obtained with Spatial Gratings or Sinusoidal Flicker

The field sensitivity of π_5 was determined with the 632.8-nm test grating presented on a 507-nm primary field of 986 td. The grating was set to 1.75 or 2.5 times its threshold value, and the radiance of a secondary field of variable wavelength was adjusted to make the grating just visible. Spectral sensitivity curves based upon the reciprocal of the radiance of the variable field for gratings of 12 and 20 cd deg^{-1} were similar. Average data obtained at these frequencies are presented in Figure 17.5 (right, circles) on a wave number scale corrected for macular and lens pigment (Wyszecki & Stiles, 1967, p. 219). The curves are the scotopic visibility function (V_λ') corrected for lens absorption (Wyszecki & Stiles, 1967, p. 584) and displaced parallel to the ordinate and abscissa.

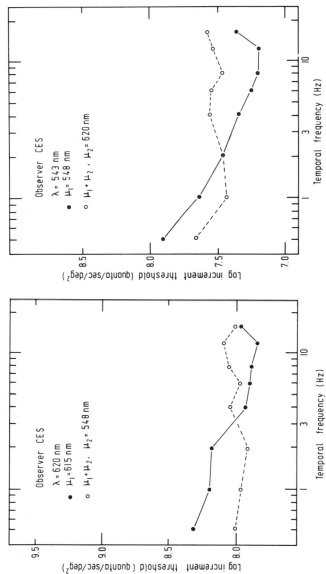

Figure 17.4. Left: Increment thresholds for a 620-nm test stimulus at different flicker frequencies upon a single adapting field (615 nm, filled circles) or a mixed adapting field (615 nm + 548 nm, open circles). Right: Increment thresholds for a 543-nm test stimulus at different flicker frequencies upon a single adapting field (548 nm, filled circles) or a mixed adapting field (548 nm + 620 nm, open circles). All fields were ~2000 td. The radiances of fields of 548, 615, and 620 nm were, respectively, 2.5×10^9, 6.3×10^9, and 7.4×10^9 quanta sec^{-1} deg^{-2}.

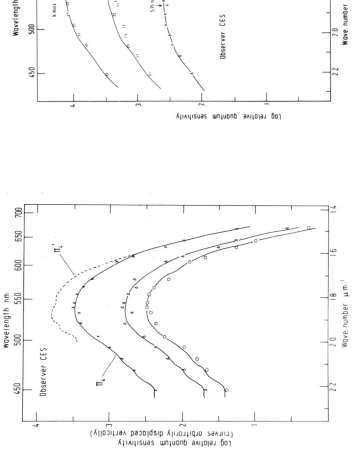

Figure 17.5. Left: Spectral field sensitivity obtained with a 514.5-nm grating superposed upon two fixed fields (689 nm and 452 nm) and one of variable wavelength and radiance. Circles, 2 cd deg⁻¹; triangles, 20 cd deg⁻¹; crosses, geometric mean of all data collected at this test wavelength. The curves for π_4 and π'_4 are based on the values tabulated by Wyszecki and Stiles (1967). Right: Spectral field sensitivity (corrected for preretinal absorption). Circles (12 and 20 cd deg⁻¹) and squares (2 cd deg⁻¹) 632.8-nm grating superposed upon a fixed 507-nm primary background and a secondary background of variable wavelength and radiance. Triangles, geometric mean of all data collected with 514.5-nm grating under conditions described for left side of figure. Curves are displaced V'_λ function corrected for lens absorption. Peak wavelengths for these curves are shown.

Field sensitivity was determined in an identical manner with a 2 cd deg^{-1} 632.8-nm grating (Figure 17.5, right, squares). There is a systematic loss of sensitivity in the middle of the spectrum compared to the displaced V'_λ function.

Field sensitivity for π_4 was determined with the 514.4-nm grating presented upon fields of 689 nm of 920 td plus 452 nm of 50 td. The grating was set at 1.75 times its threshold value and the radiance of a third field of variable wavelength was adjusted to reduce the grating to threshold. The shapes of the functions obtained with low (2 cd deg^{-1}) and high (20 cd deg^{-1}) spatial frequencies were similar (Figure 17.5, left, circles and triangles, respectively). The geometric means of all these data (Figure 17.5, left, crosses) closely fit the π_4 function given by Wyszecki and Stiles (1967). These field sensitivity data, converted to a retinal basis, fit the corrected and displaced V'_λ function (Figure 17.5, right, triangles).

The same fields were used to determine field sensitivity using 12-Hz sinusoidal flicker. This value was chosen since it was above the frequency range where

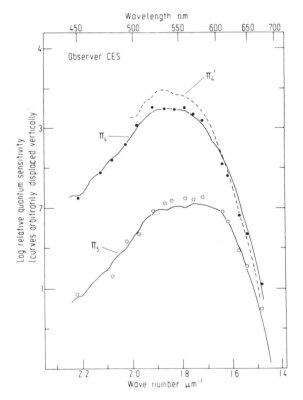

Figure 17.6. Spectral field sensitivity at 12-Hz temporal modulation. Open circles, 643-nm test upon a fixed 507-nm primary field and a secondary field of variable wavelength and radiance. Closed circles, 543-nm test upon two fixed fields (689 nm and 452 nm) and one of variable wavelength and radiance. Curves for π_4, π'_4, and π_5 are based upon values tabulated by Wyszecki and Stiles (1967).

sensitization had occurred (Figure 17.4). Test wavelengths of 643 nm and 543 nm were used to study π_5 and π_4, respectively. Figure 17.6 shows field sensitivity data in comparison to the spectral functions derived by Stiles (Wyszecki & Stiles, 1967). The data obtained with 543-nm test flicker (filled circles) match the π_4 function, whereas those obtained with the 643-nm test flicker (open circles) differ slightly from the relatively flat π_5 function.

IV. Discussion

Hue differences may serve as the basis for detection of low-frequency spatial or temporal patterns. A red grating with wide bars or a slowly flickering red light presented upon a yellow field appears as a spatially or temporally alternating red–green pattern. Hue differences were smaller for green test patterns. The sensitization effect suggests that the mechanism for detecting low-frequency patterns enhances hue differences through color opponency. Sensitization to the test pattern occurred when the yellow adapting field was a mixture of red and green, even though the combined yellow field had considerably more radiance than either of the two components. A red–green differencing mechanism adapted to a neutral yellow light may perhaps respond more vigorously to a red or green pattern than it would if adapted to a red or green light. Other investigators have also found evidence for color opponency when the test stimuli were large or of long duration (e.g., Ikeda, 1963; King-Smith, 1975; Sperling & Harwerth, 1971; Stiles & Crawford, 1933). Our high-frequency patterns were seen as a variation in brightness, and sensitization did not occur at these frequencies.

Estévez and Cavonius (1975) suggest that with the "spectral compensation method" sensitivity to temporal frequencies below 10 Hz is maintained by hue shifts. This method requires antiphase temporal modulation of lights of different spectral composition. The ratio of the intensity of the two lights is adjusted so that one class of cones is not modulated. We observed sensitization effects produced by hue differences with a uniform field that was sinusodially modulated below 4 Hz. Sensitization was greater with red than with green flicker. This may account for Green's (1969) finding of a less pronounced low-frequency falloff in sensitivity for the red mechanism compared to the green mechanism.

Stiles (1953) showed that the shape of the π_4 field sensitivity function, corrected for preretinal absorption, agreed fairly well with the shape of the similarly corrected scotopic sensitivity curve, V'_λ. The field sensitivity for green gratings (Figure 17.5) also closely matches the π_4 field sensitivity and the displaced, corrected V'_λ function. Extensive microspectrophotometric measurements of photopigments in individual cones of rhesus monkey (Bowmaker, Dartnall, Lythgoe, & Mollon, 1978) show that the "green" cones peak at about 536 nm and have spectral sensitivities closely matching the π_4 field sensitivity and Dartnall nomogram—the latter matches the displaced, corrected V'_λ function.

In the right panel of Figure 17.5 the field sensitivity for high-frequency red gratings was fitted with the displaced, corrected V'_λ function. Measurements by Bow-maker *et al.* (1978) show that the "red" cones peak at about 565 nm and have spectral sensitivities narrower than the Dartnall nomogram or the displaced V'_λ function. There is also a tendency for our data for high-frequency red gratings (Figure 17.5, circles) to be narrower than the displaced V'_λ function. If the V'_λ function was displaced rightward in Figure 17.5 to peak at 565 nm (like the "red" cones) the long-wavelength data points would definitely descend more steeply than the V'_λ function and be narrower than the Dartnall nomogram.

Field sensitivity for low-frequency red gratings differed slightly from the field sensitivity for high-frequency red gratings (Figure 17.5, right, squares and circles). In the middle of the spectrum, more background energy was required to elevate the threshold of low-frequency versus high-frequency red gratings. This difference may result from sensitization produced by hue differences when the low-frequency red grating is presented upon backgrounds that contain yellow.

Field sensitivity data obtained using red light flickering at a high frequency (Figure 17.6, open circles) differed slightly from the π_5 field sensitivity function. The π_5 mechanism may be better isolated under conditions of selective adaptation when high-frequency spatial or temporal patterns are used and hue differences are less likely. The spectral function of π_4 had a similar shape regardless of frequency. This is consistent with our finding of smaller hue differences produced by green test patterns at low frequencies.

ACKNOWLEDGMENTS

We are indebted to M. Hanser, B. Maier, and L. Thanner for help in constructing the apparatus. Thanks are extended to the Botany and Physics Departments of the University of Freiburg for loan of equipment. Professor R. Jung's interest in this work is gratefully acknowledged.

REFERENCES

Bowmaker, J. K., Dartnall, H. J. A., Lythgoe, N. N., & Mollon, J. D. The visual pigments of rods and cones in the rhesus monkey, *Macaca mulatta*. *Journal of Physiology,* 1978, *274,* 329–348.

Boynton, R. M., & Das, S. R. Visual adaptation: Increased efficiency resulting from spectrally distributed mixtures of stimuli. *Science,* 1966, *154,* 1581–1583.

Boynton, R. M., Das, S. R., & Gardiner, J. Interactions between photopic visual mechanisms revealed by mixing conditoning fields. *Journal of the Optical Society of America,* 1966, *56,* 1775–1780.

Boynton, R. M., Ikeda, M., & Stiles, W. S. Interactions among chromatic mechanisms as inferred from positive and negative increment thresholds. *Vision Research,* 1964, *4,* 87–117.

Enoch, J. M. The two-color threshold technique of Stiles and derived component color mechanisms. In D. Jameson & L. Hurvich, (Eds.), *Handbook of sensory physiology* (Vol. VIII/4): *Visual psychophysics.* Berlin: Springer-Verlag, 1972.

Estévez, O., & Cavonius, C. R. Flicker sensitivity of the human red and green color mechanisms. *Vision Research,* 1975, *15,* 879–881.

Françon, M. *Optical interferometry.* New York: Academic Press, 1966.

Green, D. G. Sinusoidal flicker characteristics of the color-sensitive mechanisms of the eye. *Vision Research,* 1969, *9,* 591–601.

Hurvich, L. M. Contributions to color-discrimination theory: Review, summary, and discussion. *Journal of the Optical Society of America,* 1963, *53,* 196–201.

Ikeda, M. Study of interrelations between mechanisms at threshold. *Journal of the Optical Society of America,* 1953, *63,* 1305–1313.

Ikeda, M., Uetsuki, T., & Stiles, W. S. Interrelations among Stiles π mechanisms. *Journal of the Optical Society of America,* 1970, *60,* 406–415.

King-Smith, P. E. Visual detection analysed in terms of luminance and chromatic signals. *Nature,* 1975, *255,* 69–70.

Sperling, H. G., & Harwerth, R. S. Red-green cone interactions in the increment-threshold spectral sensitivity of primates. *Science,* 1971, *172,* 180–184.

Stiles, W. S. The directional sensitivity of the retina and the spectral sensitivities of the rods and cones. *Proceedings of the Royal Society of London, Ser. B,* 1939, *127,* 64–105.

Stiles, W. S. Further studies of visual mechanisms by the two-colour threshold method. In *Colloquio sobre problemas opticos de la vision* (Vol. 1). Madrid: Union Internationale de Physique pure et appliequée, 1953.

Stiles, W. S., & Crawford, B. H. The liminal brightness increment as a function of wave-length for different conditions of the foveal and parafoveal retina. *Proceedings of the Royal Society of London, Ser. B,* 1933, *113,* 496–530.

Stromeyer, C. F., III, Kranda, K., & Sternheim, C. E. Selective chromatic adaptation at different spatial frequencies. *Vision Research,* 1978 (in press).

Wyszecki, G., & Stiles, W. S. *Color science: Concepts and methods, quantitative data and formulas.* New York: Wiley, 1967.

18. π-Mechanisms and Cone Fundamentals

C. R. Cavonius and O. Estévez

I. Introduction

Human color vision is demonstrably trichromatic. The implication that color vision is mediated by three mechanisms that differ in their sensitivity to energy from different regions of the spectrum was appreciated two centuries ago and was given a firm analytical foundation in the mid-nineteenth century. Since then a great deal of sound psychophysical data have been accumulated that describe the behavior of the visual system. How then have the mechanisms so successfully hidden their identities? In large measure the answer is that these data do not allow the specification of a unique set of fundamental mechanisms, since much of the data—for example, those obtained in color-matching experiments—can be accounted for by an endless series of combinations of putative fundamentals. In the 1930s, for example, Hecht proposed a system in which the three fundamentals had nearly identical spectral sensitivity functions. Although subsequent results—for example, measurements of the absorption spectra of cones—effectively rule out such a model, it was successful in accounting for a great deal of psychophysical data.

However, measurements of the spectral sensitivities of the fundamental color mechanisms are possible, and the basic method for doing these experiments—the two-color threshold method of Stiles—has been available for almost 40 years, although it has only recently received the attention that it merits. This neglect appears in part to have been due to the inaccessibility of many of the original publications; this has now been remedied by a republication of the major papers in this series, with additional comments by W.S. Stiles (Stiles, 1978). Further, although the technique is basically simple, it often appears formidable to the reader, in part because Stiles modified his method as the experiments proceeded: He initially measured an observer's sensitivity to a test flash of variable wavelength and luminance, presented on a background of fixed wavelength, but later adopted the

221

method of keeping the wavelength of the test flash fixed, while measuring the observer's sensitivity to test flashes of fixed wavelength on a background of variable wavelength and radiance. Finally, the value of Stiles' method has been questioned because it requires that the mechanisms respond independently, so that the sensitivity of each depends only upon stimulation of that mechanism and is independent of activity in the other mechanisms. This clearly is not true under all conditions (e.g., Mollon & Polden, 1977; Pugh, 1976), but probably holds to a useful approximation if these special situations are avoided.

A more serious criticism of the validity of the π-mechanisms (which is Stiles' neutral term for the processes whose spectral sensitivities are measured with the two-color threshold technique) is that they do not explain other data about color vision. The best-known example of this was Stiles' attempt to describe color-matching data by means of linear transforms of the spectral sensitivities of π-mechanisms (Stiles, 1953). Stiles did not consider the fit to be satisfactory, and concluded that an observer whose color vision was based on π-mechanisms would not be classified as a normal observer. However, the sensitivities of the π-mechanisms were not measured in the same group of observers as those who took part in the color-matching experiments. If individual differences exist among observers, it may not be wise to compare the color-matching behavior of one group of observers to the sensitivities of π-mechanisms of different observers, since small differences in the fundamentals can have a large effect when transformed to chromaticity coordinates. To investigate this possibility, we made repeated measurements of π-mechanisms in two observers (the authors) and compared their predicted and observed color-matching data. Some of these results have been presented elsewhere (Estévez & Cavonius, 1977); we now wish to extend the analysis of the data, and also to investigate the possibility of predicting hue-discrimination performance from π-mechanisms.

II. Measurement of π-Mechanisms

The original determination of π-mechanisms by Stiles was necessarily a complex procedure, since he assumed nothing about the shapes of their spectral sensitivity functions. However, once the approximate shapes of these sensitivity functions are known, their measurement in other observers can be simplified by selecting a stimulus of a wavelength to which one mechanism is relatively more sensitive than the other mechanisms, and which has a spatial contrast that can be detected by that mechanism. The spectral sensitivity of the mechanism is then measured by adding a homogeneous, monochromatic field to the stimulus and determining the radiance that is needed at each wavelength of this field to just reduce the stimulus contrast to threshold. On the basis of Stiles' data, we selected stimuli for the short-, middle-, and long-wavelength mechanisms that had maxima at about 440, 535, and >610 nm, respectively. In selecting the stimulus contrast, we found by trial that a 2.5° field filled with 1° squares, in which adjacent squares differed in contrast by 6%

(when only the stimulus, and not the monochromatic field, was present), was an effective stimulus for the middle- and long-wavelength mechanisms, whereas the same pattern, with twice the contrast, was effective for the short-wavelength mechanism. To prevent the pattern from fading, we modulated it at 1 Hz, that is, the contrast of neighboring squares was interchanged at this rate.

When measuring the sensitivity of the short-wavelength mechanism, a steady conditioning field of dominant wavelength 570 nm was added to the stimulus. This light is an effective stimulus to the middle- and long-wavelength mechanisms and should therefore reduce the contrast of the stimulus to these mechanisms, while having virtually no effect on the contrast presented to the short-wavelength mechanism. Similarly, while measuring the middle- and long-wavelength mechanisms, the contrast to the unwanted mechanism was reduced by steady fields that had dominant wavelengths of 628 and 535 nm, respectively. (It was not necessary to suppress the short-wavelength mechanism during these measurements, since its sensitivity to the stimuli was very slight.)

The spectral sensitivities of the mechanisms that were detected by these stimuli were then measured by adding steady monochromatic light to the stimuli until they were brought to threshold, thus establishing the sensitivity of the mechanism to these monochromatic fields. This is a modification of the field-sensitivity (or more accurately, field radiance versus field wavelength) method of Stiles. The advantage of this method, as opposed to those in which spectral sensitivity is measured by varying the wavelength of the stimulus, is that because the stimulus has been selected to activate selectively the mechanism that is being measured, and because an additional conditioning field has been added to suppress the other mechanisms, it is unlikely that other mechanisms will detect it, regardless of the wavelength of the monochromatic field. If, however, the stimulus wavelength were varied, there would inevitably be wavelengths that would be detected by other mechanisms, so that it would be impossible to measure the sensitivity of the desired mechanism.

The spectral sensitivities of both observers' middle-wavelength mechanism (the middle curve in Figure 18.1) generally resemble Stiles' π_4 sensitivity function at wavelengths longer than 520 nm. However, below 520 nm the sensitivities of observer DC consistently fall above those of observer OE and of π_4. We do not believe that this means that the two observers have different fundamental mechanisms, but rather that their foveas differ in the density of macular pigment, since the difference between the observers' sensitivities (shown in the inset of Figure 18.1) resembles the absorption spectrum of macular pigment. If the data for DC are corrected by this amount of macular pigment, his spectral sensitivity, as well as that of OE, resembles π_4.

The agreement between our long-wavelength mechanisms and Stiles' π_5 is less satisfactory. At wavelengths above 520 nm, our data resemble π_5, whereas at shorter wavelengths both sets of data deviate from π_5. If we again correct the data of DC for macular pigment, the two observers' data come to a common line, which between 450 and 520 nm is concave downward as compared to Stiles' measurements of π_5. The maximum difference between our functions and π_5 is only

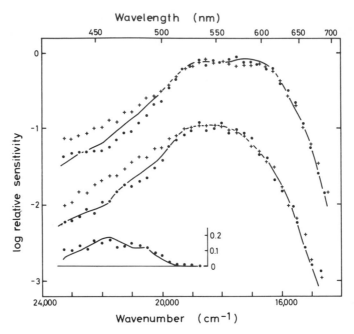

Figure 18.1. Upper data: Spectral sensitivity of two observers' (●, OE; +, DC) long-wavelength mechanisms (symbols), and Stiles' π_5 mechanism (line) displaced vertically to have the same maximum as our functions. Lower data: Same observers' middle-wavelength mechanisms and Stiles' π_4 mechanism. The middle-wavelength functions have been shifted downward by 1 log unit for clarity. Inset: Mean difference between the two observers' sensitivities (symbols), compared with the absorption spectrum of macular pigment (Wyszecki & Stiles, 1967, p. 219), given a maximum density of .2 at 458 nm.

about .1 log unit, but it shows up so regularly in our data that we do not believe that it represents random error. This difference between Stiles' data and ours means that whereas the short-wavelength branches of Stiles' π_4 and π_5 sensitivity functions follow nearly parallel courses, the short-wavelength branches of our π_5 functions are slightly concave relative to our π_4 functions, or to Stiles' π_4 or π_5 functions.

The spectral sensitivity of both observers' short-wavelength mechanism (Figure 18.2) can be adequately described by either π_1 or π_3. Since we have no way of comparing the absolute sensitivities of our mechanisms with those of Stiles, we can only compare the shapes of the π_1 and π_3 sensitivity functions. These shapes differ substantially only at wavelengths longer than 500 nm. In this region, our data tend to resemble π_1. However, we are not inclined to have too much confidence in the data in this region of the spectrum, as the monochromatic adapting fields that were needed to bring the stimulus to threshold were so bright that both observers doubted the validity of their thresholds. Thus, the question of whether we are dealing with π_1 or π_3 must remain open at present.

Unlike the other mechanisms, there is no evidence here for differential macular

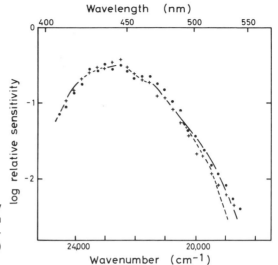

Figure 18.2. Spectral sensitivity of the short-wavelength mechanism of two observers (●, OE; +, DC) compared with Stiles' π_1 (—) and π_3 (--) mechanisms.

pigmentation in the two observers. The most plausible explanation for this (and one which is supported by the observers' impression of the way in which they made their judgments) is that they attended to more peripheral regions of the field when observing the short-wavelength stimulus, and to foveal regions, where the density of macular pigment is usually greater, when observing the medium- and long-wavelength stimuli.

III. Color Matching

Color matches were made using as primaries three light sources that resembled illuminant C, filtered by Wratten filters 47B, 29, and 61. Because the only method that we had for presenting two adjacent fields with a clean border was a Lummer–Brodhun cube, we placed the output of a monochromator, which was desaturated by one of the primaries, in the surround, and mixtures of the other two primaries in the central ellipse. Matches were made by the observers while they fixated a border of the ellipse, so that the stimulus was effectively a bipartite field. The experimenter set various ratios of the primaries in the surround, which the observer matched by adjusting the wavelength and radiance of the monochromatic beam and the radiance of the desaturating field. In this way, exact matches could be made with monochromator settings from 445 to 525 nm and from 538 to 628 nm. (The 13-nm gap represents the spectral region for which no desaturating light was available.)

During the course of these experiments, an effect was noted that supported our belief that the two observers differed in the density of macular pigmentation: They consistently used different wavelengths to match mixtures of the blue and green primaries. However, when observer OE (who presumably has more macular pigmentation) used his parafoveal retina, he accepted the matches made by observer DC.

The results of these color matches, transformed to chromaticity coordinates, are shown in Figures 18.3 and 18.4. Because we used broad-band primaries, as Guild did (cited in Wyszecki & Stiles, 1967, p. 264), our data tend to resemble his, rather than the color-matching functions of Wright (1946). Figures 18.3 and 18.4 also show linear transforms of the observers' π-mechanisms, expressed as chromaticity coordinates, using the same broad-band primaries. It can be seen that the transformed π-mechanisms reproduce the main features of the color-matching coefficients, including the negative lobe of the red color-matching function, which Stiles' functions fail to predict (Stiles, 1953). The difference between the predictions from our functions and those of Stiles is primarily due to the slight concavity in the short-wavelength branch of our π_5 sensitivity functions.

IV. Hue Discrimination

As a first step in accounting for hue discrimination in terms of π-mechanisms, we have considered the simplest case: dichromatic color vision. The normal observer is effectively a dichromat in the long-wavelength region of the spectrum, for there the sensitivity of the short-wavelength mechanism is so low that it is unlikely that it contributes to the perception of hue. Foveal hue discrimination is also effectively dichromatic when discriminations are made between small fields (e.g., 20'), pre-

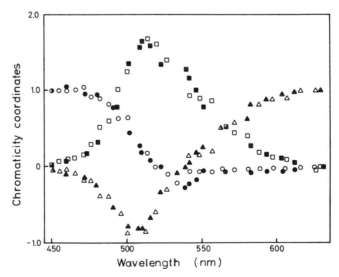

Figure 18.3. Filled symbols: Chromaticity coordinates of the spectrum colors, from the color-matching data of subject OE. Open symbols: OE's π–mechanisms, transformed using the color-matching primaries.

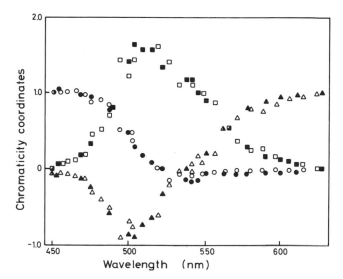

Figure 18.4. Color-matching data and π-mechanisms for subject DC, transformed as in Figure 18.3.

sumably because the short-wavelength mechanism, which is unable to detect fine detail, cannot resolve such stimuli.

Hue discrimination thresholds were measured with a 30′ field that contained a fine checkerboard pattern of 15′ squares. The adjacent squares were illuminated with light from two monochromators. The experimenter set the wavelengths of the monochromators while the observer adjusted the radiance of one beam so as to attempt to match the adjacent squares. The ranges of wavelengths that could not be discriminated from each test wavelength are shown by the data points in Figure 18.5. It is perhaps worth noting that in the region about 460 nm, in which hue discrimination was poor, the hue of the entire test field was seen to change markedly as the wavelength of one monochromator was changed, even when the adjacent checks could not be discriminated. We take this as evidence that the short-wavelength mechanism could not resolve the individual checks, although it could contribute to the hue of the entire field.

To relate hue discrimination to the sensitivities of the π_4 and π_5 mechanisms, we made the following assumption: A given wavelength elicits a certain ratio of activity in the two mechanisms; hue discrimination is possible when a second wavelength elicits a ratio of activity that differs by some threshold value. Thus, in regions of the spectrum in which the ratio of π_4/π_5 activity is changing rapidly, superior hue discrimination should be expected, since a small change in wavelength causes a large change in the relative stimulation of the two mechanisms. To relate the rate of change in π_4/π_5 sensitivity to hue discrimination, we must know how thresholds for detection of a change in the relative stimulation depend on the mean adaptation levels of the mechanisms. This can be inferred from the results of an experiment

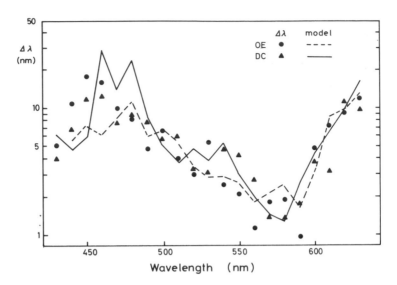

Figure 18.5. Symbols: Foveal small-field hue discrimination of two observers. Lines: Predictions of the model described in the text.

(which was done for quite different reasons) in which stimuli were presented that modulated the input of either π_4 or π_5 at 1 Hz, while the other mechanism received a constant quantum input. Detection thresholds were measured as a function of the relative adaptation levels (defined by their relative quantum catch, calculated from Stiles' sensitivity functions) of the two mechanisms. This modulation was seen as a change in hue, rather than luminance, and must have depended on the changing ratio of activity in the two mechanisms, since the measured thresholds were lower than when normal luminance modulation (i.e., in-phase modulation of the inputs to both mechanisms) was presented. The results showed that thresholds are lowest when the two mechanisms are at the same adaptation level; when the adaptation levels were changed (by means of selective chromatic adaptation), thresholds rose by $r^{1.5}$, where r is the ratio of the two adaptation levels. Using this empirical relationship and our measured π_4/π_5 sensitivity ratios (Estévez & Cavonius, 1977, Fig. 5), the expected hue discrimination behavior of the two observers was calculated at 10-nm intervals. These predicted values are shown by the lines in Figure 18.5. The predicted functions do a reasonable job of describing the hue discrimination data, whereas the same calculations, made from Stiles' π_4/π_5 ratios, predict that hue discrimination would be virtually impossible between 455 and 525 nm. This difference is again due to the fact that the short-wavelength branches of our π_5 mechanisms are slightly concave, relative to π_4, whereas Stiles' π_4 and π_5 mechanisms follow nearly parallel courses in this region of the spectrum. If hue discrimination depends, as we assume, on changes in the ratio of activity in these two mechanisms, it would be impossible to discriminate between wavelengths in the region between 455 and 525 nm. However, our observers (who were reduced to essentially tritanopic performance) and the tritanopes of Wright (1952) show rather good hue discrimination around 500 nm.

V. Discussion

With the reservation that these results are based on data from only two observers, we believe that the π_4 and π_5 mechanisms of Stiles represent (after correction for extraretinal losses) the spectral sensitivities of the middle- and long-wavelength receptors of human color vision. A similar conclusion was reached by Pugh and Siegel (1978), who found that the π_4 and π_5 mechanisms deviated less from color-matching data than any of a number of other possible fundamental sensitivity functions that they tested. Our short-wavelength mechanism appears to have a spectral sensitivity that resembles either π_3 or π_1. Of these candidates, π_3 would seem to be the more likely fundamental (Stiles, 1978; Pugh, 1976).

However, we find a small but consistent difference between our π_5 function and that of Stiles in the region between 440 and 530 nm, in which region our measured sensitivities are lower than Stiles' mean values. This discrepancy reaches a maximum of about .1 log unit at 460 nm, and resembles in shape the absorption spectrum of macular pigment. We are unable to account for the difference between Stiles' data and ours, other than the inadequate suggestion that it may represent individual differences among observers and the yet weaker possibility that it is a sex-related difference, since three of Stiles' four observers were women, whereas both of our observers were males.

It is also possible that this depression in the π_5 sensitivity function holds only for the fovea, although this does not help to explain the difference between Stiles' data and ours, since his measurements were made with a 1° central test flash. That the depression in π_5 sensitivity vanishes in the periphery can be deduced from the measurements of the sensitivity of the long- and middle-wavelength mechanisms of Wooten and Wald (1973): The ratio of sensitivities of these mechanisms, as a function of wavelength, is markedly curved at the fovea, but flattens out in the periphery. The same conclusion can be drawn from the peripheral color-matching functions of Richards and Luria (1964) in which the negative lobe of the red primary is almost absent, and which can be very well described by a transform of Stiles' π-mechanisms. These results suggest the possibility that an additional inert pigment screens the long-wavelength foveal receptors, but that it does not exist (or is reduced in density) in the periphery. Such a pigment was proposed by Smith and Pokorny (1975) to account for the fact that the spectral sensitivity of the long-wavelength mechanism of deuteranopes is more concave than that of protanopes in the spectral region about 450 nm.

If we accept π_3, π_4, and π_5 as fundamentals, we are faced with the question of whether they represent the absorption spectra (after correction for the optic media) of single visual pigments. The shapes of π_3 and π_4 have been shown by Stiles (1959) to resemble the spectra of known pigments; but π_5, with its flat peak, does not resemble closely any pigment that has been measured in solution. However, we believe that π_5 represents the absorption spectrum of a single pigment, in part because we (and many others) have been unsuccessful in attempts to alter its spectral sensitivity by selective adaptation. This negative result is not conclusive, since it could also occur if π_5 were based on two or more pigments, which might be mixed in the same receptor, or segregated in separate receptors that share a common adaptation stage.

A more compelling argument for the unitary nature of π_5 can be made if we accept that normals and deuteranopes share a common long-wavelength pigment, erythrolabe. Reflection densitometric measurements by Alpern and Pugh (1977) show that the erythrolabe of deuteranopes has the flat peak that is characteristic of π_5, and Alpern and Wake (1977) have shown that it is a single pigment, since its difference spectrum cannot be altered by selective bleaching. Similarly, microspectrophotometric measurements by Bowmaker, Dartnall, Lythgoe, and Mollon (1978) of long-wavelength cones in macaque yield spectra that resemble π_5. We can conclude that if more than one pigment is present, they occur in a fixed ratio, and act together in such a linear and inseparable manner that for the purposes of color science they may be considered as a single pigment.

REFERENCES

Alpern, M., & Pugh, E.N., Jr. Variation in the action spectrum of erythrolabe among deuteranopes. *Journal of Physiology*, 1977, *266*, 613–646.

Alpern, M., & Wake, T. Cone pigments in human deutan colour vision defects. *Journal of Physiology*, 1977, *266*, 595–612.

Bowmaker, J.K., Dartnall, H.J.A., Lythgoe, J.M., & Mollon, J.D. The visual pigments of rods and cones in the rhesus monkey, *Macaca mulatta*. *Journal of Physiology*, 1978, *274*, 329–348.

Estévez, O., & Cavonius, C.R. Human color perception and Stiles' π-mechanisms. *Vision Research*, 1977, *17*, 417–422.

Mollon, J.D., & Polden, P.D. An anomaly in the response of the eye to short wavelengths. *Philosophical Transactions of the Royal Society of London, Ser. B*, 1977, *278*, 207–240.

Pugh, E.N., Jr. The nature of the π_1 colour mechanism of W.S. Stiles. *Journal of Physiology*, 1976, *257*, 713–747.

Pugh, E.N., Jr., & Siegel, C. Evaluation of the candidacy of the π-mechanisms of Stiles for color-matching fundamentals. *Vision Research*, 1978, *18*, 317–330.

Richards, W., & Luria, S.M. Color-mixture functions at low luminance levels. *Vision Research*, 1964, *4*, 281–313.

Smith, V.C., & Pokorny, J. Spectral sensitivity of the foveal cone photopigments between 400 and 500 nm. *Vision Research*, 1975, *15*, 161–171.

Stiles, W.S. Further studies of visual mechanisms by the two-colour threshold method. In *Coloquio sobre problemas opticos de la vision*. Madrid: Union Internationale de Physique Pure et Appliquée, 1953. Vol. 1, pp. 65–103.

Stiles, W.S. Color vision: The approach through increment threshold sensitivity. *Proceedings of the National Academy of Sciences*, 1959, *45*, 100–114.

Stiles, W.S. *Mechanisms of colour vision*. London: Academic Press, 1978.

Wooten, B.R., & Wald, G. Color-vision mechanisms in the peripheral retina of normal and dichromatic observers. *Journal of General Physiology*, 1973, *61*, 125–145.

Wright, W.D. *Researches in normal and defective colour vision*. London: Kimpton, 1946.
Wright, W.D. The characteristics of tritanopia. *Journal of the Optical Society of America,* 1952, *42,* 509–521.
Wyszecki, G., & Stiles, W.S. *Color science.* New York: Wiley, 1967.

19. The Bezold–Brücke Effect and Its Complement, Hue Constancy

Tom N. Cornsweet

It is well known that the hues of most monochromatic lights change somewhat if their intensities are changed. This phenomenon, known as the Bezold–Brücke effect, has been quantified under various conditions by a number of investigators over the last 40 years, and the data play important roles in many theories of color vision. I want to suggest that perhaps the significance of the Bezold–Brücke effect has been viewed upside down. What is remarkable is not that hue varies with intensity, but rather that hue varies so little with intensity. Some careful thinking reveals that the almost perfect constancy of hue as intensity changes is just as puzzling and of just as much evolutionary significance as brightness constancy, and I will use the term "hue constancy" to refer to it. In that terminology, the Bezold–Brücke effect is a measure of departures from perfect hue constancy.[1]

Figure 19.1 shows how the hues of monochromatic lights change with intensity under two different experimental conditions. The critical difference between the conditions is the duration of stimulus exposure. In Figure 19.1A, the subject viewed each stimulus for several seconds; in Figure 19.1B the stimuli were flashed for 5 msec. The implications of the differences between these plots will be discussed later.

For both plots, if hue constancy were perfect, all of the lines of constant hue would be straight and vertical. It is evident under both conditions in Figure 19.1 that hue does change slightly as intensity is varied.

I. A Physiological Model for Hue Constancy

The neural machinery required to produce hue constancy cannot easily be built

---

[1]The term "color constancy" is commonly used to refer to a different phenomenon, namely, that the hue of an object does not change very much in spite of moderate changes in the wavelength composition of the light incident on it and its surroundings.

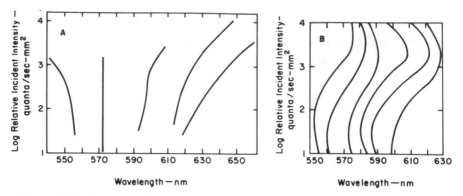

Figure 19.1. Contours of constant hue with varying intensity, for exposures of several seconds (A) and 5 msec (B). All points on any given line have the same hue. The curves in (A) are derived from the data of Purdy (1937), and those in (B) from Savoie (1973).

out of known neural elements. We will assume here that the spectral sensitivities of the three cone pigment systems are those of Wald, given in Figure 19.2. (The particular curves assumed are not important to the following arguments.) To avoid unnecessary complication, we will restrict the discussion to the long-wavelength half of the visible spectrum, from about 550 nm on, where the activity of the short-wave sensitive system can probably be neglected.

The quantum catch of any cone, that is, either the total number of quanta captured during some flash, or the rate of absorption of quanta at equilibrium for long exposures, is a reasonably linear function of the total number or rate of incident

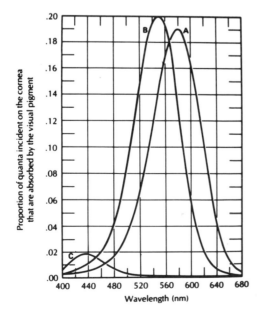

Figure 19.2. Spectral sensitivity curves for three retinal color mechanisms, derived from Wald (1964).

quanta so long as a large proportion of the pigment molecules has not been bleached. Furthermore, the immediate effect of quantum capture, that is, isomerization, almost certainly bears a fixed relationship to the quantum catch. (The quantum efficiency of isomerization is probably independent of the proportion of molecules isomerized, at least when that proportion is not large.) Therefore, for all but the highest intensities of stimuli seen in the world or the laboratory, the immediate effect of light on visual pigment varies linearly with the rate of incident quanta.

There is excellent electrophysiological evidence that a class of neural units exists in the retina that are excited by the long-wavelength-sensitive (R) system and inhibited by the middle-wavelength-sensitive (G) system, the so-called R–G opponent cells. If the action of these cells is typical of neural interactions of this kind, the output of an opponent cell is a reasonably linear function of the algebraic difference between its inputs over a usefully large dynamic range, and so it seems proper to call it an R minus G (R−G) cell.

The simplest model of the physiology of hue that is consistent with these facts is shown in Figure 19.3. It is entirely linear. Such a system would exhibit what might be called zero hue constancy. The resulting lines of constant hue can be directly calculated, and are plotted in Figure 19.4. Clearly, our visual systems do not work that way.

A very widely used model for the physiology of hue is shown in Figure 19.5, where what was called an R−G cell is now an R/G cell, that is, a ratio taker. This model predicts perfect hue constancy; all lines of constant hue are straight vertical lines. To explain the Bezold–Brücke effect within the general framework of this model, it has been assumed that the inputs to the R/G cell are nonlinearly and unequally related to quantum catch (Hurvich & Jameson, 1957). The trouble with this model is that it is not really a model because it does not describe in physiological terms just how that ratio is taken, and, as far as I have been able to determine, there is no known example of a real neural mechanism that directly calculates ratios. (It is also difficult to make an electronic device that directly calculates the ratio of its inputs. Black boxes that are called dividers always do their division indirectly, such as by successive subtractions, special forms of feedback, etc.)

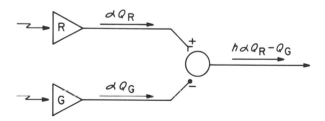

Figure 19.3. A simple model for the physiology of hue perception. A single receptor is drawn to symbolize the set of receptors containing long-wavelength-sensitive pigment (R), and another for the middle-wavelength set (G). The output of each receptor is linear with quantum catch, and the G output is subtracted from the R to obtain a signal that is monotonically related to hue.

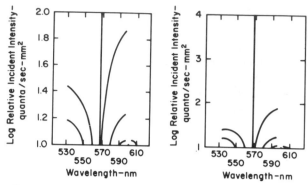

Figure 19.4. Contours of constant hue that would occur if the model in Figure 19.3 were correct. Both plots are of the same data. The plot on the right is on the same scale as the data in Figure 19.1, and the left plot is of the same data with an expanded vertical axis. Each curve represents all wavelength-intensity combinations that produce the same value of h (Figure 19.3). Each curve stops where any increase in intensity would produce a value of h that cannot be equaled by any wavelength at a relative intensity of 1.

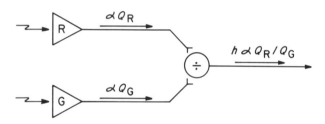

Figure 19.5. A common model for hue. The resulting constant hue contours would all be perfectly straight and vertical.

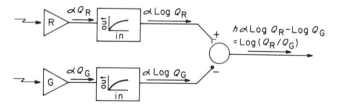

Figure 19.6. A different model that produces the same result as that in Figure 19.5. The logarithmic nonlinearity is represented here as a box separate from the receptors. However, that nonlinearity might actually reside all or in part within the receptors.

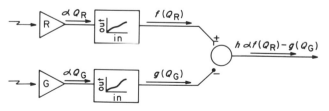

Figure 19.7. A general model for the physiology of hue.

Figure 19.6 illustrates a way of achieving an output that is related to R/G without directly performing a division. This model, again, displays perfect hue constancy. It also is significantly incomplete because it does not specify how the logarithmic transformation is performed.

However, this model suggests a more general model, shown in Figure 19.7, which I believe is very useful. Between the isomerization of pigment molecules and the input to an $R-G$ cell lies a stage whose output is some nonlinear function of its input. If that nonlinearity were perfectly logarithmic (and identical for the R and G systems, as explained later) then hue constancy would be perfect. Conversely, it is possible to deduce the shape of the nonlinearity from the relationship between intensity and hue, and then to try to determine whether or not such a nonlinearity could be the result of plausible physiological processes. Savoie (1971, 1973) did just that, using the data shown in Figure 19.1B, and obtained the functions in Figure 19.8. These functions are reasonably close to logarithmic over a wide range of intensities. He was able to fit the curves in Figure 19.8 very well by a particular combination of physiological functions that are known to exist, as will be explained.

II. The Functional Significance of Hue Constancy

If the functions in Figure 19.8 were perfectly logarithmic, they would, of course, be straight lines, since the horizontal axis is logarithmic. The functions actually resemble patchwork approaches to straight lines, almost as though evolution pulled and hammered at them until they were good enough. I believe that is a reasonable statement of what might have happened. An animal with approximate hue constancy obviously has an advantage over one without it. If ripe bananas changed from yellow to green every time the sun went behind a cloud (as they would if we were built like the model in Figure 19.3), the large amount of information contained in

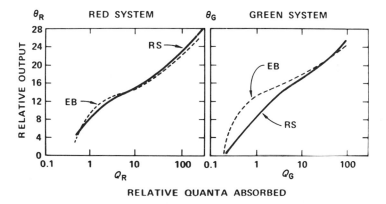

Figure 19.5. A common model for hue. The resulting constant hue contours would all be and the outputs of the R and G stages of the model in Figure 19.7. [From Savoie (1973).]

the spectral reflectance of bananas, or of any other objects, would lose its usefulness.

The functional significance of a mechanism providing hue constancy can be described in another way. It is a mechanism that responds to properties of objects. The input that corresponds to some particular object will vary strongly when the intensity of the illumination on the object is changed, but the output will not vary unless a property of the object itself, namely, its spectral reflectance, is changed.[2] In other words, the mechanism of hue constancy can be described as a mechanism that abstracts or forms the concept "hue" when spectral reflectance is constant but the intensity of the illumination changes.

Considering the powerful evolutionary forces favoring selection of species with something approximating hue constancy, and recognizing that dividers and perfect logarithmic transformations are not common biological processes, it seems plausible that the functions in Figure 19.8 are evolution's good enough tries at straight lines.[3]

III. Savoie's Physiological Model for Nonlinearity

A number of different physiological models of receptor mechanisms predict that the relationship between quantum catch and receptor output should be of the form

$$O = K_1 I/(K_2 + I), \tag{1}$$

where I is a measure of quantum catch and the Ks are constants. A number of physiological studies of receptor input–output relationships yield such a function (e.g., Normann & Werblin, 1974). Figure 19.9 shows how well Eq. (1) fits some of the data from Figure 19.8. It does not fit. The output in Eq. (1), when plotted against the log of intensity, yields an S-shaped function, but the curves in Figure 19.8 seem to form two S-shaped functions, one beginning where the other leaves off. Equation (1) does not yield even approximate hue constancy over more than about 1.5 log units of intensity.

Suppose that the visual system contained processes like those that generate Eq. (1), but with two different sets of constants so that one output begins to change when the other begins to saturate, that is, consider the following equation:

---

[2]The output would also vary if the spectral composition of the illumination were changed. The logarithmic-like transformation, followed by strong lateral inhibition within color systems, will cause the output to be relatively independent of small changes in the spectral composition of the illumination (i.e., color constancy) (Cornsweet, 1970). Strong changes in the color of the illumination were rarely encountered while the mechanism was evolving.

[3]An exactly analogous argument can be made for the evolution of brightness constancy, and since a logarithmic transformation followed by strong lateral inhibition is sufficient to account for most if not all of the data on brightness constancy (Cornsweet, 1970), the same approximately logarithmic transformation has even more utility.

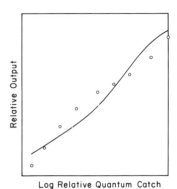

Figure 19.9. The points are from one of the curves in Figure 19.8 (Subject EB, R system), and the smooth curve is the best fit for the equation $O = (K_1 \times I)/(K_2 + I)$. The fit is poor.

Log Relative Quantum Catch

$$O = [K_1 I/(K_2 + I)] + [K_3 I/(K_4 + I)]. \tag{2}$$

Figure 19.10 shows this equation fitted to Savoie's data. The fit is excellent. A specific version of the model in Figure 19.7 that yields Eq. (2) is shown in Figure 19.11.

Of course four constants are available to arrive at the fit in Figure 19.10, and so the fit certainly cannot be taken as strong evidence that Eq. (2) is correct.[4] However, it is clearly possible to generate exactly the kinds of nonlinearities that seem to be present in the human visual system by summing the effects of processes that are known to occur in neural tissues, and I am unable to discover a simpler function that fits the data as well.

IV. Short versus Long Exposures

The lines of constant hue in Figure 19.1A are very different from those in Figure 19.1B, and the corresponding calculated nonlinearities would also necessarily be different. These differences are less puzzling when they are examined from the perspective of the model in Figure 19.7. Suppose, first, that the nonlinearity were

[4]Savoie (1971) tried to fit his data with other functions, shown in the table below, along with the best-fitting sums of squared errors. Note that Eq. (2) fits much better than the others, even when they contain as many constants.

Forms	Sum of squared errors
$K_1 \times I/(K_2 + I) + K_3 \times I/(K_4 + I) + K_5$	.18
$K_1 \times \log(K_2 + I) + K_3 \times \log(K_4 + I) + K_5$	3.53
$K_1 \times \log(I) + K_2$	11.64
$K_1 + K_2 \times I + K_3 \times I^2$	160.3
$K_1 + K_2 \times I + K_3 \times I^2 + K_4 \times I^3$	96.6
$K_1 + K_2 \times I + K_3 \times I^2 + K_4 \times I^3 + K_5 \times I^4$	47.7

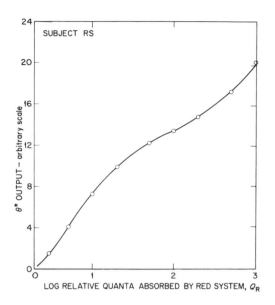

Figure 19.10. The points are the same data as in Figure 19.9, and the smooth curve is the best fit for the equation $O = (K_1 \times I)/(K_2 + I)] + [(K_3 \times I)/(K_4 + I)]$. [From Savoie (1973).]

perfectly logarithmic and identical for the R and G systems, as in Figure 19.12. The occurrence of hue constancy can be interpreted graphically as follows: Choose a wavelength that produces twice as great a quantum catch in the R as in the G system (e.g., 590 from Figure 19.2) and present it at some intensity I_1 such that its inputs to the R and the G systems are as indicated in Figure 19.12. The resulting output of the hue mechanism h_1 will be $O_{RI} - O_{GI}$. Now multiply the intensity of the stimulus by, say, 8. Since the horizontal axis is logarithmic and quantum catch is linear with

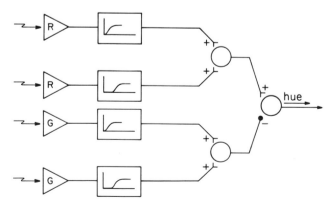

Figure 19.11. One way of modeling the equation that fits Savoie's data. It is really a particular version of the general model in Figure 19.7. [From Savoie (1971).]

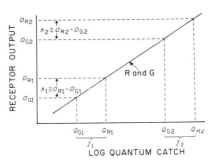

Figure 19.12. Graphical illustration of why hue would not change with intensity if the nonlinearities of both R and G systems in Figure 19.7 were perfectly logarithmic. The change in intensity from I_1 to I_2 is represented by a translation along the logarithmic horizontal axis. This produces a translation of the R and G outputs along the *linear* vertical axis. The resulting value of h is unchanged for any wavelength and any intensity change.

intensity, this will shift both the R and G inputs equally along the input axis, and the resulting hue will be $h'_2 = O_{R2} - O_{G2}$. Because the line is straight,

$$O_{R1} - O_{G1} = O_{R2} - O_{G2} \; ; 2\,h_1 = h_2,$$

that is, the new output will be identical with the old one, and thus the hue will not change. If the nonlinearities are exactly as represented in Figure 19.12, that is, identical and logarithmic for the R and G systems, the argument above will hold for any wavelength and any intensity change.

Now consider the nonlinearities in Figure 19.13, again perfectly logarithmic, but where the R and G systems are not identical. Repeating the example used above, the output

$$O_{R1} - O_{G1} \neq O_{R2} - O_{G2},$$

that is, this system does not exhibit constancy. Changes in intensity will cause changes in hue for any wavelength.

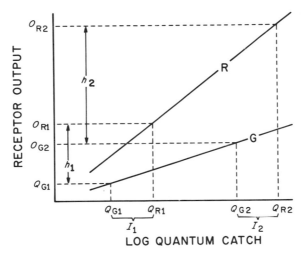

Figure 19.13. If both nonlinearities were perfectly logarithmic but not identical (i.e., of different slopes on this semilog plot), a change in intensity would produce a change in hue for every wavelength.

Now consider the model with the nonlinearities in Figure 19.14, the R and G being identical. There is a wavelength for which the quantum catches of the R and G systems are equal (565 nm in Figure 19.2), and for that one particular wavelength, the difference between the R and G system outputs will be zero for all intensities. Therefore, the hue of that wavelength will be invariant with intensity. The hues of all other wavelengths will vary with intensity depending upon the way in which the slope of this curve varies. This is illustrated for one wavelength at three intensities in Figure 19.14.

Finally, consider the general case in Figure 19.15. There is no invariant wavelength, and hue varies irregularly with intensity.

In general, for the model in Figure 19.7, contours of constant hue will vary with the relationship between the changes in slopes of the R and G input–output curves when output is plotted against the log of intensity, and no wavelength will have an invariant hue unless the input–output functions for the R and G systems either are identical or differ only by a horizontal translation.

Now reconsider the differences between the curves in Figures 19.1A and 19.1B. Suppose that a subject is completely dark-adapted, and then a pair of stimuli such as are used to measure the Bezold–Brücke effect are suddenly presented. For example, suppose that stimuli of some wavelength and intensity were presented as in Figure 19.16. The initial output of the R system would then be O_R and of the G system O_G, and the hue would be $O_R - O_G$. Now suppose that the stimuli were simply left on until adaptation was at equilibrium (i.e., the rate of isomerization of visual pigment molecules equaled the rate of regeneration). Clearly the outputs of the R and G systems would decline during this period of light adaptation, and since the irradiance is constant, the outputs would fall along the vertical lines indicated by arrows in Figure 19.16.[5] If, at the onset of the stimuli, the outputs were as the points labeled a and b, then at equilibrium, the outputs will both be smaller, as a' and b'.

In general, then, the input–output curves at equilibrium will be different from those at stimulus onset, and therefore the relationships between intensity and hue will be different for short and long flashes.[6]

But stronger statements can be made about the ways in which the input–output curves change during light adaptation. At intensities approaching zero, the decrease

[5]Obviously, at the instant the stimulus is first turned on, the outputs are at their resting levels, and they require some finite time to rise before they begin their decline during adaptation. Further, for any real system, there is some flash duration so short that the response to any shorter flash will not vary in shape. (The response is then called the impulse response.) We assume here that the 5-msec flashes of Savoie are that short.

[6]This argument leads to the prediction that the hue of a stimulus of fixed radiance and wavelength composition should change with exposure duration. Several studies of hue as a function of exposure duration have been published. For example, Nilsson (1972) found strong hue shifts with flash duration. In his report, he states that the shifts in hue he observed were in the same direction as Bezold–Brücke shifts for high luminances but contrary to them at low luminances, and he therefore believes that they are mediated by some process different from that of the Bezold–Brücke shift. His data are inconsistent with classical Bezold–Brücke data at low luminances, but are consistent with the Bezold–Brücke shifts for short flashes (see Figure 19.1B) at all luminances.

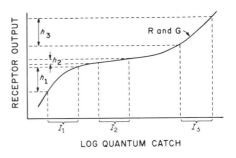

Figure 19.14. If the nonlinearities were identical but not perfectly logarithmic, hue would change with intensity depending upon the wavelength and the way in which the slope of the function changes. For any wavelength that happens to produce equal quantum catches in the two systems, the hue shift with intensity would be zero.

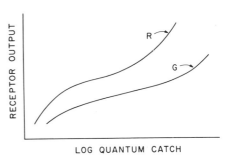

Figure 19.15. The general case, where the R and G nonlinearities are different and not perfectly logarithmic. Hue will change nonmonotonically with intensity for every wavelength.

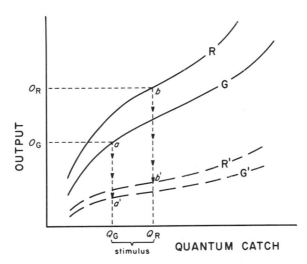

Figure 19.16. Graphical illustration of the effect of exposure duration on Bezold–Brücke hue shifts. As the exposure continues, the outputs will fall, producing new input–output nonlinearities whose slopes will be shallower than for short exposures. Therefore, Bezold–Brücke shifts will be smaller and the conditions for the production of invariant wavelengths will be approached.

in output during adaptation must also approach zero, and in general, if adaptation processes are at all well behaved, the decrease during adaptation will be greater the higher the intensity. Therefore, it is likely that the input–output curves will have shallower slopes at equilibrium for all intensities than the corresponding slopes at stimulus onset, as shown in Figure 19.16. This, in turn, means two things: First, changes in curvature will be smaller at equilibrium, thus producing smaller Bezold–Brücke hue shifts for longer exposures. Second, any differences between the R and G systems will be smaller at equilibrium, making the conditions closer to those required for the existence of an invariant hue. Comparison of Figures 19.1A and 19.1B indicates that both of these expectations are borne out. In a recent study directly comparing Bezold–Brücke shifts for 10- and 300-msec flashes, Nagy and Zacks (1977) also found results completely consistent with Savoie's data and the preceding considerations. Their 10-msec data are very similar to Savoie's, and their 300-msec data show generally smaller hue shifts and something closer to an invariant wavelength.[7]

Several researchers in color vision considered the existence of wavelengths of invariant hue when they were formulating theories, and it is easy to get the impression that data such as in Figure 19.1B, showing no invariant wavelength, somehow contradict those theories (e.g., Larimer, Krantz, & Cicerone, 1974). However, if the physiology of hue constancy is considered in terms of the very general model described in Figure 19.7, the presence or absence of invariant wavelengths is of little consequence. It is merely a question of how close to identical the nonlinearities of the various color systems happen to be.

REFERENCES

Cornsweet, T. N. *Visual perception.* New York: Academic Press, 1970.

Hurvich, L., & Jameson, D. An opponent-process theory of color vision. *Psychological Review,* 1957, *64,* 384–404.

Larimer, J., Krantz, D., & Cicerone, C. M. Opponent-process additivity. I. Red/green equilibria. *Vision Research,* 1974, *14,* 1127–1140.

Nagy, A. L., & Zacks, J. L. The effects of psychophysical procedure and stimulus duration in the measurement of Bezold–Brücke hue shifts. *Vision Research,* 1977, *17,* 193–201.

Nilsson, T. H. Effects of pulse duration and pulse rate on hue of monochromatic stimuli. *Vision Research,* 1972, *12,* 1907–1923.

Normann, R. A., & Werblin, F. S. Light and dark adaptation of vertebrate rod and cone responses. *Journal of General Physiology,* 1974, *63,* 37–61.

Purdy, D. McL. The Bezold–Brücke phenomenon and contours of constant hue. *American Journal of Psychology,* 1937, *49,* 313–315.

Savoie, R. E. *Nonlinear aspects of the human visual system derived from the variation of hue with intensity* (Tech. Rep.). California: Stanford Research Institute, October 1971.

Savoie, R. E. Bezold–Brücke effect and visual nonlinearity. *Journal of the Optical Society of America,* 1973, *63,* 1253–1261.

Wald, G. The receptors for human color vision. *Science,* 1964, *101,* 653–658.

---

[7]In Nilsson's (1972) study of hue shifts as a function of flash duration, two of his conclusions are "as pulse duration increases, hue shift magnitudes generally decrease" and "the decrease in hue shift magnitude with pulse duration is more marked at the higher illuminances [p. 1090]." Both of those results are consistent with the present analysis.

20. The Stiles–Crawford II Effect at High Bleaching Levels

B. R. Wooten, Kenneth Fuld, Margaret Moore, and Lenore Katz

I. Introduction

The hue associated with a particular colored light depends upon a number of factors other than the wavelength composition. A fairly large range of hues can result from a particular wavelength depending upon such factors as luminance level, retinal position, adaptation conditions, and surround chromaticity. One particularly subtle factor, discovered by Stiles in 1937, is the position of the light beam in the eye's pupil. Earlier, Stiles and Crawford (1933) had found that the brightness of a light diminished as a narrow beam is moved from the approximate center of the pupil to its margin. A beam of light is about five times less efficient in causing a visual sensation when it enters 3 mm off-center than when it enters through the center of the pupil. This phenomenon is known as the Stiles–Crawford effect of the first kind (S–C I). It is well known that S–C I results from the directional sensitivity of the cones; that is, rays that enter the pupil off-center, and thus impinge on the retina at an angle Θ with respect to the cone's long axis are less likely to be absorbed by the photopigment in the outer segment than if the rays entered parallel to the cone's axis. It can be calculated that Θ equals about 7.5° for a beam entering 3 mm off-center. When Stiles used monochromatic lights, he discovered that oblique rays result in slightly different hues, even after equating for brightness. This phenomenon is known as the Stiles–Crawford effect of the second kind (S–C II).

Figure 20.1 shows S–C II for one of our subjects. The ordinate represents the shift in nanometers required to bring a beam, 3 mm off-center, to the same wavelength as an on-center beam after they have been matched in hue and brightness. In the long- and short-wave portions of the spectrum, the shift is positive. For example, after adjusting for brightness, a 610-nm off-center beam looks too red compared to a 610-nm on-center beam. To equate for hue, the subject requires that the off-center light be adjusted to 604 nm. The middle-wave region shows a nega-

245

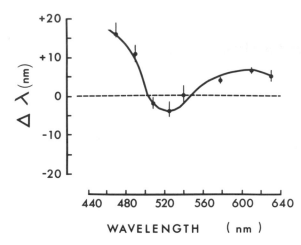

Figure 20.1. S–C II for observer BW. Δλ refers to the shift, in nanometers, required to bring an eccentric beam (3 mm off-center) to the same wavelength as an on-center beam after they were matched in hue and brightness. The circles represent the wavelength corresponding to the 50% point in the psychometric function drawn through the response versus wavelength plot. The ends of the straight lines drawn through the circles represent the wavelengths corresponding to 10 and 90% points.

tive shift; for example, a 540-nm off-center light looks too yellow before a wavelength shift is made. The results for our subject are in good agreement with earlier studies.

The cause of S–C II is not well understood, but it is clear that it involves some aspect(s) of the biophysics of cone receptors. For this reason it has received considerable attention from physiologists, physicists, and psychophysicists in the last 20 years. The strong interest in S–C II, and also S–C I, has to do with the question of how light interacts with visual receptors.

II. The Geometric Optics Account

Stiles (1937) originally suggested that S–C II may result from the three receptor classes of color vision having different degrees of S–C I. Such a proposal could account for the original hue shift, but it cannot explain Brindley's (1953) discovery that metamers are upset by decentering the beams. This aspect of S–C II requires that at least one of the cone classes has a relative spectral sensitivity that is dependent upon the angle of incidence, Θ.

It is usually held that a cell's spectral sensitivity is determined by certain aspects of its photochemistry. As light passes through the outer segment, some of it is absorbed by molecules of photopigment. The probability of absorption is wavelength dependent and is characterized by the photopigment's extinction spectrum, which may be viewed as the relative probability of absorption as a function of wavelength for a single molecule. It seems certain from single-cell spectrophotometry that there are three types of cones in the human fovea distinguished by the extinction spectra of their photopigments. From the work of Brown and Wald (1963), it is likely that these photopigments share the same chromophore as rhodopsin, that is, 11-cis retinal, but differ in some aspect of their protein moieties. From the Beer–Lambert law, it is also certain that the spectral sensitivity of the receptor is influenced by the photopigment's total absorbing power, that is, the product of the pigment's concentration and the outer segment's length. This self-screening effect was first emphasized by Dartnall (1957) and is illustrated in Figure 20.2 for human rhodopsin. The curves show the relative spectral absorption for solutions of various optical density. As can be seen, the relative absorption becomes broader as optical density increases. Various direct (Dobelle, Marks, & MacNichol, 1969; King-Smith, 1971) and indirect (Miller, 1972) methods indicate that human cones probably have an optical density at the peak wavelengths of between .30 and .45.

The self-screening effect can provide a satisfactory account of S–C II provided certain assumptions are made (Walraven & Bouman, 1960). The key proposition is that cone receptors act as light guides due to their greater refractive index compared to the extracellular environment. Light that impinges on the receptor at a slightly oblique angle will be wholly transmitted down the length of the outer segment due to total internal reflection. As obliquity increases, however, more and more light is leaked out, thus reducing the effective transmission path through the outer segment. The shorter pathlength means that the effective optical density is reduced and, hence, self-screening is reduced. From Figure 20.2, it can be seen that this has the effect of narrowing the relative spectral absorption curve. The magnitude of the narrowing is, of course, a function of the photopigment's maximum optical density and the amount of path shortening.

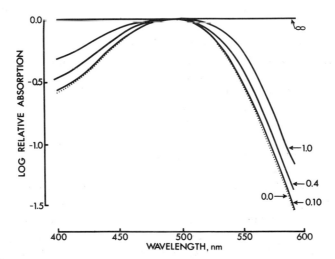

Figure 20.2. The self-screening effect based on Wald and Brown's (1958) extinction spectrum (dotted line) for human rhodopsin. The smooth lines show the relative absorption for solutions with peak optical density indicated to the right.

III. The Physical Optics Account

A strikingly different account of how visual receptors and light interact was first suggested by Toraldo di Francia (1949). He pointed out that when the diameter of a receptor is close to the wavelength of light, the manner in which light is propagated through the receptor must be considered from the point of view of physical optics. Since the diameter of human cones is only slightly greater than the wavelength of visible radiation, he suggested that the cones may act as dielectric waveguides. If this idea is correct, it means that light energy is nonuniformly distributed within the receptor in a way that is somewhat analogous to the standing waves in organ pipes. The precise form of these patterns, called modes, is dependent upon a number of physical properties such as the diameter of the receptor and its refractive index relative to that of the extracellular environment.

Of particular interest with respect to S–C I and II is that the amount of light energy contained within a waveguide, and thus available for absorption by a photo-pigment, is critically dependent upon the angle of incidence and the wavelength. Thus, waveguide principles potentially offer a unified explanation of both S–C I and II. In fact, Snyder and Pask (1973) have shown that S–C II may be interpreted as successfully by waveguide principles as by self-screening. Modes have been observed in glass fiber optics with diameters similar to foveal cones (Kapany & Burke, 1961; Osterberg, Snitzer, Polanyi, & Hilberg, 1959). In addition, Enoch (1961a, 1961b, 1961c) has observed what appear to be modal patterns in excised primate retinas. Brindley and Rushton (1959), however, have offered evidence that seems to rule out strong waveguide effects in human vision. They showed that monochromatic light passed transscleraly has about the same hue as light entering through the pupil.

In summary, while waveguide theory can in principle account for S–C II, it is by no means required on the basis of available data. Self-screening offers an equally plausible and considerably simpler explanation with fewer assumptions and fewer free parameters. The purpose of this study was to test the generality of the self-screening effect as an explanation of S–C II.

IV. Experimental Rationale and Method

In order for the self-screening effect to account for S–C II, two conditions must be met. First, the oblique rays must have an appreciably shorter pathlength through the pigment-containing outer segments. Second, the photopigment must be present in considerable concentration. The latter condition is the key to our experiments and deserves some amplification. Assume, for the moment, that the three types of cone photopigments have a concentration such that, given an outer-segment length of 30 μm, the optical density at the wavelength to which they are most sensitive is .40. Also assume that an oblique incidence of 7.5°, corresponding to an entry beam 3 mm off the pupil's center, results in a reduction of the pathlength by a factor of 5.

The maximum optical density for the oblique rays would then be .08. From Figure 20.2, it can be seen that these conditions would result in considerable differences between the corresponding relative absorption functions; that is, the spectral sensitivities of the three receptor types would be considerably different for the normal and oblique conditions. Now consider the case where the photopigments are in relatively low concentrations such that for normal incidence the maximal optical densities are .01. For the $7.5°$ oblique ray, the maxima would be .002. For such small values, as can be inferred from Figure 20.2, there is no appreciable self-screening and, thus, no important difference in relative spectral absorption between the normal and oblique conditions. The limit illustrates the point well: For a single molecule of photopigment the relative spectral absorption function, that is, the extinction spectrum, is totally independent of the light's angle of incidence. If S–C II is totally explainable on the basis of self-screening, a simple and strong prediction can be made: The magnitude of S–C II should be inversely proportional to photopigment concentration. In the limit, when photopigment levels are near zero, S–C II should be abolished. In the present study, we test these predictions by manipulating photopigment concentration.

The S–C II proper is the dependency of hue per se on the position in the pupil of the monochromatic light beam. A concomitant effect, mentioned previously, is the effect of pupil-entry position on metamerism. This latter aspect of S–C II is actually the more important phenomenon, since a change in metameric color matches strongly implies that one or more of the visual receptors has a relative spectral sensitivity that varies with pupil-entry position.

In Experiment I, we studied the metameric aspect of S–C II at various photopigment concentration levels by adapting the eye with a white light provided by a xenon lamp and attenuated with Inconel filters that had flat absorption spectra. The subjects were adapted to the white light for 4 min. Thereafter, the $10°$ adapting field followed a sequence of 3 sec off and 10 sec on. The matching fields were 20 min in visual angle and were presented for 1 sec at the end of the 3-sec dark period. The resulting levels of photopigment bleaching were calculated from Rushton and Henry's (1968) reflection densitometry measurements and pigment kinetic equations. They ranged from 0 to 88% in approximately 10% increments. Subjects were asked to make a Rayleigh match. The standard field was 580 nm. The variable field consisted of a mixture of 540 and 630 nm, the intensities of which the subject adjusted to match perfectly the 580-nm standard. The luminance level of these fields was adjusted by the subject so that color was clearly visible for each adapting level. Both subjects had normal color vision.

The purpose of Experiment II was to determine the effect of photopigment bleaching on the actual S–C II hue shift. As discussed, the hue shift should be abolished at near total bleach levels according to the self-screening explanation. Adaptation conditions were identical to those in Experiment I. The hue shift was measured with a constant stimulus procedure. Each standard field was of fixed wavelength and luminance. The matching field was varied in 1- to 3-nm steps by the experimenter, depending on the spectral region. The subject's task was first to adjust the luminance of the matching field until it matched the standard in brightness. Then the subject was required to indicate whether the matching field had a hue associated with a shorter or a longer wavelength than the standard. Each wavelength was presented five times in random order. A graph was then constructed plotting percentage response versus wavelength. The wavelength corresponding to the 50% point was taken to indicate the hue match.

The apparatus for the experiments was a four-channel Maxwellian-view system. An achromatizing lens located at a point conjugate to the pupil corrected for the chromatic aberration of the eye. The entry beam was circular with a diameter of 1 mm. The subject's eye was dilated to about 7 mm with 1 to 2 drops of .5% Mydriacil. An auxiliary channel allowed direct viewing of the pupil for precise alignment and monitoring. A preliminary determination was made for each subject to locate the peak of his or her S–C I function. Hereafter, when we refer to the center or on-axis position, we actually mean the pupillary position for maximum luminous efficiency. For BW, this was 1 mm nasal to the geometric center; for LK, it was 1 mm temporal. Eccentric or off-axis position was always 3 mm from the peak position.

V. Results and Discussion

Figure 20.3 shows the results for the Rayleigh matches of Experiment I. Filled and open circles refer to the on- and off-axis conditions, respectively. The lines were drawn through the points by eye. The ordinate is plotted as the log of the 630/540 ratio (on a quantal basis) required to match the 580-nm standard. The abscissa is our estimate of the photopigment bleach states for various adaptation levels. Both subjects show the same overall trend with only small quantitative differences. At the 0% bleach level BW and LK require, respectively, about .12 and .16 log unit more 630-nm compared to 540-nm light for the off- than the on-axis condition. As the bleaching level increases, the difference in the ratios decreases up to about a 70% bleach. Up to this level, the data are at least qualitatively in accord with the self-screening prediction. Beyond the 70% level, however, the difference in the ratios seems to remain approximately constant.

At this point, one might ask whether the overall form of the data corresponds in a quantitative way to the self-screening predictions. In order to answer this question with certainty, we need to know the extinction spectra of the middle- and long-wave photopigments (the short-wave one may be ignored in this part of the spectrum), the concentration of the photopigments, the length of the outer segment, and the pathlength of the oblique rays. With the exception of the outer segment's length, these values are only approximately known. It is possible, however, to make a good estimate of the match points if certain assumptions are made.

First, consider the on-axis condition. If we assume a set of spectral sensitivity functions for the receptors that are linear combinations of the CIE color matching data, then we should be in accordance with the experimental points at the 0%

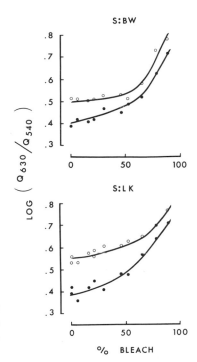

Figure 20.3. Rayleigh matches for observers BW and LK. Filled and open circles refer to on- and off-axis (3 mm) beams, respectively. The smooth lines were drawn through the data points by eye.

bleach. We have used the Vos and Walraven (1971) primaries for this purpose. As can be seen in Figure 20.4, these functions give a 630/540 ratio in good agreement with our subjects' values at the 0% bleach. To derive the other points, however, it is necessary to assume some value of optical density that matches one of the ratio values. We have chosen a value of .50 at the most sensitive wavelength for each of the two receptors. This value was chosen because it fits the experimental data for both subjects at the 88% bleach level. Once the 0 and 88% levels are satisfactorily fit, it is possible to calculate all the intermediate values from the Beer–Lambert expression. The resulting function is linear and is shown by the lower of the two straight lines for each subject in Figure 20.4. The predicted function does not provide a good fit to the experimental points. The data are positively accelerated compared to the linear prediction.

A similar account can be made for the off-axis condition. It is only necessary to assume some value for the pathlength reduction of the oblique rays. If we assume that the oblique rays pass through only 30% of the outer segment, we achieve a good fit to the 0% bleach level. The upper straight line for each subject in Figure 20.4 represents the predicted 630/540 ratios. As for the on-axis condition, the data are considerably bowed compared to the linear prediction.

There are really two difficulties associated with the foregoing self-screening analysis. The obvious one is, of course, that the predicted functions do not provide a good fit to the experimental analysis. Another problem is that the assumed

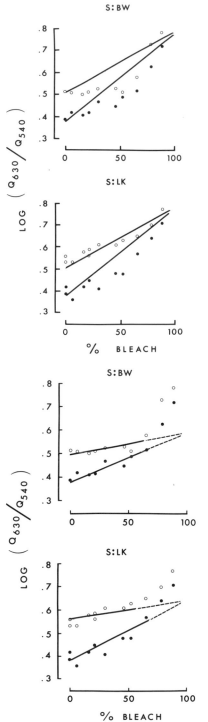

Figure 20.4. Same data as in Figure 20.3. The lower and upper lines in each plot represent the Rayleigh matches as predicted by self-screening for on- and off-axis beams, respectively. The predictions assume the Vos and Walraven primaries and a maximum optical density of .50.

Figure 20.5. Same data as in Figure 20.3. The lines are as in Figure 20.4, except that the maximum optical density is assumed to be .25 for BW and .35 for LK.

maximum optical density of .50 is somewhat higher than available direct estimates. King-Smith (1971), for example, has calculated a value of about .4 on the basis of reflection densitometry. If we take Dobelle, Marks, and MacNichol's (1969) single-cell photometry estimate of .0079 optical density unit per micrometer of outer segment, we come up with a value of .31, given a 40-μm outer-segment length. While it must be admitted that these estimates are rough, the fact remains that a value of .50 is clearly on the high side.

Given these difficulties, we considered the possibility that the self-screening analysis may hold only over the low and intermediate bleach levels. Consequently, we recalculated the predicted 630/540 ratios assuming lower values of optical density. These predicted linear functions had a smaller slope, as shown in Figure 20.5. We found that the two subjects required slightly different densities, .25 for BW and .35 for LK. Nevertheless, each subject's data were well described by the linear prediction up to about a 70% bleach level. In addition, we regarded the values of .25 and .35 as in better agreement with existing estimates than the previous value of .50.

In summary, we find, on the basis of manipulating the concentration of photo-pigment, that the alteration in Rayleigh equations caused by decentering the entry beam can only be partially explained by self-screening. The explanation holds well over the low and intermediate bleach levels. That self-screening is a factor in S–C II should not be too surprising since it derives from a simple physical principle, the Beer–Lambert law. What is perhaps more interesting is that it fails at all. This partial failure raises the important question of whether waveguide effects can provide a supplementary account.

Before discussing possible waveguide effects, one possible confounding factor should be considered. Although there is little evidence in its favor, a buildup of semistable, colored photoproducts by the bleaching light is possible. If this happens, it would alter the Rayleigh matches in a way that is predictable only if the spectral absorption properties of these photoproducts are known. This possibility seems unlikely since departures from the simple self-screening prediction would be expected much earlier than at the 70% bleach level. One reason for doing Experiment II, however, was to check on the possible confounding effects of stable, colored photoproducts.

The S–C II hue shift involves the comparison of monochromatic lights. If self-screening is the sole cause of the effect, then the magnitude of the shift should diminish as bleaching level increases. At a near total bleach, the hue shift should be immeasurably small. Unlike the effect on metamers, this prediction holds even if a colored photoproduct is generated by the bleaching light. This is true because isomers, unlike metamers, are unaffected by colored filters, that is, two lights of the same spectral composition will still be identical after the same selective filtering. For this reason, as well as our intrinsic interest in the hue shift itself, we measured S–C II in Experiment II at the highest bleaching level that allowed for stable hue matches.

The open circles in Figure 20.6 show the result for subject BW at the 88% bleach level. For comparison, the filled circles represent the 0% bleach level and are the same data as in Figure 20.1. The lines have been drawn through the data points by eye. The striking aspect of the high bleach results is that they depart dramatically from the prediction of zero shift. The 470- and 490-nm points are consistent with the self-screening prediction in that the hue shift is greatly reduced at the high bleach level; one could argue that an even higher bleach might have reduced the shift to zero. At all other spectral regions, however, there is actually a shift in the opposite direction from the 0% bleach level. This reversal is particularly large at 610 nm where the shift goes from +6.5 nm at a 0% bleach to −17 nm at an 88% bleach. We should again emphasize that the self-screening model unambiguously predicts a near-zero shift at such a low level of pigment concentration. Self-screening simply cannot accommodate the observed reversals.

In order to examine intermediate bleaching levels, we selected the 610-nm region for further study. Figure 20.7 shows the results for the same subject at various bleaching levels. Notice that at low and intermediate levels, there is a gradual decline in the shift toward zero that is consistent with self-screening. At about 60%, however, the data depart from the self-screening prediction, which is shown by the dotted line. The data reach zero shift at about 70%, which is much too soon according to self-screening. At higher levels, the reversal, apparent in Figure 20.6, is seen.

VI. Summary and Conclusions

In general, we feel that a strong statement is justified from our data: Self-screening alone can account for the S–C II only at low and intermediate bleaching levels. This conclusion is contrary to that reached by Brindley (1953) on the basis of some fragmentary observations. We have calculated that Brindley's highest bleach

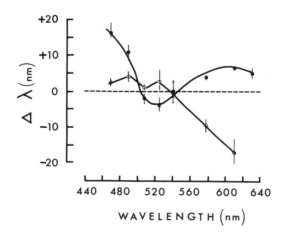

Figure 20.6. S–C II for 0% bleach (filled circles; same data as in Figure 20.1) and 88% bleach (open circles). Subject BW.

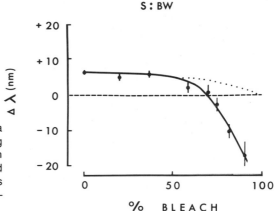

Figure 20.7. S–C II for BW with a 610-nm standard at various bleaching levels. The continuous line was drawn through the data by eye. The dotted line represents the expected results based on self-screening over the 50–100% bleach range.

level corresponded to our 70% condition. Thus, his measurements are consistent with ours, but are of limited generality. We are currently extending our experiments by repeating our measurements and studying more subjects.

Results from the high bleach conditions of Experiments I and II strongly indicate that self-screening is an inadequate explanation. What, then, is required to explain these data? Unless there is some factor of which we are unaware, we must conclude that the only available framework that is capable of accounting for our high bleach measurements is waveguide theory. We consider it plausible that there are relatively weak waveguide effects that become important only when the photopigment is severely depleted; that is, at low bleach levels a receptor's spectral sensitivity is determined almost entirely by the absorption properties of the photopigment. As bleaching increases, however, the wavelength-dependent waveguide effects become more important. At high bleach levels, that is, where pigment concentration is low, the wavelength selective effects of the receptor acting as a waveguide may become dominant. We are currently attempting to evaluate quantitatively this possibility based on waveguide principles.

REFERENCES

Brindley, G. S. The effects on colour vision of adaptation to very bright lights. *Journal of Physiology,* 1953, *122,* 332–350.

Brindley, G. S., & Rushton, W. A. H. The colour of monochromatic light when passed into the human retina from behind. *Journal of Physiology,* 1959, *147,* 204–208.

Brown, P. K., & Wald, G. Visual pigments in human and monkey retinas. *Nature,* 1963, *200,* 37–43.

Dartnall, H. J. A. *The visual pigments.* New York: Wiley, 1957.

Dobelle, W. H., Marks, W. B., & MacNichol, E. F. Visual pigment density in single primate foveal cones. *Science,* 1969, *166,* 1508–1510.

Enoch, J. M. Nature of the transmission of energy in the retinal receptors. *Journal of the Optical Society of America,* 1961, *51,* 1122–1126. (a)

Enoch, J. M. Visualization of waveguide modes in retinal receptors. *American Journal of Ophthalmology,* 1961, *51,* 1107–1118. (b)

Enoch, J. M. Waveguide modes in retinal receptors. *Science,* 1961, *133,* 1352–1354. (c)

Kapany, N. S., & Burke, J. J. Fiber optics. IX. Waveguide effects. *Journal of the Optical Society of America,* 1961, *51,* 1067–1078.

King-Smith, P. E. The optical density of erythrolabe determined by retinal densitometry. *Journal of Physiology,* 1971, *218,* 101–102P.

Miller, S. S. Psychophysical estimates of visual pigment densities in red–green dichromats. *Journal of Physiology,* 1972, *223,* 89–107.

Osterberg, H., Snitzer, E., Polanyi, M., & Hilberg, R. Optical wave-guide modes in small glass fibers. *Journal of the Optical Society of America,* 1959, *49,* 1128.

Rushton, W. A. H., & Henry, G. H. Bleaching and regeneration of cone pigments in man. *Vision Research,* 1968, *8,* 617–631.

Snyder, A. W., & Pask, C. The Stiles–Crawford effect—Explanation and consequences. *Vision Research,* 1973, *13,* 1115–1137.

Stiles, W. S. The luminous efficiency of monochromatic rays entering the eye pupil at different points and a new colour effect. *Proceedings of the Royal Society of London, Ser. B,* 1937, *123,* 90–118.

Stiles, W. S., & Crawford, B. H. The luminous efficiency of rays entering the eye pupil at different points. *Proceedings of the Royal Society of London, Ser. B, 112,* 428–450.

Toraldo di Francia, G. Retinal cones as dielectric antennas. *Journal of the Optical Society of America,* 1949, *39,* 324.

Vos, J. J., & Walraven, P. L. On the derivation of the foveal receptor primaries. *Vision Research,* 1971, *11,* 799–818.

Wald, G., & Brown, P. K. Human rhodopsin. *Science,* 1958, *127,* 222–226.

Walraven, P. L., & Bouman, M. A. Relation between directional sensitivity and spectral response curves in human cone vision. *Journal of the Optical Society of America,* 1960, *50,* 780–784.

21. VECP: Its Spectral Sensitivity[1]

John B. Siegfried

I. Introduction

This chapter compares electrophysiological visual evoked cortical potential (VECP) measures of spectral sensitivity with psychophysical measures of spectral sensitivity. In contrast to the electroretinogram (ERG), which remains largely scotopic regardless of the retinal area or location of the stimulus due to the effects of stray light (unless strong measures are taken to eliminate or minimize their effects), the VECP reflects largely photopic function (see Armington, 1964). This is thought to be the result of primarily two causes: (*a*) a "neural amplification" of the fovea resulting from much less convergence in the projection pathways for foveal cones than in those for rods and (*b*) greater proximity of the foveal cortical projection to the scalp recording electrode, the projection from the peripheral retina lying within the calcarine fissure at a greater distance from the scalp (Riggs & Wooten, 1972). While it has been demonstrated that if large stimulus fields are employed at scotopic levels of illumination the VECP exhibits scotopic spectral sensitivity (Klingaman, 1976; Wooten, 1972), this chapter will concentrate on the spectral sensitivity of the VECP under photopic conditions.

II. Methods

A. Electrophysiological Considerations

In psychophysical measurements, generally the subject is instructed to use a constant criterion, namely, to say "yes" if he can see the light flash and "no" if he

[1] Some of the research reported here was supported by National Science Foundation Research Grant GB 37665.

257

cannot. From these data, the threshold is abstracted, which is usually defined as a statistical point such as the value of stimulus energy that on one-half of the trials yields a response of yes, and on one-half of the trials a response of no. With electrophysiological data, we also utilize a constant response criterion; in this case, an electrical one.

A common way to abstract spectral sensitivity information from the VECP is as follows:

1. Select a number of stimulus wavelengths that adequately represent the visible spectrum.
2. Arrange a series of graded stimulus intensities.
3. For each wavelength, obtain the VECP in response to each level of intensity (presenting a sufficient number of flashes for adequate computer signal-to-noise enhancement).
4. Plot VECP amplitude or implicit time (latency to peak) as a function of log stimulus intensity for each wavelength.
5. Select a criterion amplitude or implicit time that is able to cut across the linear portions of these intensity functions.
6. At each wavelength, determine the stimulus energy necessary to elicit the criterion response.
7. Finally, plot the reciprocal of the energy required to elicit the criterion response as a function of wavelength.

This method produces a spectral sensitivity function defined in terms of equal stimulus–response effectiveness.

In practice, this procedure works well with implicit time measurements. However, such often is not the case for amplitude measurements due to the tendency of the response amplitude to "saturate" above moderate levels of retinal illuminance. Additionally, while VECP implicit time is closely controlled by stimulus parameters, amplitude tends to fluctuate with varying states of attention.

B. Stimulus Considerations

VECP spectral sensitivity has been studied by means of at least five procedures. These are:

1. Brief flashes of light presented against an otherwise dark field, with or without an adapting surround field
2. Temporal alternations of a test light and a standard or reference light
3. Sinusoidally modulated light
4. Spatial contrast reversal of a barred pattern
5. Brief flashes of light presented as increments upon a steady background light

Some of the results these various methods have produced will now be discussed.

III. Results of VECP Spectral Sensitivity Measurements

A. Brief Flashes of Light Presented against an Otherwise Dark Field

Brief flashes of light presented upon a dark background and viewed centrally lead to entoptic scatter to large portions of the retina, no matter how restricted the geometrical image. Thus, even though the retinal illuminance will be greatest within the geometrical image, which may be restricted to the fovea, great numbers of rod receptors will also be stimulated with flashing stray light. While the VECP is dominated by the projection from the fovea under these conditions, it is nevertheless possible that such stimulation of large areas of the peripheral retina can lead to rod intrusion in the VECP. Thus, one runs the risk of obtaining a spectral sensitivity curve that mixes cone and rod spectral sensitivities if the effects of stray light are not dealt with, and if the geometrical image is not limited to the rod-free fovea. VECP spectral sensitivity curves obtained using this procedure have tended to have broader shapes, and to be generally higher in the blue region of the spectrum than one would predict for an exclusively photopic function on the basis of psychophysical results (Cavonius, 1965).

B. Temporal Alterations of Test and Standard Light

Temporal alternation of a test and a standard or reference light in such a way that no overlap or dark interval exists between them reduces somewhat the effects of scattered light if the retinal illuminance of the two members of the temporally alternated pair is not too different. Then the major change from test to reference light will be one of spectral composition. An experiment employing this method (Siegfried, 1971) utilized a 750-msec reference white light, temporally alternated with a 250-msec narrow-band spectral light. Luminance of the reference light was held constant, while luminance of the test light was manipulated over a small range surrounding the luminance of the reference light. For test lights from a series of narrow wavelength bands representing the visible spectrum, luminances were found for which VECP amplitude produced by the transition from reference white light to test chromatic light equaled that produced by the transition from test chromatic light to reference white light. Psychophysical data were obtained in the same experimental sessions by determining which test light luminance setting produced a perception of brightness equal to that of the reference. Figure 21.1 reproduces the major results of this experiment, showing the excellent agreement between VECP and psychophysical data for each of two subjects.

C. Sinusoidally Modulated Light

Sinusoidally modulated light is employed to elicit "steady-state" evoked potentials. An overall adaptation level, or mean luminance level, is established around

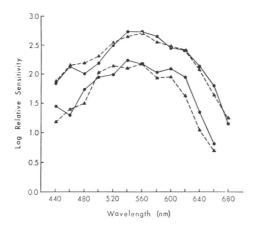

Figure 21.1. Mean log relative spectral sensitivity curves determined from evoked cortical potential data (solid lines and circles) and from psychophysical data (broken lines and triangles) obtained in the same experiment. The curves for one subject have been arbitrarily displaced downward .5 log unit for clarity. [From J.B. Siegfried, Spectral sensitivity of human visual evoked cortical potentials: A new method and a comparison with psychophysical data. *Vision Research*, 1971, *11*, 405-417.]

which the intensity of the light is modulated as a sinusoidal function of time. Because the input to the visual system is confined to a single temporal frequency, information concerning the temporal transfer function can be obtained. When employed to determine spectral sensitivity, mean luminance level is maintained at a constant value. In one experiment employing this method (Regan, 1970), a standard white and a spectral light were modulated at 100% depth and a frequency of 24 Hz, and were 180° out of phase. Luminance of the spectral light was varied, and the amplitude of the second harmonic of the stimulus modulation frequency was measured in the electroencephalogram (EEG). Using eight different spectral lights, Regan ascertained the amount of energy of the spectral light necessary to cause the second harmonic to fall to a minimum. The reciprocal of these energies, when plotted as a function of wavelength, yielded a spectral sensitivity curve that agreed to within .07 log unit of psychophysical settings of minimum flicker. The possibility of a relationship between psychophysical settings of minimum flicker and minimum VECP amplitudes had also been demonstrated in a more limited study (Siegfried, Tepas, Sperling, & Hiss, 1965).

D. Spatial Contrast Reversal of a Barred Pattern

Spatial contrast reversal of a barred pattern, as developed by Johnson, Riggs, and Schick (1966), is produced by optical shifting of a vertically oriented square-wave grating image horizontally on the retina by precisely the width of one bar. The resulting perception is one of a sharply focused grating whose adjacent bars instantaneously replace each other. In one experiment utilizing this stimulus technique to obtain spectral sensitivity information (May & Siegfried, 1970), the grating was composed of alternate black and colored bars. The wavelength of the colored bars was changed, and the grating was superimposed upon a steady white (xenon) background. For each wavelength, a series of stimulus intensities produced a graded series of VECP responses when amplitudes and implicit times were measured. Both criterion amplitude and criterion implicit time plots were constructed and employed

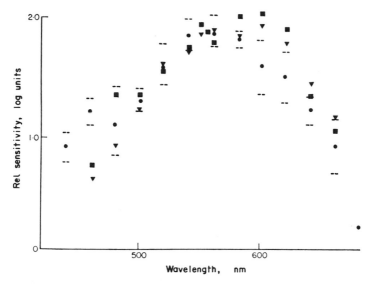

Figure 21.2. A comparison of spectral sensitivity data from subject JS derived from criterion amplitude difference (Siegfried, 1971) (circles) and criterion amplitude (squares) and criterion implicit time (triangles) data of May and Siegfried (1970). Horizontal bars denote the range of data points for the data of Siegfried. The curves in this figure were normalized at 560 nm. [From J.G. May & J.B. Siegfried, Spectral sensitivity of the human VER obtained with an alternating barred pattern. *Vision Research,* 1970, *10,* 1399–1410.]

to plot spectral sensitivity curves. Results were in close agreement with psychophysical results obtained in the same experiment. Figure 21.2 shows some of the results of this study.

E. Brief Flashes of Light as Increments on a Steady Background Light

A small incremental test light may be superimposed upon a large, steady background adapting field. VECPs are obtained to the test lights, which are of brief duration. In one such study (Siegfried, 1975), psychophysical increment thresholds were obtained for a 1° visual angle 50-msec duration test light superimposed upon a 20° steady white (equal energy) background. At each of a series of test light wavelengths, VECPs were elicited to a graded series of luminances, beginning with psychophysical increment threshold value. The criterion implicit time method was employed to derive a spectral sensitivity curve. Results for one subject are shown in Figure 21.3. The VECP curve based on criterion implicit time measurements is in excellent agreement with that obtained with the same subject by the psychophysical procedure of increment threshold adjustment.

In summary, it can be stated in general that when stimulus conditions are appropriately manipulated, it is possible to elicit VECPs whose properties are exclusively

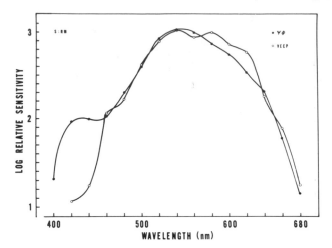

Figure 21.3. Mean log relative spectral sensitivity curves determined from the VECP criterion implicit time data (open circles) and from psychophysical data (filled circles) obtained in the same experiment. Test flashes presented superimposed upon a white (equal energy) background. Curves were adjusted vertically by inspection for best agreement over the middle- and long-wavelength region of the spectrum.

photopic. These conditions include (*a*) test target limited to the fovea; (*b*) photopic levels of illumination; and (*c*) steady adaptation of the peripheral retina. Under these conditions, psychophysical and VECP spectral sensitivity are both photopic and agree with each other whether the electrophysiological curve is derived from implicit time or from amplitude measures (see also DeVoe, Ripps, & Vaughan, 1968; Dobson, 1976). Under neutral background adaptation conditions, the results of most studies show that implicit time is the preferred measure, exhibiting less variability than results based on amplitude measures.

IV. Spectral Adaptation

Three systems underlie human chromatic vision. These originate in three photopigments with differing action spectra residing in different cone receptors. Since spectral adaptation of these systems is largely independent, selective chromatic adaptation results in complex changes in the spectral sensitivity function. In psychophysical work, experiments based on the two-color threshold technique of Stiles (1949) have demonstrated complex changes resulting from spectral adaptation. However, attempts to demonstrate comparable effects in the human ERG have been largely disappointing (see Cavonius, 1962). Small effects have been observed, but they do not compare in magnitude with those observed for psychophysical methods. In contrast to ERG results, relatively strong selective adaptation effects have been shown in VECP records. Burkhardt and Riggs (1967) superimposed a 10° narrow-band flickering stimulus (17.6 Hz) upon a 16° narrow-band background.

They found that the greatest amplitude VECP was observed when the wavelengths of the test flash and the background differed by a large amount. They also found wavelength-dependent temporal effects and observed temporal phase shifts in the VECP of up to 180°. It has also been shown that the effects of selective adaptation of the VECP are strongly dependent upon modulation frequency (Regan, 1968), suggesting that different underlying mechanisms have different time constants.

Numerous additional studies have reported data showing that the VECP is susceptible to strong modification by spectral adaptation backgrounds (Estévez, Spekreijse, van den Berg, & Cavonius, 1975; Huber, 1972; Kaneko, Nakajima, Akamatsu, Sugimachi, Kanbayashi, & Hatada, 1966; Kellerman & Adachi-Usami, 1972/1973; White, 1976; Yamanaka, Sobagaki, & Nayatani, 1973). The existence of specific "color channels" in human pattern vision has, in addition, been suggested by Regan (1973, 1974). Thus, under certain conditions, VECP amplitude and phase are dependent upon the wavelength of the background light.

An experiment was recently carried out to assess the effects of narrow-band spectral adaptation upon the VECP spectral sensitivity function (Siegfried, 1975). In this experiment a psychophysical increment threshold spectral sensitivity curve was first obtained by the method of adjustment for two narrow-band spectral background conditions: yellow (585 nm) and blue (460 nm). The test stimulus was a superimposed 1° visual angle centrally fixated flash, of 100-msec duration, presented at a frequency of 1 Hz. Then, with the same testing conditions and the same subjects, VECP spectral sensitivity curves were obtained for each of these background conditions using the method of criterion implicit time. The results for the

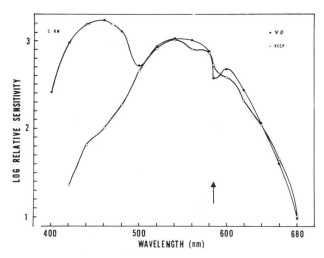

Figure 21.4. Mean log relative spectral sensitivity curves determined from VECP criterion implicit time data (open circles) and from psychophysical data (filled circles) obtained in the same experiment. Test flashes presented superimposed upon a yellow (585 nm) background. Curves were adjusted vertically by inspection for best agreement over the middle- and long-wavelength region of the spectrum.

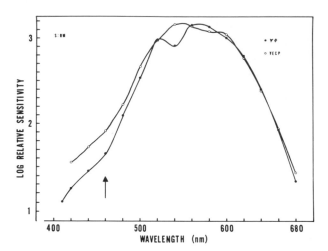

Figure 21.5. Mean log relative spectral sensitivity curves determined from VECP criterion implicit time data (open circles) and from psychophysical data (filled circles) obtained in the same experiment. Test flashes presented superimposed upon a blue (460 nm) background. Curves were adjusted vertically by inspection for best agreement over the middle- and long-wavelength region of the spectrum.

yellow and blue background conditions are shown in Figures 21.4 and 21.5, respectively. While there is good agreement between the psychophysical curve and the VECP curve for the blue background condition (Figure 21.5), the same is not the case with the yellow adaptation condition. With the yellow background (Figure 21.4), agreement is excellent in the long- and middle-wavelength regions of the spectrum, but the VECP curve does not exhibit the relatively high sensitivity in the short-wavelength region noticed in the psychophysical curve. Additional experiments have demonstrated that the short-wavelength-sensitive mechanism has longer implicit times than mechanisms operating in the middle- and long-wavelength regions of the spectrum (Siegfried, 1976, unpublished data; Krauskopf, 1973). This would explain why the VECP spectral sensitivity curve derived from criterion implicit time data would fail to agree with the psychophysical increment threshold curve in the short-wavelength region of the spectrum when yellow adaptation has been employed to partially isolate the short-wavelength-sensitive mechanism. The work of Boynton and Whitten (1972), who investigated selective chromatic adaptation in primate photoreceptors, suggests that these longer implicit times can already be seen at the receptor level. In addition, it has been shown that lights stimulating primarily the short-wavelength-sensitive mechanism are associated with longer psychophysical reaction times than are characteristic of those associated with light flashes in other regions of the visible spectrum (Mollon & Krauskopf, 1973). It has recently been demonstrated that under the same conditions that produce unexpectedly long implicit times in the VECP, the resulting amplitudes of VECP responses are also decreased (Zrenner, 1976, pp. 241–246; Siegfried, unpublished data).

V. Conclusion

It has been clearly demonstrated that the VECP spectral sensitivity function is photopic under well-controlled stimulus conditions designed to assure stimulation of photopic mechanisms only. It is also becoming clear that under conditions of narrow-band spectral adaptation, VECP spectral sensitivity agrees with psychophysical spectral sensitivity under identical conditions when either criterion amplitude or criterion implicit time is employed, except when the short-wavelength-sensitive mechanism is the primary origin of the electrophysiological response. Then, because of its longer implicit time and smaller amplitude, the VECP curve indicates a lower sensitivity than the psychophysical curve in the short-wavelength region of the spectrum.

REFERENCES

Armington, J. C. Relations between electroretinograms and occipital potentials elicited by flickering stimuli. *Documenta Ophthalmologica*, 1964, *28*, 194–206.

Boynton, R. M., & Whitten, D. N. Selective chromatic adaptation in primate photoreceptors. *Vision Research*, 1972, *12*, 855–874.

Burkhardt, D. A., & Riggs, L. A. Modification of the human visual evoked potential by monochromatic backgrounds. *Vision Research*, 1967, *7*, 453–459.

Cavonius, C. R. *The effects of chromatic adaptation upon the human electroretinogram.* Unpublished doctoral dissertation, Brown University, Providence, Rhode Island, 1962.

Cavonius, C. R. Evoked response of the human visual cortex: Spectral sensitivity. *Psychonomic Science*, 1965, *2*, 185–186.

DeVoe, R. G., Ripps, H., & Vaughan, H. G., Jr. Cortical responses to stimulation of the human fovea. *Vision Research*, 1968, *8*, 135–147.

Dobson, V. Spectral sensitivity of the 2-month infant as measured by the visually evoked cortical potential. *Vision Research*, 1976, *16*, 367–374.

Estévez, O., Spekreijse, T. J., van den Berg, T. P., & Cavonius, C. R. The spectral sensitivities of isolated human color mechanisms determined from contrast evoked potential measurements. *Vision Research*, 1975, *15*, 1205–1212.

Huber, C. Visual evoked responses during exposure to strong colored lights. *Ophthalmic Research*, 1972, *3*, 55–62.

Johnson, E. P., Riggs, L. A., & Schick, A. M. L. Photopic retinal potentials evoked by phase alternation of a barred pattern. In H. M. Burian & J. H. Jacobson (Eds.), *Clinical electroretinography*. Third International Society for Clinical Electroretinography (ISCERG) Symposium. *Vision Research*, 1966, *6* (suppl.).

Kaneko, H., Nakajima, A., Akamatsu, T., Sugimachi, T., Kanbayashi, S., & Hatada, T. Clinical application of VEP (VEP by monochromatic color flicker stimuli). In H. M. Burian & J. H. Jacobson (Eds.), *Clinical electroretinography*. Third International Society for Clinical Electroretinography (ISCERG) Symposium. *Vision Research*, 1966, *6* (suppl.).

Kellerman, F. J., & Adachi-Usami, E. Spectral sensitivities of colour mechanisms isolated by the human visual evoked response. *Ophthalmic Research*, 1972/1973, *4*, 199–210.

Klingaman, R. L. The human visual evoked cortical potential and dark adaptation. *Vision Research*, 1976, *16*, 1471–1477.

Krauskopf, J. Contributions of the primary chromatic mechanisms to the generation of visual evoked potentials. *Vision Research*, 1973, *13*, 2289–2298.

May, J. G., & Siegfried, J. B. Spectral sensitivity of the human VER obtained with an alternating barred pattern. *Vision Research,* 1970, *10,* 1399–1410.

Mollon, J. D., & Krauskopf, J. Reaction time as a measure of the temporal response properties of individual colour mechanisms. *Vision Research,* 1973, *13,* 27–40.

Regan, D. Chromatic adaptation and steady-state evoked potentials. *Vision Research,* 1968, *8,* 149–158.

Regan, D. Objective method of measuring the relative spectral luminosity curve in man. *Journal of the Optical Society of America,* 1970, *60,* 856–859.

Regan, D. An evoked potential correlate of colour: Evoked potential findings and single-cell speculations. *Vision Research,* 1973, *13,* 1933–1941.

Regan, D. Electrophysiological evidence for colour channels in human pattern vision. *Nature,* 1974, *250,* 437–439.

Riggs, L. A., & Wooten, B. R. Electrical measures and psychophysical data on human vision. In D. Jameson & L. M. Hurvich (Eds.), *Handbook of sensory physiology* (Vol. VII/4): *Visual psychophysics.* New York: Springer-Verlag, 1972.

Siegfried, J. B. Spectral sensitivity of human visual evoked cortical potentials: A new method and a comparison with psychophysical data. *Vision Research,* 1971, *11,* 405–417.

Siegfried, J. B. Effects of spectral adaptation on the spectral sensitivity function of the visual evoked cortical potential. Association for Research in Vision and Ophthalmology, Spring Meeting Program, 1975 (abstr.).

Siegfried, J. B. VECP implicit time and narrow band spectral adaptation. Association for Research in Vision and Ophthalmology, Spring Meeting Program, 1976 (abstr.).

Siegfried, J. B., Tepas, D. I., Sperling, H. G., & Hiss, R. A. Evoked potential correlates of psychophysical responses: Heterochromatic brightness matching. *Science,* 1965, *149,* 321–323.

Stiles, W. S. Increment thresholds and the mechanisms of colour vision. *Documenta Ophthalmologica,* 1949, *3,* 138–165.

White, C. T. Personal communication, 1976.

Wooten, B. R. Photopic and scotopic contributions to the human visually evoked cortical potential. *Vision Research,* 1972, *12,* 1647–1660.

Yamanaka, T., Sobagaki, H., & Nayatani, Y. Opponent-colors responses in the visually evoked potential in man. *Vision Research,* 1973, *13,* 1319–1333.

Zrenner, E., & Kojima, M. Visually evoked cortical potential (VECP) in dichromats. In E. B. Streiff (Ed.), *Modern problems in ophthalmology* (Vol. 17). Basel: S. Karger, 1976.

22. Studies of Form-Contingent Color Aftereffects[1]

Keith D. White

I. Background

Form-contingent color aftereffects (CAEs) are perceptual changes that are seen as an appearance of hues on particular black and white patterns. Notable features that distinguish CAEs from classic visual aftereffects such as ordinary afterimages include (*a*) the fact that the appearance of CAEs depends to an unusual degree upon shared pattern attributes (such as the orientations, or slants, of lines present on patterns used to establish and to test CAEs), and (*b*) the long-lasting persistence of the perceptual changes.

General methods for demonstrating CAEs were originated by McCollough (1965) and are still widely used today. CAEs may be established by a few minutes' inspection of two oppositely colored patterns presented alternately; for example, one pattern is a grating composed of red and black vertical lines and the other pattern is a grating of green and black horizontal lines. The vertical grating is viewed for a few seconds, then the horizontal one is viewed. The subject alternates between the gratings throughout the period of inspection. Following their establishment, CAEs may be revealed when the subject sees black and white test lines that appear subjectively colored. Vertical test lines look faintly greenish and horizontal ones look pinkish. Oblique lines, however, still appear white. The colors seen as aftereffects are contingent upon (though complementary to and less saturated in appearance than) the particular color-orientation pairings that had been used to establish them. But the most striking distinction of CAEs is their time course for

[1]This research was conducted at the W.S. Hunter Laboratory of Psychology at Brown University, and was supported by a NSF predoctoral fellowship to K. White and by USPHS Grants EY00744 and EY00030 to L.A. Riggs.

decay; they can often be revealed in tests made many hours, or days, or sometimes even weeks after they were established.

Early work on CAEs generated both considerable experimental interest and a variety of theoretical accounts, with models ranging in emphasis from neurophysiological constructs to classic conditioning or memorylike processes (for reviews, see Anstis, 1975; Harris, in press; Skowbo, Timney, Gentry, & Morant, 1975; Stromeyer, in press). This theoretical diversity can be attributed in part to the very features distinguishing CAEs in that dependence upon such pattern attributes as line orientation seems akin to known receptive field arrangements (e.g., Hubel & Wiesel, 1965; McCollough, 1965; White & Riggs, 1974), whereas long-lasting persistence seems more nearly akin to learning and remembering (e.g., Riggs, White, & Eimas, 1974). But also contributing to this theoretical diversity was a manner of explication prevailing in the Zeitgeist, an approach to the study of sensory coding that can be called *heuristic neuromythology.*[2] The approach was heuristic in that neurophysiologists studying single units and psychophysicists studying aftereffects read one another's work enthusiastically, and attempted to identify in their respective findings those data that were able to be plausibly interrelated; yet it sometimes became neuromythology in that no compelling proof showed that the activity of single neural units gave rise to elementary percepts or, conversely, that particular perceptual findings had to imply the presence in the brain of a corresponding class of individual neurons (Barlow, 1972; Erickson, 1974; Sherrington, 1941). The zealous use of this manner of explanation perhaps led at first to an electric feeling of anticipation that deep secrets of the brain were soon to be revealed, but later, given complex results, led to an extreme lack of reliance on any specific neurophysiological evidence that explained CAEs. Still the focal issue, whether CAEs are thought of as cells or as recollections, is to ask what the nervous system does and how it does it.

Inasmuch as aftereffects are perceptual changes that persist in the absence of the specific stimulation that produced them, the relevant perceptual information must be retained within the nervous system. Our selective vulnerability to aftereffects indicates that these neural mechanisms must be somehow specialized in their abilities for information transfer. Important questions about the mechanisms underlying CAEs are whether they are comprised of one or many classes of neurons, how they acquaint the brain with their transferred information, and in what ways they are specialized to do so. These questions make use of the principle that, at some point in the nervous system, the distinction between receptive fields underlying pattern vision and neural substrates of learning or memory becomes less pronounced (Gross, Bender, & Rocha-Miranda, 1974; Hubel & Wiesel, 1965, 1968; Kluver &

---

[2]I first heard this phrase in a colloquium given by Dr. Jacob Nachmias. Although the term "mythology" sometimes connotes lack of a truthful basis, the word is used here in stricter accord with the definition of myth as a "story . . . that serves to unfold part of the world view . . . or explain a . . . natural phenomenon [Webster's Seventh New Collegiate Dictionary]."

Bucy, 1939; Mishkin, 1972; Penfield & Milner, 1958; Zeki, 1971, 1974). The rationale we follow in our psychophysical studies of CAEs is to define them operationally through manipulation of stimulus parameters; first, we measure the selective character of the responses, and second, we seek to enable neurophysiological explorations that can make use of the same stimulus variables and similar methods of assessment.

II. Assessment of Aftereffects

Let us turn now to methods devised for operational studies of CAEs. These are similar to McCollough's (1965) in the inspection procedure but differ with regard to testing in that colorimetric test procedures are used to secure more objective and quantitative assessments of CAE strengths. Riggs, White, and Eimas (1973, 1974) developed a color-cancellation procedure in which the test gratings themselves are adjusted in chromaticity to attain a point of subjective equality for color. Physical chromaticities produced on a bipartite test pattern serve to cancel out (or titrate) the subjective colorations of the aftereffects so that a color match between two test gratings of different orientations can be achieved. At the point of color match the two gratings (which are present in top and bottom halves of the test pattern) typically appear nearly neutral in color, ensuring that the test pattern can be made to look essentially the same whether CAEs are vivid or weak,[3] thereby reducing the subject's awareness of his own CAE strengths. This is accomplished by a special color-mixing device that enables chromaticities produced on the test gratings to lie on a particular complementary axis in the CIE chromaticity specification system (see White, 1976a). Our cancellation procedure relies on the assumptions that (a) the colors seen as aftereffects would be complementary to the colors viewed during the inspection period and (b) subjective colorations would obey laws of color mixture not radically different from those for chromatic lights. An important constraint in practice is that chromatic lights actually used for inspection and for

---

[3]Since both the pinkish and greenish aftereffects are being canceled simultaneously on different areas of the test pattern, an imbalance in the relative vividness of the subjective colorations (or an imbalance in the canceling chromaticities) would fail to ensure the same judgmental endpoint throughout the course of measurements. Such imbalances are revealed as a fairly uniform wash of color over the whole test pattern when its top and bottom halves have been set to match; the overall color can be judged relative to the achromatic surround (White, 1976a). Most subjects frequently judge the appearance as a neutral gray at the match point, evidence that all the relative balances are fairly good. Less often the test pattern is tinged with hue, reported as greenish more frequently than pinkish, bluish, or yellowish. Nearly the same sorts of hue reports are obtained from pretests in the absence of CAEs as from tests of vivid CAEs, suggesting that the relative balance of the subjective colorations is not much worse than the relative balance of the cancellation chromaticities. Pilot work indicated the importance of choosing inspection pattern chromaticities whose additive mixture appeared achromatic (White, 1976a) to achieve proper balance of the CAEs, but we have not applied this stringent criterion for each individual subject.

testing be sufficiently complementary to one another for satisfactory attainment of the criterion appearances.

Systematizing the manner of eliciting the subject's report can allow valid comparisons of results from different individuals and even from different laboratories by the use of standardized chromaticity units to score the color judgments. Colorimetric testing procedures are therefore powerful empirical tools (see also Fidell, 1970; Hepler, 1971; MacKay & MacKay, 1974; Shute, 1977; Sigel & Nachmias, 1975; Skowbo, Gentry, Timney, & Morant, 1974). Nevertheless, chromaticity scores give only *indirect* measures since CAEs themselves must be a state of the nervous system. Evidence that CAEs are present comes from altered color reports but, of course, the reports are not the aftereffects per se. Inferences about CAE strengths based on chromaticity scores are accordingly constrained in two important ways. First, color judgments depend on many factors in addition to the presence of CAEs, and the absence of appropriate controls for them serves to alter the nature of the measuring instrument itself (e.g., the lights would certainly be less effective for color cancellation if viewed only scotopically). For further discussion see White (1976b). Second, chromaticity scores must be expressed so as to yield useful estimates of the strengths of CAEs themselves. The CIE specification system provides many standard measures by which to assign numerical values to the test results, yet it is not really clear how any of those numbers must represent the actual amounts of CAEs. There would be little debate that as the CAEs become more vivid, chromaticity measures that correlate with subjective saturation would be expected to increase in an ordinal fashion. But would each unit of the chromaticity score represent the same amount of CAE? Studies addressing this question found that the chromaticity measure of *excitation purity* (the index used on all figures here) can be treated as approximately linearly representative of CAE strengths, based on evidence of (*a*) the ability to predict qualitative as well as quantitative changes in the colors of CAEs through linear summation and (*b*) the ability to translate target measures from high scale ranges to low ones (White, 1977). We therefore use units of excitation purity (P_e) to provide the "index of CAE strength."

Application of our colorimetric testing procedure has used a typical sequence of experimental steps carried out for each individual subject. Before CAEs are built up, the subject is light-adapted for at least 1 min, and then is presented the bipartite test pattern to make 10 color-matching judgments (called pretests). The subject's task is to adjust the chromaticities produced by the color-mixing device until the pair of gratings present on the test pattern appear to be matched in color (and nearly neutral). These pretests serve to measure possible small biases for color on the test gratings before building up CAEs. Next, a period of inspection establishes the CAEs using alternate presentations of two complementary colored gratings. After the inspection phase, a series of test sessions is begun. Each test session is comprised of 10 judgments made in the same way as the pretests but, because of the presence of CAEs, the test judgments require a change in chromaticities to yield a matched appearance on the testing pattern. The required change in chromaticity,

ΔP_e, provides our index of CAE strength.[4] Test sessions are usually made at progressively longer times after inspection until the CAEs have largely decayed away.

III. Experimental Results

A. Time Courses for Establishment and Decay

Riggs *et al.* (1973, 1974) first used this approach to study the time courses for establishment and decay of CAEs, finding that: (*a*) Pretest scores for some subjects showed small but reliable differences from the point of objective equality for color on the test gratings (see also MacKay & MacKay, 1974; White, 1976b). (*b*) Individual subjects differed in the strength of CAE established by a particular period of inspection. (*c*) CAE strength increased with duration of the inspection period over the range from 15 sec to at least 150 min of inspection. The increase showed diminishing returns; the square root of inspection duration was a good predictor of the score for CAE strength. (*d*) CAE strengths declined with time after inspection, tracing time courses for decay such as those illustrated in Section III,B. The functional relationship between CAE strengths and time after inspection was poorly described as a simple exponential decay. The persistence of CAEs, as judged by significant differences in the scores for pretests and tests made late in decay, ranged from as little as 2 hr following 15 sec of inspection (Subject PE) to as much as 15 days following 150 min of inspection (Subject KW). (*e*) The most strikingly regular feature in the data was a high correlation between strengths measured soon after inspection and the subsequent rates of decline with time. Unlike our other observations, this one required no specific regard either to individual differences or to the particular inspection durations that had established the CAEs (see Section III,E).

---

[4]To take as a measure the change in scores relies on pretests providing a stable indication of the "baseline." We gauged pretest score stability using sequences like a typical experiment, but with no inspection period and hence no buildup of CAEs. Results indicate suitable reproducibility over a period of 2–3 hr, but stability declines for times as long as a day. Statistically significant fluctuations in the pretest scores over time occur in the absence of specifically produced CAEs. Other statistical considerations we have evaluated are (*a*) the distributions of scores within a test (or pretest) session; (*b*) the stochastic independence of judgments made within a session; and (*c*) the reliability of establishing identical CAEs with separate but otherwise identical periods of inspection (see White, 1976b, 1977). By examining samples of up to 2000 judgments, we found that (*a*) the mean and standard deviation adequately represent scores within a test session, even though the sample size is small (i.e., 10 judgments); (*b*) the covariance of successive judgments within each test session is only a small proportion of the total test session variance (i.e., though not truly independent, the repeated measures do serve to reduce uncertainty); and (*c*) estimated standard errors of the means based on individual test sessions tend to be too low, but obtained standard errors are still suitably reliable (based on 11 runs using the same type of inspection made over a period exceeding 1 year, the obtained standard errors had values of about P_e = .005).

B. Comparison of Testing Procedures

Our within-subject repeated-measures design is simple to implement but may yield confounded results from successive induction or reduction influences exerted by the test procedure itself on CAE decay. We evaluated this possibility by comparing the results from our repeated-tests procedure with those obtained in a different procedure using delayed discrete test sessions (see also Jones & Holding, 1975).[5] Each of our seven subjects participated individually in at least four separate but otherwise identical periods of inspection, presented in different months to minimize carryover of CAEs. Following one of the inspections there were repeated tests so that a session of 10 judgments was made at each of five elapsed times: immediately, and about 1, 4, 16, and 96 or more hours after the end of inspection. Following the other inspection periods no test was made until a delay interval had elapsed; then there was one discrete test session of 10 judgments. Sample results from one subject (PG) are shown in Figure 22.1.

The graph in Figure 22.1 shows the index of CAE strength (in percentage units of ΔP_e for the test judgments) as a function of time after inspection (shown in minutes on a logarithmic scale) in order to compare the results of repeated versus delayed test procedures. Each plotted point represents the mean P_e for 10 judgments at the indicated mean time after inspection. Vertical bars mark off 1 SD (standard deviation) of the scores on either side of the mean. Each of the five different symbols stands for a separate period of inspection that had preceded the tests. Open circles with connecting lines plot results from the repeated-tests procedure. Each filled symbol plots results from a delayed discrete test, each made after its own inspection. For the filled upright triangle, the delay between end of inspection and testing was about 1 hr, for the filled circle about 17 hr, and for the filled square about 100 hr. Subject PG's results are representative of all seven subjects in showing that scores on delayed and repeated tests declined with time along similar courses. Her results are not representative of the sizes or directions of differences between conditions, however. Across all subjects, scores on the delayed discrete tests were "too low" or "too high" relative to repeated tests about equally often for each decay time. Even though these results cannot prove the absence of systematic differences due to the testing

---

[5]Jones and Holding (1975) also compared repeated-tests versus delayed discrete test procedures, but concluded that CAEs decay little if at all in the absence of testing. Important differences between their experiment and ours include their use of a between-subject (or groups) design, and of a psychophysical task like that of Fidell (1970) (i.e., making a single test grating appear subjectively neutral, rather than our matching task). Reservations in generalizing Jones and Holding's conclusions to our methods are the following: (a) Because of significant individual differences, averaging the results of a group of subjects does not necessarily represent the behaviors of any particular individual. (b) The repeated-tests group differed from the delayed-test groups in the accumulated amount of practice for making the test judgments (Jones, personal communication), potentially yielding differences in reliability. (c) Jones and Holding's largest averaged scores correspond approximately to $P_e = .034$ (Jones, personal communication) with unreported reliability measures. Fidell's (1970) estimates of reliability using a similar task (although different equipment, etc.) reported a range of *pretest* scores exceeding $P_e = .05$, about 1.6 times larger than Jones and Holding's (1975) largest reported values.

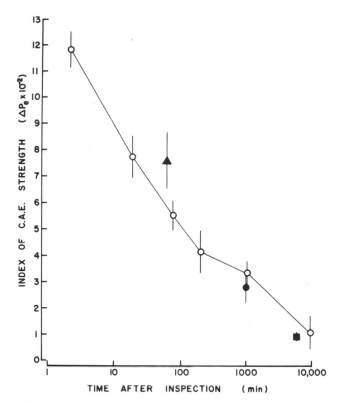

Figure 22.1. Comparison of repeated-testing and delayed discrete testing procedures. Scores on the index of CAE strength ($\Delta P_e + 10^{-2}$) are shown as a function of time after inspection (in minutes, on a log scale) for Subject PG. Open symbols and their connecting lines are from the repeated-tests procedure, while each closed symbol represents a delayed discrete test. Each plotted point shows the mean P_e and vertical bars mark off ± 1 SD for the 10 test judgments. Similar courses of CAE decay were found whether scores were obtained in repeated-testing or in delayed discrete testing procedures.

procedure, they demonstrate that induction or reduction effects must either be small or else equally potent and mutually offsetting. We concluded that repeated testing, clearly a much more rapid way to obtain the data, seems valid for a first approximation to measuring the time course for CAE decay.

C. Parameters of Inspection

Several of us have gone on to apply the same basic repeated-tests procedure in studying parameters of the inspection and testing stimulation. The reasoning we follow to decide whether manipulation of the *inspection* stimuli influenced CAE establishment is simply the following: If exactly the same test pattern is used for assessment but subjects require different amounts of chromatic change to yield a matched appearance for it (depending upon the preceding inspection conditions), and if reliable changes in the chromaticities persist throughout the course of decay, then we conclude that the observed persistent changes must have been due to a change in the CAEs themselves as a result of the targeted stimulus manipulation.

1. LUMINANCE

The first study of this kind examined luminance as a variable, finding that inspection of high-luminance patterns evoked systematically larger test scores than did inspection of otherwise similar low-luminance patterns. These results, and others on luminance as a parameter of the testing stimulation, are detailed elsewhere (White, 1976a).

2. PRESENTATION RATE

We also measured the influence of presentation rate of the inspection patterns on the establishment of CAEs. Procedures and equipment were similar to those detailed by White (1976a) with the exceptions that (a) the luminances used for inspection patterns and for the test pattern were held constant (in all but one case, see the following); (b) all tests were made on the same, steadily presented test pattern; (c) each of the separate periods of inspection was of 15-min duration (White had used 25 min); and (d) in separate periods of inspection, the magenta and green inspection patterns were alternated at different speeds. The total number of inspection pattern presentations covaried exactly with their presentation rate.

Figure 22.2 presents sample results showing the decline in index of CAE strength (in percentage units of ΔP_e) with the lapse of time after inspection (in minutes on a log scale). Each plotted point in Figure 22.2 stands for the same measures as in Figure 22.1, that is, mean ΔP_e and ± 1 standard deviation for 10 test judgments. These results are from one subject (JR). Each symbol shape represents a different pattern presentation rate used during the preceding inspection period. Clearly, there are reliable and persistent changes in the indexed CAE strengths that can be attributed to pattern presentation rate. The smooth functions drawn through each data set, lines fitted by the method of least squares, pass near the observed values throughout the range of elapsed times (tests were made for about 1 day following inspection). We have used smooth functions like these to derive an index of initial CAE strength which serves as a reduced description of each data set. Because the scores are declining over time, the changes in strength due to decay must be partialed out in order to examine the influences on strength that were due to the presentation rates. The index of initial strength is one way to partial out decay since we define it as the expected value of ΔP_e at 1 min after inspection (i.e., $t = 1$ min or $\log t = 0$). This is simply the calculated value for a regression coefficient, the intercept in our particular fitted functions (see also White, 1976b, 1977). The index of initial strength for the data set shown by triangles in Figure 22.2 is represented at the leftmost endpoint of the dotted line. Usually, specifying only one of the two regression coefficients

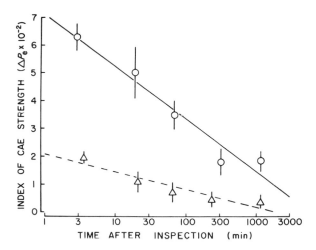

Figure 22.2. Influence of inspection pattern presentation rate on CAE establishment. Scores on the index of CAE strength ($\Delta P_e \times 10^{-2}$) for Subject JR are shown as a function of time after inspection (in minutes on a log scale). Each plotted point represents the same measures as in Figure 22.1 (mean and ± 1 *SD* of P_e for 10 judgments). The two curves represent different pattern presentation rates used in the preceding inspection periods. Circles show test results following inspection at a low rate (.0082 cycle sec^{-1}), while triangles were obtained after inspection at a high rate (18.2 cycles sec^{-1}). Smooth lines were fitted to the data by the method of least squares. The intercept of each line at $t = 1$ min (i.e., log $t = 0$) provides the respective index of initial strength (see text).

would not be adequate, but here their values are so highly correlated as to provide the key information in a single number (see Section III,E).

The overall relationships found between inspection pattern presentation rate and established CAE strengths are shown in Figure 22.3A as a highly condensed representation of 1260 observations (3 subjects $\times$ 7 periods of inspection $\times$ 60 judgments each). Figure 22.3A shows the index of *initial* strength (in percentage units of ΔP_e) as a function of inspection pattern presentation rate (cycles per second on a log scale). Small dots show the derived initial strengths, with lines of different textures used to connect the derived measures for different subjects. Individual subjects differ in their initial strengths but show qualitatively similar relationships between their scores and the pattern presentation rate. For all 3 subjects, scores were moderate following inspection at the lowest rate (one 7½-min presentation of each colored grating, or 1 cycle during the 15-min inspection period), and were higher for somewhat faster rates but went down again for rates above 1 cycle sec^{-1}. The highest rate used (18.2 cycles sec^{-1}, or 16,400 presentations of each colored grating) was definitely flickering. Points beyond the break in the abscissa mimicked a presentation rate above the flicker fusion frequency; we projected the inspection patterns simultaneously, adding neutral filters of density .3 to approximate the Talbot level brightness. Strengths following this simultaneous, luminance-attenuated presentation showed little further change, suggesting that 18.2 cycles sec^{-1} had

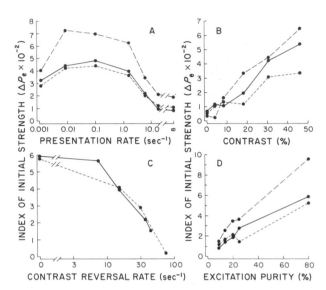

Figure 22.3. Some parametric influences of inspection stimulation on CAE establishment. (A) Index of initial strength ($\Delta P_e + 10^{-2}$) shown as a function of inspection pattern presentation rate (cycles per second on a log scale). Each dot represents a derived measure, the expected value of ΔP_e at $t = 1$ min, obtained from least-squares fits (see text). Lines connect the derived values for different individuals (— —,JR; ———,SE; ---,LR). (B) Index of initial strength as a function of inspection pattern contrast. Lines again connect the derived measures for individual subjects (— —,JR; ———,SE; ---,DP). (C) Index of initial strength as a function of rate of contrast reversal (cycles per second on a log scale). Individual subjects are represented as in the other panels (---,KW; ———,JF). (D) Index of initial strength as a function of excitation purity of the chromatic lights that illuminated the inspection patterns (— —,TD; ———,TA; ---,AP).

nearly reached the practical upper limit of presentation rates. We concluded that inspection pattern presentation rate has a small but measurable influence on the establishment of CAEs, a broad range of moderate rates being more efficient to build up CAEs than either higher or lower ones. The influence of presentation rate (or of total number of presentations per se) is not large, however, since initial strengths changed only about a factor of 3 while the rates changed by a factor of 16,400.

3. CONTRAST, RATE OF CONTRAST REVERSAL, AND EXCITATION PURITY

Other parameters of the inspection stimulation have been studied using basically the same approach. Summaries of these results are shown in Figure 22.3B–D. Figure 22.3B shows that inspection pattern contrast (calculated as the maximum minus the minimum luminance, divided by twice the space-averaged luminance) exerts a systematic and nearly linear influence on the scores of initial strength. Figure 22.3C shows the initial strengths for a range of rates of temporal contrast reversal. Contrast reversal was produced on inspection patterns having equal stripe widths for which the dark and the bright stripes appeared to exchange places (see Harris & Gibson, 1968); actually, stripes were luminance-modulated sinusoidally over time but the even-numbered stripes were in antiphase relative to the odd-numbered ones. Figure 22.3D shows the influence on CAE establishment of the excitation purity of chromatic lights used to illuminate the inspection gratings. Purity of the chromatic lights is akin to the apparent saturation of the colors. Results in Figure 22.3D show that even low-purity, rather desaturated colors used on the inspection patterns can still produce CAEs, though much less efficiently than high-purity ones. All the results shown in Figure 22.3 demonstrate that CAE strengths depend upon inspection stimulation, and suggest that control of parameters such as these is required for valid comparisons of CAEs, especially comparisons involving different laboratories using their own methods.

D. Parameters of Testing

We have also studied parametric influences of the testing stimulation using a slightly different rationale. As a general scheme for the experiments, specific CAEs were established with a single period of inspection and then were tested using several different test patterns. The way the test patterns differed from one another depended upon the specific study (luminance, contrast, rate of contrast reversal, or orientation of test gratings). Basic results are not presented here but, when graphed, looked similar to those shown in Figures 22.1 and 22.2 except that different curves represented different patterns used to test the same CAEs. In some studies, variables of the inspection and of the testing stimulation showed strong evidence of interaction (e.g., White, 1976a), whereas in other studies the interaction was minimal. These complex results may not be surprising since, not only may the different test patterns probe CAEs themselves in different ways, but also judgments are determined by many factors in addition to the presence of CAEs and those extra factors could be altered in an unwanted fashion by test stimulus manipulation. The net effect is that parameters of the testing stimulation are not easily summarized.

E. Uniformity of Decay

How similar were the observed time courses for decay in these several studies? Qualitatively, each of the more than 200 curves looks nearly linear when plotted on semilogarithmic coordinates such as those of Figures 22.1 and 22.2. Regularity in the form of decay for all of our subjects and for various ways of establishing and testing CAEs is displayed in a highly condensed manner in Figure 22.4. The ordinate of this graph is an indicator of the rates of decline in CAE strengths over time,[6] which are specifically derived as regression coefficient b in our fitted empiri-

---

[6]The rate of decline in CAE strength is indicated by regression coefficient b in the form $dP_e/d \ln(t)$ rather than as dP_e/dt. It can be shown that $dP_e/d \ln(t)$ is proportional to $(1/t) \times (dP_e/dt)$ for positive values of b, and to $t \times (dP_e/dt^{-1})$ for negative values of b. Regression coefficent b represents a uniform relation between decay rate and time after inspection.

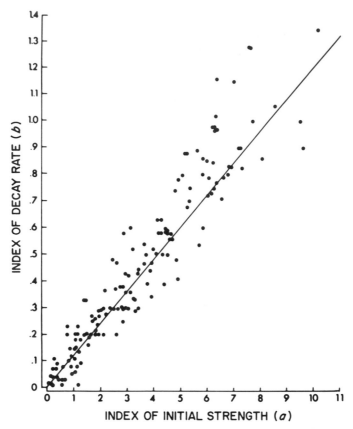

Figure 22.4. Similarities in the time courses for CAE decline. Index of decay rate (*b*) is shown as a function of index of initial strength (*a*). Each dot is derived from plotting *b* against *a*, obtained by fitting the expression $\Delta P_e = a - b \ln(t)$ to data such as those shown in Figures 22.1 and 22.2. This graph is a highly condensed summary of results across studies in which various manipulations of inspection and testing stimulation took place (luminances, presentation rates, contrasts, excitation purities, and relative orientations of lines). Although large differences were found in the values of *a* and *b*, attributed to parameters of stimulation and to individual differences, the ratio of *b* to *a* is nearly constant.

cal functions $\Delta P_e = a - b \ln(t)$ (where t is time after inspection). The abscissa in Figure 22.4 is a, the other regression coefficient, whose values give the index of initial strength. Each dot on the graph plots the values of b against a, derived by least-squares fit to a data set comprised of 60 or more judgments. The smooth line drawn through the points represents the proportionality $b = .12a$, the regularity first observed by Riggs *et al.* (1974). The summary relationship shown in Figure 22.4 emphasizes the correlation between initial strengths and subsequent rates of decay of the CAEs. This is not meant to show that CAEs always decay in an identical fashion, but rather to point out similarities in the time courses that are resistant to stimulus manipulations and to individual differences. Even though initial strengths and rates of decline both vary in their values, the ratio of one to the other stays nearly fixed.

IV. Conclusions

How have these operational studies improved our understanding of CAEs? Research described here aims more directly at empirical rather than specific theoretical impact. Measures of how selected parameters alter the efficiency of building up or testing CAEs have utility in devising experimental procedures, and serve as needed background for the design of crisp experiments to validate theoretical models. Another series of our studies detailed elsewhere (White, Petry, Riggs, & Miller, in press) attains theoretical importance through manipulating intrasubject variables, such as the subjective appearances of stimuli, to compare the relative salience of peripheral sensory events and higher order processes. Further empirical impact arises from the functional relationships found between stimulus parameters and CAE strengths, as relationships of the same kinds can be looked for in the presence of drugs or diseases, or using animal psychophysics or neurophysiological preparations. The relationships also constrain modeling of the hypothetical mechanisms that seem to be required; for example, theorists on pattern vision might find it intriguing that CAE strengths are related linearly, rather than exponentially, to the contrasts of gratings. From a broader perspective, the body of studies from this and other laboratories has begun to disclose the signatures of neural mechanisms underlying CAEs. Although CAEs behave in some ways like pattern vision and in other ways like learning or remembering, they are less ephemeral than the stuff that dreams are made of and thus are more amenable to scientific examination. In short, we have kept the electric feeling of anticipation that secrets of the nervous system are eventually to be revealed, and we believe that objectively based studies of CAEs may accomplish that goal.

ACKNOWLEDGMENTS

Coinvestigators included P.D. Eimas, S.R. Ellis, J.L. Miller, and H.M. Petry. Invaluable assistance was given by K. Castellan, J. French, A. Graves, D. Hirsch, J. Kass, and E. Rathjen. I thank W. A. H. Rushton and P. E. King-Smith for mathematical assistance.

REFERENCES

Anstis, S. M. What does visual perception tell us about visual coding? In M. S. Gazzaniga & C. Blakemore (Eds.), *Handbook of psychobiology*. New York: Academic Press, 1975.

Barlow, H. B. Single units and sensation: A neuron doctrine for perceptual psychology? *Perception,* 1972, *1*, 371–394.

Erickson, R. P. Parallel "population" neural coding in feature extraction. In F. O. Schmitt & F. G. Worden (Eds.), *The neurosciences: Third study program*. Cambridge, Massachusetts: Massachusetts Institute of Technology Press, 1974.

Fidell, L. S. Orientation specificity in chromatic adaptation of human "edge-detectors." *Perception & Psychophysics*, 1970, *8*, 235-237.

Gross, C. G., Bender, D. B., & Rocha-Miranda, C. E. Inferotemporal cortex: A single-unit analysis. In F. O. Schmitt & F. G. Worden (Eds.), *The neurosciences: Third study program*. Cambridge, Massachusetts: Massachusetts Institute of Technology Press, 1974.

Harris, C. S. Insight or out of sight?: Two examples of perceptual plasticity in the human adult. In C. S. Harris (Ed.), *Visual coding and adaptability*. Hillsdale, New Jersey: Lawrence Erlbaum Association, in press.

Harris, C. S., & Gibson, A. R. Is orientation-specific color adaptation in human vision due to edge-detectors, afterimages, or "dipoles"? *Science*, 1968, *162*, 1506-1507.

Hepler, N. K. Motion-contingent color aftereffects: A lasting modification of perception. Unpublished doctoral dissertation, McGill University, Montreal, Canada, 1971.

Hubel, D. H., & Wiesel, T. N. Receptive fields and functional architecture in two non-striate visual areas (18 and 19) of the cat. *Journal of Neurophysiology*, 1965, *28*, 229-289.

Hubel, D. H., & Wiesel, T. N. Receptive fields and functional architecture of monkey striate cortex. *Journal of Physiology*, 1968, *195*, 215-243.

Jones, P. D., & Holding, D. H. Extremely long-term persistence of the McCollough effect. *Journal of Experimental Psychology: Human Perception and Performance*, 1975, *1*, 323-327.

Kluver, H., & Bucy, P. C. Preliminary analysis of functions of the temporal lobes in monkeys. *Archives of Neurology and Psychiatry (Chicago)*, 1939, *42*, 979-1000.

MacKay, D. M., & MacKay, V. The time course of the McCollough effect and its physiological implications. *Journal of Physiology*, 1974, *237*, 38-39P.

McCollough, C. Color adaptation of edge-detectors in the human visual system. *Science*, 1965, *149*, 1115-1116.

Mishkin, M. Cortical visual areas and their interactions. In J. Karczmar & J. Eccles (Eds.), *The brain and human behavior*. New York: Springer-Verlag, 1972.

Penfield, W., & Milner, B. Memory deficit produced by bilateral lesions in the hippocampal zone. *American Medical Association Archives of Neurology and Psychiatry*, 1958, *79*, 475-497.

Riggs, L. A., White, K. D., & Eimas, P. D. Encoding and decay of orientation-contingent aftereffects of color. *Journal of the Optical Society of America*, 1973, *63*, 1287.

Riggs, L. A., White, K. D., & Eimas, P. D. Establishment and decay of orientation-contingent aftereffects of color. *Perception & Psychophysics*, 1974, *16*, 535-542.

Sherrington, C. S. *Man, on his nature*. Cambridge, U.K.: Cambridge University Press, 1941.

Shute, C. C. D. Strength and decay of McCollough effects (ME). *Journal of Physiology*, 1977, *268*, 36-38P.

Sigel, C., & Nachmias, J. A re-evaluation of curvature-specific chromatic aftereffects. *Vision Research*, 1975, *15*, 829-836.

Skowbo, D., Gentry, T., Timney, B., & Morant, R. B. The McCollough effect: Influence of several kinds of visual stimulation on decay rate. *Perception & Psychophysics*, 1974, *16*, 47-49.

Skowbo, D., Timney, B. N., Gentry, T. A., & Morant, R. B. McCollough effects: Experimental findings and theoretical accounts. *Psychological Bulletin*, 1975, *82*, 497-510.

Stromeyer, C. F. Form-color aftereffects in human vision. In H. Teuber & R. Held (Eds.), *Handbook of sensory physiology* (Vol. 8). New York: Springer-Verlag, in press.

White, K. D. Luminance as a parameter in establishment and testing of the McCollough effect. *Vision Research*, 1976, *15*, 297-302. (a)

White, K. D. Studies of orientation-contingent color aftereffects. Unpublished doctoral thesis, Brown University, Providence, Rhode Island, 1976. (b)

White, K. D. Summation of successively established orientation-contingent color aftereffects. *Perception & Psychophysics*, 1977, *22*, 123-136.

White, K. D., Petry, H. M., Riggs, L. A., & Miller, J. Binocular interactions during establishment of McCollough effects. *Vision Research*, in press.

White, K. D., & Riggs, L. A. Angle-contingent color aftereffects. *Vision Research*, 1974, *14*, 1147-1154.

Zeki, S. M. Convergent input from the striate cortex (area 17) to the cortex of the superior temporal sulcus in the rhesus monkey. *Brain Research,* 1971, *28,* 338–340.

Zeki, S. M. Functional organization of a visual area in the posterior bank of the superior temporal sulcus of the rhesus monkey. *Journal of Physiology,* 1974, *236,* 549–573.

23. On Identifying Detectors

John Krauskopf

I. Introduction

Some readers may be misled by the figures contained herein into believing that this chapter is primarily about a method of measuring the spectral sensitivity of cone mechanisms. Although this line of experimentation did begin with that goal, the theoretical and experimental methods that have been developed are of greater importance than the data obtained.

In 1959, working in Lorrin Riggs' laboratory, I had the naive idea that one might be able to determine the spectral sensitivity of single cone receptors by measuring the variation with wavelength of the detection threshold for small spots stabilized on the retina. Even though the image would be blurred and fall on a number of cones, I thought it might be detected by the cone in the center of the blur, the one that received the most light. My appreciation of the importance of the quantum nature of light was increased when I discovered (or rather rediscovered—see Holmgren, 1884) that small stimuli varied in color from trial to trial. Thus, even if stabilization were perfect, the actual distribution of light on the retina must vary from trial to trial enough, evidently, for different populations of cones to be activated on one trial and another. The goal of my experiments could not be achieved since thresholds were not determined by the action of a single class of cones. I concluded this because I accepted Müller's Doctrine of Specific Nerve Energies: The quality of a sensation is determined by the nerves that are activated and not by the quality of the stimulus evoking the activity.

The very reasons that led me to conclude that these experiments were futile led to the development of a new theory about detectors and to a method of identifying the nature of the detectors. In 1965 R. Srebro and I published a preliminary account of the application of this method to the determination of the spectral sensitivity of red

283

and green cones (Krauskopf & Srebro, 1965). This chapter presents the theory and experiments in more detail together with newer corroborative evidence.

II. Methods

In my abortive stabilized image experiments, subjects reported that the same small spot appeared "red," "green," "blue–green," "blue," or "white." Although the colored flashes on different trials usually appeared strikingly saturated, they sometimes appeared desaturated. We wanted to test the idea that the stimulus generated a small number of categories of experience, and if so to find the best method for studying the variation in frequency of experience with stimulus parameters. We tried both color matching and color naming.

A. Color Matching

In a typical experiment, 1.3' diameter spots of seven monochromatic lights varying in wavelength from 502 to 650 nm were presented for 10 msec. In each of seven sessions detection thresholds for tests at three wavelengths were first measured by an up–down procedure. Then in the main experiment, stimuli at five intensity levels approximately .1 log unit apart arrayed around the threshold were presented in a completely random order. Following a test flash, the observer adjusted the wavelength of a 1° disc until it matched the hue of the test flash. The observer was excused from this duty under two circumstances: if the test was invisible or if it appeared white.

Results for one observer are presented in Figures 23.1 and 23.2 in the form of histograms of the frequency of matches as a function of matching wavelength. Figure 23.1 plots the 829 matches that were made in 2625 trials, summed over all test wavelengths. Clearly, the matches fall within two well-defined categories. Figure 23.2 plots the same matches separately for each test wavelength. In both figures the distributions are bimodal. The central values of the two distributions are at about 500 and 625 nm and do not seem to depend on test wavelength.

These results strengthened our conviction that experiences were categorical and suggested that only two hues were seen. Complete trivariant color matching would have been required to investigate the locus of the white and desaturated experiences, but such experiments are very time consuming.

B. Color Naming

Color naming is a more efficient way of investigating the experiences. Tests can be made of the number of categories necessary to describe the experiences. For example, in early experiments observers were allowed to use the hue names "red," "green," "blue–green," and "blue," but it was found that the ratios of the fre-

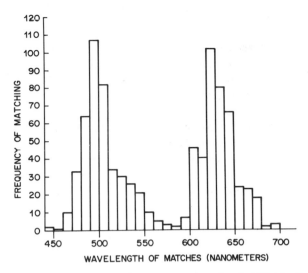

Figure 23.1. Frequency distribution of matches to near threshold lights. Pooled results for 829 matches to test lights distributed over the spectrum from 502 to 650 nm. Abscissa: Matching wavelength in nanometers.

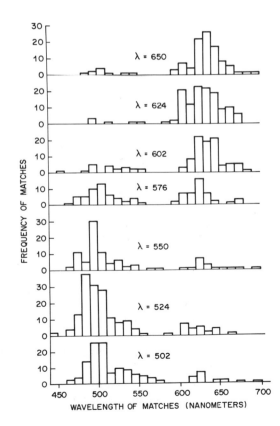

Figure 23.2. Frequency distribution of matches in Figure 23.1 plotted separately for each test wavelength.

quencies of the last three classes were invariant with stimulus wavelength, implying that the observers were using these words to describe the same experience.

In the sample color-naming experiment presented here, 10 test wavelengths ranging from 517 to 650 nm were used as test stimuli. In a session, detection thresholds were measured by use of an up–down procedure for half of the test wavelengths. Five test intensities about .1 log unit apart straddling the threshold were chosen as test stimuli for each wavelength. One of the 25 stimuli so defined was randomly chosen for presentation on a trial. The observer named the stimuli using a push-button code. A session included 625 such trials. The judgments were easily made and using modern computer controlled equipment a session was completed in less than 45 min. Data were collected in 20 sessions; a total of 12,500 judgments were made.

Figure 23.3 plots at each wavelength the percentage of flashes judged red, green, desaturated red, desaturated green, and white interpolated at 50% frequency of seeing. The frequency of each class of judgment varies independently with wavelength. This shows that there were at least five categories of experiences. Although only five categories seemed apparent, one could test for other hypothesized categories by applying the test of independent variation of category frequencies with stimulus parameters.

III. Theory

At this point R. Srebro and I, partly on the basis of the results and partly on theories of color vision, made some guesses about the detection process. Our results suggested a quantizing of responses. We supposed that the visual system had a number of independent detectors and that very few were activated on each trial when the stimulus intensity was near threshold and in fact that often only one detector was activated. We guessed that some of the detectors in our situation consisted only of long-wave cones and some only of middle-wave cones. If only those detectors served by long-wave cones were activated the observer would see red; if only those served by the middle-wave cones were activated he would see green. If both were activated he would see white or desaturated red or desaturated green depending on the ratio of activation of red and green detectors. It is important to note that the hypothesis that the detectors are homogeneous with respect to cone type is a specific hypothesis. In principle the method of analysis of the data does not require this homogeneity.

Three particularly important results emerged when we examined the consequences of a detailed theory of independent detectors:

1. Only one detector is activated on a large fraction of the trials in the probabilistic range of intensities.
2. The variation with intensity of single detector events is qualitatively different from that of multiple detector events.

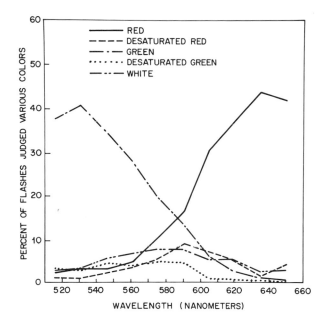

Figure 23.3.   Color naming (at 50% seeing) as a function of test wavelength.

3. A measure of the effect of a stimulus on one detector independent of its effect on other detectors was found.

These results lead directly to a method of measuring the sensitivity of detectors, which we used to determine the spectral sensitivity of the long- and middle-wave cones.

Consider a detection surface consisting of a large number N of statistically independent detectors. First, take the case in which all the detectors are of the same class, that is, have an equal probability of being "activated." We can apply simple probability theory. Equation (1) gives the probability of activation of k units $[P_a(k)]$ as a function of the probability P of activating any of the units:

$$P_a(k) = \{N!\,/\,[k!\,(N-k)!]\}\,P^k(1-P)^{N-k}. \tag{1}$$

Further assume that the activation of any single detector is sufficient for seeing. Then the probability of seeing is given by

$$P_s = 1 - (1-P)_N. \tag{2}$$

The fraction of detections due to k hits $[P_a(k)/P_s]$ is of particular interest and may be approximated for large N ($N \to \infty$) by

$$P_a(k)/P_s \simeq (1/k!)\,[-\ln(1-P_s)^k\,(1-P_s/P_s). \tag{3}$$

Figure 23.4 plots $P_a(k)/P_s$ as a function of P_s using Eq. (3) for $k = 1$ to 5. Two important features are revealed: (*a*) Only the curve for detections mediated by single

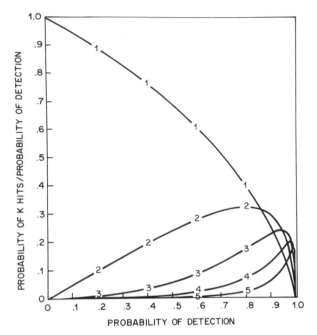

Figure 23.4. Theoretical plot of the fraction of detections resulting from activation of exactly one to five detectors as a function probability of detection.

unit activations is monotonically decreasing, and (*b*) on a large fraction of the trials on which the target is detected, only *one* unit is activated. For example, at $P_s = .50$ $P_a(1)/P_s = 1n\ 2$, or .69.

A. Some Results

Figures 23.5–23.7 plot the fraction of those stimuli seen which were called red and green, desaturated red and green, and white, respectively, as a function of total fraction seen. Only the data for the four central wavelengths are plotted. Only for saturated color judgments does this fraction decrease with increasing frequency of seeing; the fractions for desaturated colors and white increase. This is in accord with our speculation that red and green alone are due to single detector events. This result has been confirmed several times.

B. More Theory

Consider a retina with three classes of detectors, one composed of red cones alone, the second, green, and the third, blue. The probability that only one class of cones, say red (P_r'), is activated is given by:

$$P_r' = P_r(1 - P_g)\ (1 - P_b),\tag{4}$$

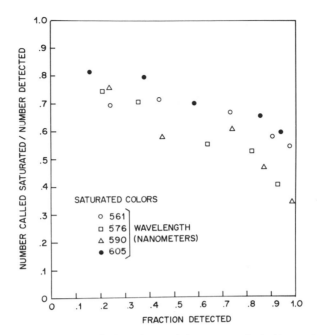

Figure 23.5. Fraction of the flashes detected that were called either red or green as a function of fractions detected.

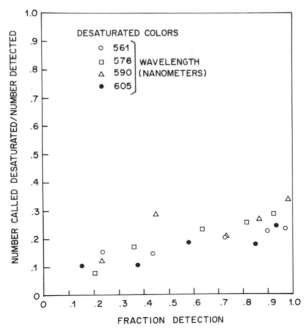

Figure 23.6. As in Figure 23.5 but for desaturated red or desaturated green.

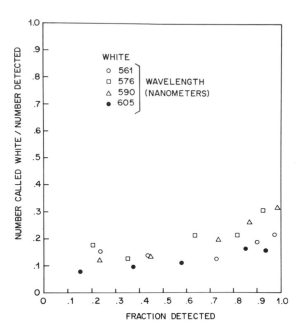

Figure 23.7. As in Figure 23.5 but for white.

where P_r, P_g, and P_b are the probabilities of activating any number of members of the red, green, or blue classes of cones. The probability of not activating any of the three classes is the probability of not seeing and is given by

$$P_{ns} = (1-P_r)(1-P_g)(1-P_b). \tag{5}$$

Equation (4) divided by Eq. (5) yields

$$P'_r/P_{ns} = P_r/(1-P_r). \tag{6}$$

The left-hand term is a function only of P_r. This is a powerful result. It implies that a ratio of observable quantities is dependent only on the effect of the stimulus on one class of detectors.

We can use Eq. (6) to estimate the spectral sensitivity $S_r(\lambda)$ of the red cone receptors. Assume that the probability of activating the red receptors (P_r) is a monotonically increasing function (f_r) of the photons caught, $[S_r(\lambda)E(\lambda)]$, that is,

$$P_r = f_r[S_r(\lambda)E(\lambda)], \tag{7}$$

where $S_r(\lambda)$ is the spectral sensitivity function for the red cones. By hypothesis P'_r/P_{ns} can be estimated by taking the ratio (F_c) of the number of flashes called red to the number not seen. For each λ studied the reciprocal of that energy $E(\lambda)$ at which F_c is a constant may be used to estimate the spectral sensitivity of the red cones.

C. More Results

Figure 23.8 is a sample plot of the ratios of the number of flashes called red and called green to the number not seen as a function of test energy and illustrates the method of measuring sensitivity. The upper curves of Figure 23.9 plot spectral sensitivity curves for red and green cones derived from color-naming data using this method. An overall spectral sensitivity curve and one derived using the white judgments are also plotted.

This shows that our method produces reasonable looking spectral sensitivity curves. If, in fact, the sensitivity curves we have labeled red and green result from activation of homogeneous classes of cones they should be invariant in shape under chromatic adaptation. To test this hypothesis the experiment that produced the upper set of curves in Figure 23.9 was repeated with one important change. The eye was strongly red-adapted before the experimental session and between trials. At these times the observer was exposed to a circular patch of tungsten light that had been passed through a No. 70 Wratten filter and was extinguished only for an interval .5 sec before and .5 sec after presentation of test flash. The lower set of curves in Figure 23.9 was derived from the color-naming data obtained under these conditions. The change in sensitivity for the red, green, and white mechanisms and the

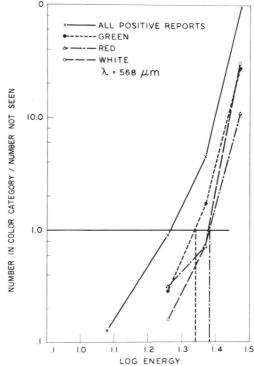

Figure 23.8. Example of plots used to estimate sensitivities. The ratio (F_c) of the number of flashes called a particular color divided by the number not seen is plotted as a function of stimulus energy. An arbitrary criterion ratio of 1 was chosen. Sensitivity is defined as the reciprocal of the energy required to achieve this ratio.

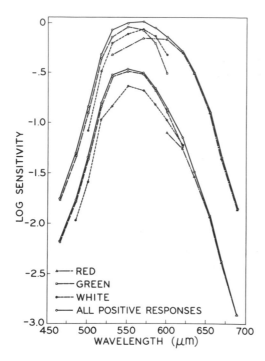

Figure 23.9. Spectral sensitivities derived from color-naming experiments. Upper curves dark-adapted. Lower curves red-adapted.

differences in overall sensitivity are plotted in Figure 23.10. Overall sensitivity is decreased by between .4 and 1.1 log units, depending on wavelength. The white sensitivity also is not invariant under adaptation. But the red and green sensitivities are each shifted by a constant amount from the dark-adapted to red-adapted state. Except for the end points of the red difference curve, which are uncertain due to the insufficient number of observations, each difference curve is constant to within .1 log unit.

The Stiles method of deriving the field sensitivities of the π-mechanisms is quite different from the color-naming method (Stiles, 1939). The interpretation of Stiles' field sensitivity curves in relation to photopigments is controversial (Boynton, Ikeda, & Stiles, 1964). There is clear evidence that π_1 is not independent of the long-wave mechanisms (Krauskopf, 1974; Mollon & Polden, 1977; Pugh, 1976). The short-wave mechanisms probably have little effect in the present experiments because the stimuli are small, brief, and foveal. In an extensive study of the detection of mixtures of monochromatic lights, I found no sign of interaction between π_4 and π_5 (Krauskopf, 1970). Detection thresholds could be completely accounted for by two independent classes of detector. Therefore, it seemed worthwhile to compare the spectral sensitivities derived by the two methods.

Increment threshold for 510- and 650-nm test flashes of the same size and duration (1.3′ and 10 msec) as those used in color-naming experiments were measured on backgrounds varying from 450 to 675 nm. The background intensities necessary to raise the threshold for the 650-nm test by 1 log unit were used to estimate the π_5

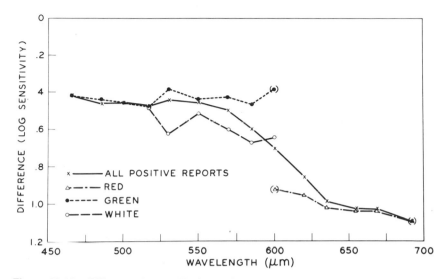

Figure 23.10. Difference in sensitivities estimated under dark-adapted and red-adapted conditions.

field sensitivity, and the π_4 field sensitivity was similarly estimated using the 510-nm test flash. Results of these experiments and of color-naming experiments are plotted in Figure 23.11. The differences between π_4 and π_5 and between green and red sensitivities are plotted as well. This method of plotting eliminates the effects of preretinal absorption and allows between and within observer comparisons. The difference curves are similar enough to one another to draw the conclusion that the two procedures are measuring the same processes in both observers.

The only other extensive data on the appearance of small stimuli are those of Bouman and Walraven (1957). Their results are similar to ours with one important exception. Their observers reported that some flashes appeared "colorless," a category that they distinguished from white. Only 1 of the 10 observers I have studied has ever used that category. Perhaps some observers have a class of detector with a broad spectral response that generates the colorless experience. One could easily imagine detectors that generate no visual experience but nevertheless allow the observer to report the occurrence of a stimulus reliably. It does not follow from the assumption of independent detection and of the Müller doctrine that detectors would have the spectral sensitivity of individual classes of cones. More than one class of cones might provide the input to a detector. This is not true for the detectors of small foveal stimuli in our experiments, but is true for some detectors of larger stimuli, which is suggested by the fact that such stimuli do not exhibit the sort of trial-to-trial variation in appearance that small stimuli do. Further, antagonistic interaction has been demonstrated in the detection of mixtures of blue and red light (Krauskopf, 1974), which means that the detectors must receive inputs from at least two types of cones.

This chapter is entitled "On Identifying Detectors" to emphasize its main point,

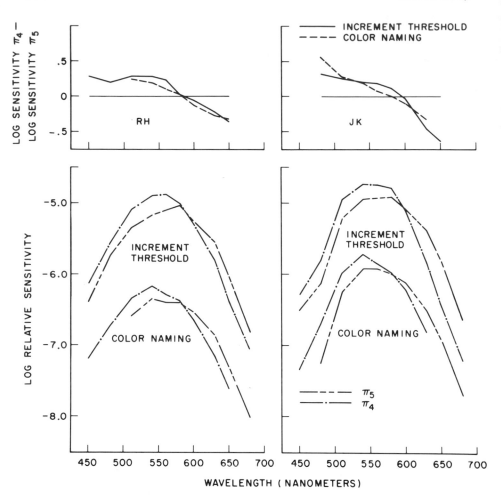

Figure 23.11. Comparison of relative spectral sensitivities (lower) derived by color-naming and increment threshold procedures for π_4 and π_5 or red and green. Placement of pairs of curves on ordinate is arbitrary. Upper curves differ in sensitivity for each procedure.

namely, that application of the Müller doctrine alerts one to the existence of detectors. For example, people confidently mislabel incremental and decremental *luminance* pulses when the pulses are as much as five times bigger than those whose presence is reliably reported. This fact led me to hypothesize that independent detectors signaled increases and decreases in brightness. The hypothesis was supported by a demonstration that thresholds for detecting incremental and decremental changes in light can be independently manipulated (Krauskopf, 1976). The methodology is very different in this case than in the experiments discussed here: Application of the Müller doctrine to the problem of identification of detectors is the principal link. Whether the specific methods used in the present experiments will be generally useful remains to be seen.

ACKNOWLEDGMENTS

This work has been done intermittently over quite a few years; I may forget to mention all who helped. Richard Srebro collaborated on the early color-naming experiments. Mohan Sondhi gave valuable mathematical assistance. George Shortess assisted in the stabilized image experiments. Virgil Graf, Virginia Turner, and Jean Benisch assisted in the color-matching and color-naming experiments. Adam Reeves made valuable editorial comments. Charles S. Harris, a master of illusion, has helped on this occasion, as on others, to create the impression that I write better than I do and in so doing has improved my understanding of my work. To all of them my thanks.

REFERENCES

Bouman, M. A., & Walraven, P. A. Some color naming experiments for red and green lights. *Journal of the Optical Society of America,* 1957, *47,* 834–839.

Boynton, R.M., Ikeda, M., & Stiles, W.S. Interactions among chromatic mechanisms as inferred from positive and negative increment thresholds. *Vision Research,* 1964, *4,* 87–117.

Holmgren, F. Über den Farbensinn. *Compt Rendu du Congrès International de Science et Medecine (Vol. 1. Physiology).* Copenhagen, 1884. Pp. 80–98.

Krauskopf, J. Probability summation in cone mechanisms. Paper presented at the meeting of the Association for Research in Vision and Ophthalmology, Sarasota, Florida, 1970.

Krauskopf, J. Interaction of chromatic mechanisms in detection. In G. Verriest (Ed.), *Modern problems in ophthalmology, 13,* 1974, 92–97.

Krauskopf, J. Further evidence that independent mechanisms detect increases and decreases in brightness: Selective adaptation. Paper presented at the meeting of the Association for Research in Vision and Ophthalmology, Sarasota, Florida, 1976.

Krauskopf, J., & Srebro, R. Spectral sensitivity of color mechanisms: Derivation from fluctuation of color appearance near threshold. *Science,* 1965, *150,* 1477–1479.

Mollon, J.D., & Polden, P.G. An anomaly in the response of the eye to light of short wavelength. *Philosophical Translations of the Royal Society of London,* 1977, *278,* 207 210.

Pugh, E. N. The nature of the π_1 mechanism of W. S. Stiles. *Journal of Physiology (London),* 1976, *257,* 713–747.

Stiles, W.S. The directional sensitivity of the retina and the spectral sensitivity of rods and cones. *Proceedings of the Royal Society of London, Ser. B,* 1939, *127,* 64–105.

Acuity, Contrast, and Movement

24. A Discourse on Edges[1]

Floyd Ratliff

> *Be it the edge of time or space, there is nothing so awe-inspiring as a border.*
>
> —YUKIO MISHIMA, *Spring Snow*

I. Introduction

An *edge,* in the sense used here, is the line where a visible object or area begins or ends. The ability to discriminate such transitions and to locate them with some precision is fundamental for vision.

To identify and to locate an edge require some kind of comparison; that is, in order to find the line where one thing ends and another begins, some attribute or another—such as intensity, color, or texture—must somehow be selected, evaluated in neighboring areas, and the separate evaluations compared or contrasted with one another. If there is a consistent and significant difference along a line of such comparisons, then that line is the locus of an edge. However, prominent edges may sometimes appear visually where there are none of any significance physically. Also, the apparent visual locus of an edge may be displaced somewhat from the actual physical locus. Such uncertainties and discrepancies are generally of little significance in everyday visual experience, but they can be very troublesome in exact work—both practical and scientific. In science, especially, one must take care to make a proper distinction between light (in the physical sense) and sight (in the psychophysiological sense).

For example, visual edge effects (Mach bands) were mistaken for physical X-ray diffraction patterns (Fomm, 1896) shortly after the discovery of X rays by Röntgen. [For the correction of this mistake see Haga and Wind (1899).] Indeed the first evidence of the periodic nature of visible light, published by Grimaldi in 1665, appears to have been a misinterpretation of a visual edge effect of this sort (see Mach, 1926). The apparent enlargement of the earth's shadow on the moon, which

[1]Preparation of this chapter was supported in part by Grants EY 188, EY 1428, and EY 1472 from the National Eye Institute, National Institutes of Health.

299

had greatly troubled astronomers and led to innumerable conflicting theories during the eighteenth and nineteenth centuries, turned out to be a displacement due to a visual edge effect (Seeliger, 1899). In the not too distant past it was puzzling to find that electron diffraction patterns appeared visually to contain maxima and minima that did not appear in the physical densitometer tracings (cf. Pirenne, 1946; Burnham & Jackson, 1955). Such problems are by no means behind us, even though we now have some (but far from complete) knowledge of the underlying mechanisms. Very recently radiologists have become increasingly aware of the role of edge effects in the purely visual interpretation of clinical X rays (Lane, Proto, & Phillips, 1976). Although such effects may facilitate perception of density changes in a radiograph, misinterpretation of their significance may lead to errors in diagnosis.

Such edge effects are not restricted to the visual system. Indeed, they occur in a large number of diverse systems for storing, transmitting, and processing information—both natural and man-made. The underlying mechanisms may differ greatly, but the basic processes are all of a kind—in a formal sense, at least. All are "comparators"; that is, by one means or another a local sample is taken from a restricted area and somehow compared or contrasted with samples taken from a larger surrounding area. In the following section several different systems for handling information are compared. In no two are the specific mechanisms the same, but similar logical operations are performed by the different mechanisms and the end effects are much the same in all.

II. Comparison of Several Diverse Comparators

The archetype of all the several systems to be considered is illustrated in Figure 24.1. A narrow Gaussian field of excitation (which samples a local region) is opposed by a larger Gaussian field of inhibition (which samples a widespread region). This particular function describes (approximately) the steady-state interaction of excitation and inhibition in the retina of the compound lateral eye of *Limulus*—a system that has been in existence for some three or four hundred million years. In a formal sense this invertebrate neural network is almost identical to, and the effects it produces almost the same as, a wide variety of other systems or processes. These include fields of opposed excitation and inhibition in vertebrate visual systems, fields of local photochemical reactions and of widespread diffusion of by-products of those reactions in photographic processes, electrostatic fields of opposite polarity in xerographic copying systems, fields of opposite sign in mathematical functions of the form $\sin x/x$, and negative feedback among coupled electronic circuits operating in parallel. Some examples are shown in Figure 24.2. The basic principle is the same in all (except the $\sin x/x$ function): What is coextensive with a widespread area is rejected; what is found only in a local area is accepted. Insofar as such a system is linear, it may be represented in the spatial domain by the *line-spread function*, or in the frequency domain by its Fourier transform, the *modulation transfer function*. This kind of "filtering" (low-

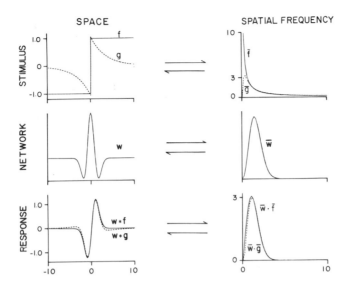

Figure 24.1. A one-dimensional representation of a linear neural network with a totally compensatory inhibitory surround. The network is the difference between a narrow positive Gaussian and a broad negative Gaussian. The two columns represent Fourier transform pairs (as indicated by the double half-arrows). The left-hand column traces the passage of two dissimilar spatial stimulus patterns, f and g, through the neural network represented by the line-spread function w; that is, f and g are convolved with w to obtain the two responses w∗f and w∗g. The right-hand column shows the corresponding distribution of spatial frequencies, $\bar{f}$ and $\bar{g}$, and the corresponding modulation transfer function $\bar{w}$. Here $\bar{f}$ and $\bar{g}$ are multiplied by $\bar{w}$ to give the two responses $\bar{w} \cdot \bar{f}$ and $\bar{w} \cdot \bar{g}$. Note that the differences in the two stimuli lie mainly in the low-frequency range. Since low frequencies are strongly suppressed by this network, the responses to the dissimilar stimuli are similar. Both show marked and nearly identical edge effects. [From Ratliff & Sirovich (1978).]

frequency attenuation, high-frequency cutoff) results in characteristic and well-known edge effects (Figures 24.1 and 24.2).

When the "inhibitory surround" (or its equivalent) is diminished somewhat or removed altogether by some means or another, the pronounced edge effects are correspondingly diminished or abolished. For example, in the vertebrate visual system low-frequency attenuation and its attendant edge effects are pronounced at high intensities, moderate at moderate intensities, and weak or absent at low intensities. In photography low-frequency attenuation depends upon the contrast sensitivity of the film, the type of developer used, and the amount of agitation of the film during the development.[2] In xerography the low-frequency attenuation varies with the thickness of the photosensitive plate and with the location of the electrode with respect to the plate. The edge effect in mathematics (which is known as the Gibbs

---

[2]The so-called unsharp mask technique of making etching-like photographs is essentially a low-frequency attenuation method.

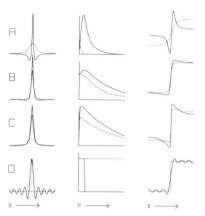

Figure 24.2. Edge effects in vision (A), in photography (B), in xerography (C), and in mathematics (D). The left-hand column shows line-spread functions, the center column shows corresponding modulation transfer functions, and the right-hand column shows the *calculated* output of each system in response to a rectilinear step input. For ease of comparison all functions are plotted on similar scales. (A) *Human vision.* the calculations are based on measurements of contrast sensitivity of human observers at a high level (solid lines) and a low level (dashed lines) of light adaptation by De Valois *et al.* (1974). I have made the assumption that modulation transfer functions would have essentially the same form as the contrast sensitivity curve. Note that the low-frequency attenuation and the corresponding edge effects are absent at low levels of adaptation. (B) *Photography.* The calculations are based on modulation transfer functions measured at the same density level for film processed in Kodak D-76 developer (solid lines) and in Kodak D-19 developer (dashed lines). [The modulation transfer functions are redrawn after Barrows and Wolfe (1971).] Note that the D-76 developer, which has a greater low-frequency attenuation than the D-19, produces the strongest edge effects. (C) *Xerography.* Solid lines: Method with strong edge effect produced by the opponent center-surround shape of the electrostatic field on the photosensitive plate. Dashed lines: Method with edge effects removed by changing thickness of plate and by bringing toner particles closer to plate during development. [Redrawn after Neugebauer (1967).](D) *The Gibbs phenomenon.* Solid lines: The Fourier transform of a spatial distribution of the form sin x/x (left-hand column) is a rectangular function (center column). Note that there is no low frequency attenuation. The missing high-frequency components give rise to an overshoot, an undershoot, and adjacent damped undulations (with the form of a sine integral) in the output to a rectilinear step input (right-hand column). These edge effects (the Gibbs phenomenon) diminish in width, but not in amplitude, as the rectangular spectral function extends out to higher frequencies, the corresponding spatial distribution becomes very narrow, approaching a delta function centered on $x = 0$ (left-hand column). As a result, the overshoot, undershoot, and adjacent undulations become very narrow, and the output to a rectilinear step input (right-hand column) approaches a perfect reproduction of that step (see Jennison, 1961).

phenomenon) becomes very narrow (and thus quite insignificant) if the function sin x/x is extended out to very large values of x.[3]

The diminution or dropping out of the inhibitory surround has a profound effect on the response of each and every one of the systems or processes illustrated in Figure 24.2. For one thing the "gain control" inherent in negative feedback is lost. Most obvious in the examples shown, however, is the diminution of the edge effects as the low-frequency attenuation or filtering becomes less pronounced. Not shown is the effect of a strong filter as an "equalizer." In Figure 24.2 the inputs are all the same (rectilinear steps) so it is not surprising that the outputs (strong edge effects) are all similar when there is strong low-frequency attenuation. Let us consider a more interesting case: dissimilar stimuli that evoke similar responses.

[3]The amplitudes of the first overshoot and the first undershoot are always 9%, however.

III. Equivalence Classes of Edge Stimuli

If dissimilar inputs yield similar outputs, we generally attribute this to nothing more complicated than a transmission of features that the two inputs have in common and a filtering out of those features that differ. In vision, however, questions of a seemingly different nature about the relation between the form of a given response in the visual pathway and the form of the corresponding visual appearance have frequently been raised. The question comes up, for example, in the study of the so-called Craik–O'Brien–Cornsweet effects (Craik, 1940, 1966, pp. 94–97; O'Brien, 1958; Cornsweet, 1970). These particular edge-dependent effects are very striking. For example, an antisymmetric combination of two gently falling exponentials "looks like" a rectilinear step—this is the familiar "Cornsweet illusion." Many persons assume that the neural response and the visual appearance must be isomorphic. Since the Cornsweet stimulus "looks like" a rectilinear step the suggestion has frequently been made that the usually observed neural response to such a stimulus (pronounced maxima and minima adjacent to the edge) must somehow be "filled in" in order to produce a rectilinear appearance. For this reason, the supposed neural mechanisms underlying these edge-dependent effects have frequently been represented as a "two-stage process" (Fleischer, 1939; Fry, 1948; Walls, 1954; Hood & Whiteside, 1968; Gerrits & Vendrick, 1970; Ratliff, 1971). In the first stage, lateral inhibition (principally) is supposed to produce the edge effects and in the second stage, a "filling in" or "homogenization" of the pattern is supposed to take place. For example, in discussing a similar problem in brightness contrast, Fry (1948) concluded that "although the mechanism of inhibition sharpens the contrast, it is necessary in addition to postulate a [nerve impulse] frequency-equalizing mechanism which smooths out the [impulse] frequency difference on each side of the border . . . [p. 173]."

Our intuition may tell us that such a filling in process is necessary, but logic does not compel us to believe so. At least it is unnecessary to postulate filling in as an active process. A much simpler interpretation based on the concept of *equivalence classes* of visual stimuli is adequate (Ratliff & Sirovich, 1978). For example, in the theoretical calculations shown in Figure 24.3 the rectilinear step stimulus as well as a wide range of other edge stimuli with curvilinear and rectilinear components (first column) all belong to the same equivalence class of visual stimuli; that is, they all result in effectively the same neural activity (second column). According to this view, the perceived illumination of each and every member of this equivalence class would be essentially the same simply because the neural responses are essentially the same (compare Mach, 1865; Cornsweet, 1970; Campbell, Howell, & Robson, 1971; Ratliff, 1971; Tolhurst, 1972; Shapley & Tolhurst, 1973).

Any question about equivalence is two-sided, and so is the answer. For example, we are all struck by the fact that Craik–O'Brien–Cornsweet stimuli (and all other members of that equivalence class of stimuli) look like rectilinear step stimuli, and many find this mysterious. But, conversely, it is equally true and equally mysterious that rectilinear step stimuli look like Craik–O'Brien–Cornsweet stimuli (and also

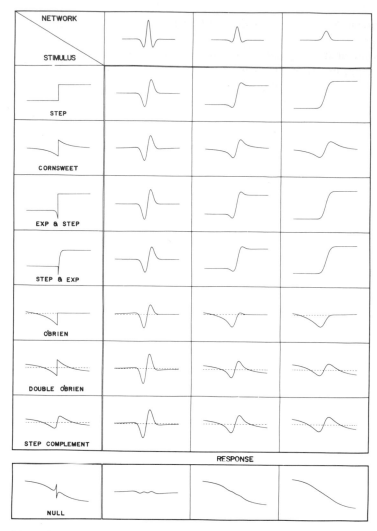

Figure 24.3. Responses of model linear networks to a variety of edge stimuli. The network on the left has a totally compensatory inhibitory surround (inhibition equals excitation); the network in the center has a partially compensatory surround (inhibition is weaker than excitation); the network on the right has no inhibitory surround (zero inhibition). To facilitate comparison of responses, the amplitudes of the line-spread functions representing the networks were adjusted so that the peak-to-peak amplitudes of the responses to the step stimuli are approximately the same for all three networks. [From Ratliff & Sirovich (1978).]

like all other members of that equivalence class). In other words, no one of the stimuli in this equivalence class is the "ideal" or "standard" stimulus. Some—it is true—may be more familiar, less complicated, more likely to occur in nature, or may have some rather distinctive physical attribute. But no one is more effective as a visual stimulus than is any other. All belong to the same equivalence class; all appear the same; all supposedly yield the same or similar neural responses.

Logically, nothing more than similarity of neural responses is required to explain the equivalence. Nevertheless, one cannot by any reasoning eliminate a priori some higher order stage or filling in process (whether it be the "frequency-equalizing" process of Fry or any of the manifold other possibilities one might imagine for this purpose). But parsimony demands that any such additional stage or process be considered only if neurophysiological evidence for it should appear.

IV. Effects of Adaptation on Equivalence Classes

Heggelund and Krekling (1976) found that one of the Craik–O'Brien–Cornsweet effects depends on adaptation level and that it appears only in photopic vision. They state that "the results . . . are . . . contrary to the model of Ratliff (1972) according to which level of adaptation should make no difference . . . [p. 495]." Heggelund and Krekling note that their results "might indicate that the Craik effect only occurs under adaptational conditions where the retinal receptive fields have an antagonistic center-surround organization [p. 495]." If—as they suggest—these edge-dependent effects disappear at adaptational levels at which the opponent surround also disappears, then this is consistent with rather than contrary to the model of Ratliff (1971, 1972). But whether the suggestion by Heggelund and Krekling and the simple linear *Limulus* model used by Ratliff are consistent with the actual physiology of the vertebrate visual system is another question. The answer is probably no in the first case and certainly no in the second (see Section VI). Nevertheless, there is some heuristic value in these simple ideas. Let us consider them further.

The line-spread function of the human visual system (Figure 24.2) is known to pass in stages from having a large opponent surround at high light levels to the complete loss of the surround at low light levels (see Patel, 1966; Kelly, 1972; De Valois, Morgan, & Snodderly, 1974). Such a transition is represented in a simplified form by the three line-spread functions shown on the top row of Figure 24.3. These represent networks with a totally compensatory inhibitory surround, a partially compensatory inhibitory surround, and no inhibitory surround. For simplicity and ease of calculation the functions are superpositions of Gaussians. The first column contains seven different stimulus patterns and the associated rows show the transition of the responses at the three stages. The responses are the convolution product of the stimulus with the various line-spread functions shown.

Each of the several stimulus patterns can be regarded as a combination of steps and exponentially falling functions. For example, the "Cornsweet" pattern is the antisymmetric combination of two gently falling exponentials (each of which can be regarded as a separate "Craik" pattern); the "exp & step" stimulus is a step function with a sharply falling exponential subtracted on the left. The "O'Brien" pattern is also of this form but has a left starting point higher than the right and contains a gently falling exponential. For obvious reasons the sixth pattern is given the name of "double O'Brien." The "step complement" differs from the step the most of all the patterns—indeed, as much as possible while still belonging to the same equivalence class.

The next column of this figure shows that to good approximation all seven stimuli produce very nearly the same response after passing through the first of these line-spread functions. They all belong to the same equivalence class of stimuli—for the first line-spread function. The O'Brien, double O'Brien, and step complement stimuli differ from all the others in that they exhibit a relative contrast exchange; that is, although the light intensity at the left is greater than at the right the response under the first line-spread function is essentially the same as that of a step (first stimulus) *with opposite relative intensity*. (Note relationship to dotted lines.)

The equivalence class is split under the loss of opponency. The second line-spread function (third column) has half as much inhibition as excitation and is therefore less able to produce pronounced edge effects. The third line-spread function (fourth column) has no inhibitory surround and hence merely results in a "blurred" copy of the stimulus. All three line-spread functions show high-frequency suppression. This accounts for the continued equivalence of the step, exp & step, and step & exp stimuli in the transition from one to another of all three line-spread functions. For the same reason the double O'Brien and step complement stimuli also remain equivalent under all three line-spread functions.

For a linear system the difference of any two members of an equivalence class is a null stimulus, which gives rise to an effectively null response. This is illustrated in the bottom part of Figure 24.3, where the null stimulus is the difference between the step and step complement stimuli in the upper part of the figure. Passage of the null stimulus through the first line-spread function yields a nearly uniform (null) response. Actually, by further sculpturing the null pattern a more nearly zero response can be obtained. This was deliberately avoided to show the location of the vanishing response and to underline the notion that nearly zero responses appear as nulls as they enter the noise.[4] Note that the step and step-complement stimuli do not yield equivalent responses under the second and third line-spread functions. Therefore, the stimulus which *is* a null for the first line spread function is *not* a null for the second and third functions.

In summary, stimuli that differ objectively may produce equivalent neural responses (and visual appearances) simply because the visual system "filters" out those features of the stimuli that differ and transmits some of those features the stimuli share in common. Such stimuli form an equivalence class. For a linear system, the difference between any two members of the same equivalence class is a null stimulus.

---

[4]The effects shown in Figure 24.3 result from calculations using a *model* network. There is no implication that equivalence classes of stimuli for this particular network would appear equal to a human observer. However, given a sufficiently exact measurement of the line-spread function or modulation transfer function of the human visual system, one might be able to calculate equivalence classes of stimuli and null stimuli for the human observer—at least in the neighborhood of any operating point.

V. Moving Edges

One basic principle stands out in the preceding analysis of a simple *Limulus* type of model network: What is coextensive with a widespread area is rejected; what is found only in a local area is accepted. This kind of filtering by linear systems in the steady-state results in characteristic and well-known edge effects. What is not as well known or as completely understood is that a similar comparison or contrast of local and remote events in both space *and* time can have much more pronounced effects than do the steady-state interactions to which so much attention has been given. Indeed, the steady-state contrast effects in the *Limulus* retina are the weakest of all. They have been the most intensively studied merely because they have been the most accessible—in terms of stimulus control, response measurement, data analysis, and theoretical treatment.

The reason for the stronger dynamic effects is simple. The excitation has a relatively rapid time course, the inhibition a relatively slow time course. Thus for a brief transient period the opposed influences of excitation and lateral inhibition can be completely separated in time so that the full effects of each can occur separately. Also, the "tuning" that results from the delay of the inhibition with respect to the excitation can lead to a substantial "amplification" of the response under certain circumstances (Ratliff, Knight, & Graham, 1969; Ratliff, Knight, & Milkman, 1970). Furthermore, since there is no significant temporal phase shift of inhibition with distance (Ratliff, Knight, Dodge, & Hartline, 1974), the separate inhibitory effects exerted on any particular point by synchronous excitation of neighbors (no matter what their location) are synchronous too, and thus may sum to yield a very strong effect in combination.

A complete mathematical model of the dynamic behavior of the *Limulus* retina was formulated some time ago (Knight, 1973). But the direct test of the model (Brodie, Knight, & Ratliff, 1978) awaited several new developments in methods of stimulus control and data analysis. A novel and more powerful form of Wiener analysis (Victor, Shapley, & Knight, 1977) was one of the most important advances. This form of analysis uses a simple signal instead of conventional Wiener "white" noise. The input signal consists of the sum of a few sinusoids chosen to span the whole modulation transfer function with an adequate sampling mesh. This has the advantage that the entire temporal modulation transfer function can be obtained in one run of a minute or two instead of in an hour or two. Furthermore, one can measure one point on the spatial transfer function at the same time. In addition (see Section VI) one can measure nonlinearities at the same time.

New electro-optical methods for stimulus control (Shapley & Rossetto, 1976) were used to illuminate the eye with a spatial sinusoid. This sinusoid was used as a phase contrast reversal stimulus, that is, it was centered on the test receptor and "rotated" about the mean so as to alternate the peaks and troughs. But this rotation was not done with a simple periodic temporal signal—rather the sum of sinusoids signal just described was used. The response of the optic nerve to the noisy reversal of the spatial sinusoid was measured for a period of approximately 60 sec.

This measurement was repeated at several spatial frequencies sufficient to span the spatial modulation transfer function. The response to the input stimuli looks like "trash," but it is not. From such a jumble of data one can extract the entire spatiotemporal transfer function for this eye with all amplitude and phase information for all relevant spatial and temporal frequencies.

Once the information is obtained one should be able to predict in advance the response of *any* arbitrary spatiotemporal stimulus. Figure 24.4 shows that this can indeed be done quite successfully. Responses to a square wave at two velocities are shown. Note how the edge effect increases with increasing velocity and becomes more and more asymmetrical. At high velocity, it is large and asymmetrical. Since the lateral inhibition is delayed by a (nearly) fixed amount of time with respect to the excitation that produces it, the leading edge of the inhibitory field falls farther behind as the velocity increases. At high velocity the result is an almost purely excitatory transient that is then quickly shut off by the trailing inhibition. In the limit of an infinitely high velocity there would be no leading inhibition at all, and the response would be the same as for a full field increment and decrement (see Ratliff *et al.*, 1974, Figure 8).

Some might complain that a square wave is not an "arbitrary" stimulus and we should test our theory with something more complicated. Actually, for a linear

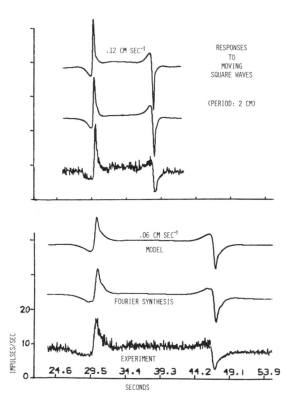

Figure 24.4. Response of optic nerve fiber of *Limulus* retina to moving square waves of light imaged on the cornea. (Eye is about 1 cm wide.) Lowest trace in each frame: Observed response. Middle trace (offset 15 impulses sec⁻¹): Prediction (Fourier synthesis) based on empirical spatiotemporal transfer function. Upper trace (offset an additional 15 impulses sec⁻¹): Prediction from model of retina. [Redrawn after Brodie *et al.* (1978).]

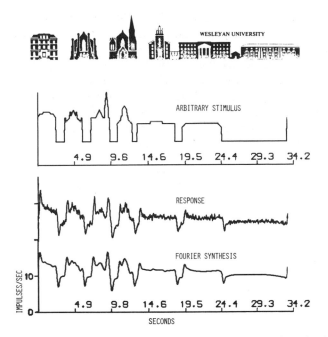

Figure 24.5. Response of optic nerve fiber of *Limulus* retina to a moving stimulus of arbitrary form. Velocity: .6 cm sec^{-1}. Upper trace: Arbitrary stimulus. Middle trace: Observed response. Lower trace: Predicted response. [Redrawn after Brodie *et al.* (1978).]

system, a square wave is just as arbitrary as any other wave form. But to satisfy Doubting Thomases the profile shown in Figure 24.5 was chosen as an arbitrary test stimulus. Theory and experiment agree as well as before.

VI. Nonlinear Analysis of Neural Networks

The modulation transfer function or its Fourier transform (the line-spread function in space or impulse function in time) provides a simple, convenient, and universal characterization for a linear system. But no visual system is strictly linear. (Even the *Limulus* retina is only piecewise or segmentally linear in the first approximation.) Unfortunately, the characterization of a nonlinear system depends on a complex input ensemble and a more cumbersome theory is required to treat this dependence.

Wiener's (1958) Gaussian white noise technique has recently been applied to the analysis of nonlinear biological systems. Although Wiener's technique is elegant from a theoretical point of view, the practical problems it poses severely limit its use. To circumvent these problems other analytical methods using input signals somewhat less complex than white noise have been devised (e.g., Krausz & Friesen, 1975, pp. 125–146; Marmarelis, 1975, pp. 106–124; Spekreijse & Oosting, 1970). A new method developed by Victor, Shapley, and Knight (1977) allows one to use a more practical input—namely, the sum of sines referred to in Section IV—without abandoning the theoretical advantages of Wiener's technique.

The new method uses a superposition of nearly incommensurate sinusoids. This forms an input signal that is periodic, yet rich enough to provide a useful characterization of a nonlinear system. The characterization is based on Fourier components of the response at harmonics and combinations of the frequencies in the input. If the frequencies are chosen properly, Fourier analysis alone resolves the first- and second-order components; that is, fundamental frequencies may be chosen such that they are not equal to any of their next-order sum, difference, or harmonic frequencies (for example: .7, 1.5, 3.1, and 6.3). This small sample shows that the frequencies are discrete and that the nonlinearities (harmonics and combination frequencies) may therefore be easily identified if they appear in the response:

Fundamental	.7	
Difference	.8	(1.5 − .7)
Harmonic	1.4	(2 × .7)
Fundamental	1.5	
Difference	1.6	(3.1 − 1.5)
Sum	2.2	(.7 + 1.5)
Difference	2.4	(3.1 − .7)
Harmonic	3.0	(2 × 1.5)
Fundamental	3.1	
Difference	3.2	(6.3 − 3.1)
Sum	3.8	(.7 + 3.1)
Sum	4.6	(1.5 + 3.1)
Difference	4.8	(6.3 − 1.5)
Difference	5.6	(6.3 − .7)
Harmonic	6.2	(2 × 3.1)
Fundamental	6.3	
Sum	7.0	(6.3 + .7)
Sum	7.8	(6.3 + 1.5)
Sum	9.4	(6.3 + 3.1)
Harmonic	12.6	(2 × 6.3)

Victor, Shapley, and Knight (1977) have analyzed the responses of cat ganglion cells to spatial sinusoids that are modulated in time by such a sum of sinusoids. The input signal spanned a range of about .3 to 30 cycles per second—sufficient to sample fully the temporal modulation transfer function of such cells. Compare the cat X and Y ganglion cells shown in Figure 24.6. The X ganglion cell is practically as linear as the *Limulus* retina. (It would not be stretching the point to call it a "cat ommatidium.") There is a strong response to the fundamental frequencies in the midrange, flanked by the familiar low-frequency attenuation and high-frequency cutoff. However, the half-plane showing the next-order combination frequencies (the nonlinearities) is barren—there is essentially no response there.

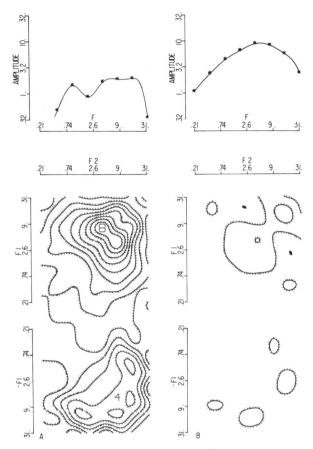

Figure 24.6. Linear response (top) and second-order frequency kernel (bottom) from a typical cat retinal ganglion Y cell (left) and a typical X cell (right). The spatial pattern was a .5 cycle deg^{-1} sinusoidal grating in the position that produced a maximal linear response. The temporal modulation signal (see text) was deterministic, consisting of a sum of eight sinusoids, each with a peak contrast of .05. Note that the amplitude of the linear response (impulses per second) is plotted on a log scale. The peak response of the Y cell (about one impulse per second) is not significant. In the plots of the second-order frequency kernels each contour line represents one impulse per second; the tick marks point downhill. Frequency is measured in cycles per second. [From Victor *et al.* (1977).]

The Y ganglion cell shown, on the other hand, yields practically no linear response at this particular location of this particular spatial frequency. But there is an enormous nonlinear component. Note the large "hill" of sum frequency nonlinearity in the upper part of the half-plane and the somewhat smaller hill of difference frequency nonlinearity in the lower part of the half-plane.

When there is an observable linear component, Y cells are found to have the familiar linear center and surround mechanisms. But the linear and nonlinear mechanisms that drive the Y cell do not have similar spatial properties. In addition

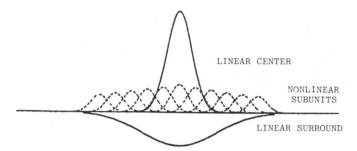

Figure 24.7. One dimensional spatial model for the Y cell receptive field. There is a broad linear surround and a narrow linear center (solid curves). Overlapping the entire receptive field is an ensemble of nonlinear subunits (dashed curves), each of which is narrower than the linear center. [From Hochstein & Shapley (1976).]

to the usual linear center-surround, in every Y cell there appears to be an ensemble of smaller nonlinear spatial subunits extending over the entire receptive field (Figure 24.7). The linear mechanisms dominate the Y cell's response to sinusoidal gratings of low spatial frequency while the nonlinear subunits are the dominant input when the grating has a high spatial frequency. This arrangement is not unique to the cat—a similar combination of relatively large linear center-surround units and a widely distributed ensemble to relatively small nonlinear subunits have also been found in the frog retina (see Chapter 25 by Gordon and Shapley).

We are just beginning to exploit this novel sum of sines version of Wiener analysis. It appears to offer a powerful method by means of which new principles of great generality may be elucidated—principles akin to but more complex than our old ideas about the integrative activity of the visual system. Old and fruitful concepts, such as the simple summation of opposed center-surround influences, will not have to be abandoned altogether, but in many cases they will have to be greatly modified.

ACKNOWLEDGMENT

I thank Abraham Z. Snyder for technical assistance.

REFERENCES

Barrows, R. S., & Wolfe, R. N. A review of adjacency effects in silver photographic images. *Photographic Sciences and Engineering,* 1971, *15,* 472–479.
Brodie, S.E., Knight, B.W., & Ratliff, F. The response of the *Limulus* retina to moving stimuli: A prediction by Fourier synthesis. *Journal of General Physiology,* 1978 (in press).
Burnham, R.W., & Jackson, J.E. Mach rings verified by numerical differentiation. *Science,* 1955, *122,* 951–953.
Campbell, F.W., Howell, E.R., & Robson, J.G. The appearance of gratings with and without the

fundamental Fourier component. *Journal of Physiology*, 1971, *217*, 17P–19P.

Cornsweet, T. *Visual perception*. New York: Academic Press, 1970.

Craik, K.J.W. Visual adaptation. Unpublished doctoral thesis, Cambridge University, Cambridge, England, 1940.

Craik, K.J.W. *The nature of psychology: A selection of papers, essays, and other writings* (S.L. Sherwood, Ed.). Cambridge University Press, 1966.

De Valois, R.L., Morgan, H., & Snodderly, D.M. Psychophysical studies of monkey vision. III. Spatial luminance contrast sensitivity tests of macaque and human observers. *Vision Research*, 1974, *14*, 75–81.

Fleischer, E. Zur Physiologie des Flaechensehens. *Zeitschrift der psychologischen Physiologie der Sinnesorgane*, 1939, *I*, Abt.145, 45–111.

Fomm, L. Die Wellenlaenge der Roentgen Strahlen. *Sitzungsberichte der mathematisch–physikalischen Classe der koeniglichen bayrischen Akademie der Wissenschaften*, 1896, *XXVI/II*. (Reprinted in *Annalen der Physik*, 1896, *59*, 350–353.)

Fry, G.A. Mechanisms subserving simultaneous brightness contrast. *American Journal of Optometry and Archives of the American Academy of Optometry*, 1948, *25*, 162–178.

Gerrits, H.J.M., & Vendrick, A.J.H. Simultaneous contrast, filling-in process and information processing in man's visual system. *Experimental Brain Research*, 1970, *11*, 411–430.

Haga, H., & Wind, C.H. Die Beugung der Röntgenstrahlen. *Annalen der Physik und Chemie*, 1899, *68*, 844–895.

Heggelund, P., & Krekling, S. Edge-dependent lightness distribution at different adaptation levels, *Vision Research*, 1976, *16*, 493–496.

Hochstein, S., & Shapley, R. M. Linear and nonlinear spatial subunits in Y cat retinal ganglion cells. *Journal of Physiology*, 1976, *262*, 265–284.

Hood, D.C., & Whiteside, J.A. Brightness of ramp stimuli as a function of plateau and gradient widths. *Journal of the Optical Society of America*, 1968, *58*, 1310–1311.

Jennison, R.C. *Fourier transforms and convolutions for the experimentalist*. New York: Pergamon Press, 1961.

Kelly, D.H. Adaptation effects on spatio-temporal sine-wave thresholds. *Vision Research*, 1972, *12*, 89–101.

Knight, B.W., Jr. *Some questions concerning the encoding dynamics of neuron populations*. International Union for Pure and Applied Biophysics, Academy of Sciences of the USSR. Symposial Papers, International Biophysics Congress, 1973. Pp. 422–436.

Krausz, J., & Friesen, W.O. Identification of discrete input nonlinear systems using Poisson impulse trains. *Proceedings of the First Symposium on Testing and Identification of Nonlinear Systems*. Pasadena: California Institute of Technology, 1975.

Lane, E.J., Proto, A.V., & Phillips, T.W. Mach bands and density perception. *Radiology*, 1976, *121*, 9–17.

Mach, E. Ueber die Wirkung der raeumlichen Vertheilung des Lichtreizes auf die Netzhaut. *Sitzungsberichte der mathematisch–naturwissenschaftlichen Classe der kaiserlichen Akademie der Wissensschaften*, 1865, *52*, 303–322.

Mach, E. *The principles of physical optics* (John S. Anderson & A.F.A. Young, trans.). London: Methuen, 1926. [Originally published in 1921, Leipzig: Johann Ambrosius Barth. Reprinted by Dover Publications, 1953.]

Marmarelis, V.Z. Identification of nonlinear systems through multilevel random signals. *Proceedings of the First Symposium on Testing and Identification of Nonlinear Systems*. Pasadena: California Institute of Technology, 1975.

Neugebauer, H.E.J. Development method and modulation transfer function of xerography. *Applied Optics*, 1967, *6*, 943–945.

O'Brien, V. Contour perception, illusion and reality. *Journal of the Optical Society of America*, 1958, *48*, 112–119.

Patel, A.S. Spatial resolution by human visual system. The effect of mean retinal illuminance. *Journal of the Optical Society of America*, 1966, *56*, 689–694.

Pirenne, M. *The diffraction of X-rays and electrons by free molecules.* Cambridge, England: Cambridge University Press, 1946.

Ratliff, F. Contour and contrast. *Proceedings of the American Philosophical Society,* 1971, *115*, 150–163.

Ratliff, F. Contour and contrast. *Scientific American,* 1972, June, 91–101.

Ratliff, F., Knight, B.W., Dodge, F.A., & Hartline, H.K. Fourier analysis of dynamics of excitation and inhibition in the eye of *Limulus:* Amplitude, phase, and distance. *Vision Research,* 1974, *14*, 1155–1168.

Ratliff, F., Knight, B.W., & Graham, N. On tuning and amplification by lateral inhibition. *Proceedings of the National Academy of Sciences,* 1969, *62*, 733–740.

Ratliff, F., Knight, B.W., & Milkman, N. Superposition of excitatory and inhibitory influences in the retina of *Limulus:* The effect of delayed inhibition. *Proceedings of the National Academy of Sciences,* 1970, *67*, 1558–1564.

Ratliff, F., & Sirovich, L. Equivalence classes of visual stimuli. *Vision Research,* 1978 (in press).

Seeliger, H. Die scheinbare Vergrösserung des Erdschattens bei Mondfinsternissen, *Abhandlungen der mathematisch–physikalischen Classe der königlichen bayerischen Akademie der Wissenschaften,* 1899, *19*, 385–499.

Shapley, R.M., & Rossetto, M. An electronic visual stimulator. *Behavior Research Methods and Instrumentation,* 1976, *8*, 15–20.

Shapley, R.M., & Tolhurst, D.J. Edge detectors in human vision. *Journal of Physiology,* 1973, *229*, 165–183.

Spekreijse, H., & Oosting, H. Linearizing: A method for analyzing and synthesizing nonlinear systems. *Kybernetik,* 1970, *7*, 22–31.

Tolhurst, D.J. On the possible existence of edge detector neurons in the human visual system. *Vision Research,* 1972, *12*, 797–804.

Victor, J.D., Shapley, R.M., & Knight, B.W. Nonlinear analysis of cat retinal ganglion cells in the frequency domain. *Proceedings of the National Academy of Sciences,* 1977, *74*, 3068–3072.

Walls, G. The filling-in process, *American Journal of Optometry,* 1954, *31*, 329–340.

Wiener, N. *Nonlinear problems in random theory.* New York: The Technology Press of Massachusetts Institute of Technology and Wiley, 1958.

25. Contrast Sensitivity and Spatial Summation in Frog and Eel Retinal Ganglion Cells[1]

James Gordon and Robert M. Shapley

I. Introduction

It has long been known by visual psychophysicists that the visual system can sum the effects of lights falling on different retinal areas. The first direct physiological evidence that this spatial summation could take place in the retina was from the recording of optic nerve activity of the Conger eel by Adrian and Matthews (1927a, 1927b, 1928). They showed that increasing the area of a stimulus caused a decrease in response latency. Later, Hartline (1938, 1940a, 1940b), recording from single optic nerve fibers of the frog, showed that each fiber responded to lights within a discrete retinal area he termed the receptive field of that fiber. Furthermore, the effects of lights within the receptive field could sum, and this summation was sometimes linear; that is, there could be an exact trade-off between area and intensity of the lights so that, as long as a certain number of quanta were presented within equisensitive retinal areas, the fiber's threshold would be surpassed.

The idea of linear spatial summation was explored in the cat retina by Enroth-Cugell and Robson (1966) using sinusoidal grating stimuli in which lights falling on different parts of the receptive field were increasing or decreasing in intensity 180° out of phase with each other. The purpose of such a stimulus was to produce clashing between the responses to light onset and offset. In a linear system the light onset and offset responses are the inverses of each other. Their sum, if they are of the same magnitude, is zero. The responses to this temporally modulated grating, a stimulus similar to that which we used extensively in the experiments to be de-

[1]This work was supported, in part, by Grants EY 1472, EY 188, and EY 1428 from the U.S. National Eye Institute.

scribed in this chapter, indicated clearly that while many cells did indeed show linear spatial summation (X cells) many cells did not (Y cells). Another nonlinear feature of Y cells was the "on–off" or frequency-doubled responses (of the same sign) they gave to fine contrast-reversal gratings.

This highly nonlinear behavior of at least one class of cat ganglion cells brings us back to the earlier work on eels and frogs. Recording multiunit activity in the eel optic nerve, Adrian and Matthews (1927a, 1927b, 1928) had shown that there were responses both to the onset and offset of light. In his single-fiber frog recording in the frog retina, Hartline found that some fibers respond at light onset, others at light offset, and many fibers respond both at light onset and offset. We have shown in earlier work (Gordon & Graham, 1973) that the responses of the frog on–off cells must be the result of a nonlinearity in the retina that is not due simply to a rectification caused by the lack of a spontaneous discharge at the ganglion cell level. Rather it must be due to nonlinearities at an earlier retinal stage.

The major aim of the present experiments was to use contrast-reversal as well as drifting gratings (see Section II) to explore the nature of spatial summation in eel and frog retinas. We will show that the eel has both linear or X cells and nonlinear cells, but that the nonlinear cells differ significantly from the nonlinear Y cells of the cat described extensively by Hochstein and Shapley (1976a, 1976b). They are probably more like the on–off W cells of the cat (Stone & Fukuda, 1974), and we will call them $\bar{X}$. We will show in addition that while the frog has linear X cells it also has both types of nonlinear cells, $\bar{X}$ (or W) and Y. Furthermore, these classes appear to cut across the previous classifications. We will use the results of these experiments to suggest some models for possible ways in which the retina might be organized.

Some mention should be made about our choice of experimental subjects. The frog was used because extensive work by many investigators has shown a multiplicity of cell types, a number of which are clearly nonlinear (see Gordon & Hood, 1976, pp. 29–86, for a review). We wanted to see if by studying spatial summation in frog ganglion cells we could find similarities to the growing number of classes in the cat retina. Underlying this was the hope that we might gain insights into some general principles about the organization of vertebrate retinas. The eel was used because we wanted to use the same techniques on a fish retina, and Adrian and Matthews had shown this eye to be very hardy and to have relatively few optic nerve fibers. We could not obtain the same eel they studied, *Conger vulgaris,* and so used the common American eel *Anguilla rostrata*. This eel has the additional interesting feature that when it matures and migrates out to sea to spawn, its eye undergoes dramatic changes. These include a large hypertrophy and a shift in its visual pigment from a primarily a_2-based porphyropsin with a peak absorption at about 523 nm to a rhodopsin with a peak absorption at about 480 nm (Carlisle & Denton, 1959; Beatty, 1975). All of our work to date has involved the use of the immature yellow eel which lives in rather shallow coastal waters. We intend to extend our studies to the mature migrating eel to find out how its retina changes to adapt it for life as a deep sea fish.

II. Experimental Techniques

The excised eyecups of eel (*Anguilla rostrata*) and frogs (*Rana catesbeiana*) were used in these experiments. Low-resistance micropipettes were mounted on a hydraulic microdrive and lowered to the surface of the retina. In the eel eyes the electrode tip was placed on a fiber bundle as it crossed the surface of the retina and recording was generally from fibers. In the frog eyes the retina was penetrated and recording was usually from ganglion cell bodies. Amplified, discriminated nerve impulses were led to the microprocessor–stimulator–averager to be described. Using a single lens and a mirror, we imaged the face of a cathode ray tube (CRT) onto the eyecup with a reduction of 2:1 or 4:1. In most cases neutral density filters were used to reduce the stimulus intensity so that the illuminance in the retinal plane was .2 lum · m^{-2}.

The stimulus pattern on the CRT consisted of a 512-line raster presented at 200 frames per second. A temporal waveform, synchronized with the raster and fed into the z axis of the oscilloscope, produced a variety of displays. A contrast-reversal sinusoidal grating was used to test the cells' linearity of spatial summation. The number of bars (or spatial frequency), position of the grating relative to a cell's receptive field (or spatial phase), contrast, and temporal frequency of this stimulus could be varied.

A contrast-reversal grating is one in which the grating is stationary, but the intensity of adjacent bars is modulated (in this case sinusoidally) so that the dark bars become light as the bars become dark. This alternation continues at a predetermined temporal frequency. The contrast of the stimulus is

$$(I_{max} - I_{min})/(I_{max} + I_{min}),$$

and in our display it was linear with z axis voltage up to contrasts of .5. In a cell with linear spatial summation and with excitatory and inhibitory processes having similar temporal dynamics, there should be a position of the grating in which the processes exactly cancel and there is no response—the null position (Enroth-Cugell & Robson, 1966). Furthermore, the cell's sensitivity to the sinusoidal grating away from the null position should be a sinusoidal function of position (Hochstein & Shapley, 1976a).

Drifting sinusoidal gratings in which spatial frequency, temporal frequency, and contrast could be varied were used to determine the spatial modulation transfer function of the cells. Contrast of the drifting gratings was defined in the same way as for the contrast-reversal gratings. A given temporal frequency meant that the number of bars of the grating passing a fixed point was the same regardless of the spatial frequency of the grating. Single bars, which were modulated sinusoidally in intensity above and below the mean background level, and which were placed at various positions with respect to the cell's field, were used to determine neural linespread functions.

All of these patterns were produced by a stimulus generator that was operated under microprocessor control. The system was designed by Milkman, Shapley, and

Kocsis, and built in the Rockefeller University electronics shop. The duration of a run was usually 15 sec except for low temporal frequencies (less than 1 Hz) where the duration was increased to 30 sec. The microprocessor ran a signal averager that was locked to the stimulus. Upon discrimination, nerve impulses were binned and averaged over one cycle of the stimulus. Fourier analysis of the responses was performed on a PDP 11/20 computer, off-line.

III. X Cells

In both the eel and the frog there are cells that show linear spatial summation. In Figure 25.1 the responses of one of these cells for the eel is shown for three positions of a contrast-reversal grating. It is clear that the cell has a null position (0°) where there is no response and that 90° away from this position there are large responses that look approximately sinusoidal. The responses, in order to be quantified, were Fourier analyzed into their fundamental and harmonic components. The ratio of the second harmonic to the fundamental is small (less than .1) for all spatial frequencies. Thus, in X cells, the fundamental component of the response dominates regardless of the spatial frequency of the grating.

If the contrast of the grating is varied at a given position then the response amplitude as a function of contrast can be plotted, as in Figure 25.2. The responses are typically linear with contrast up to some value where the response begins to saturate. Since most of our contrasts are relatively low and produce responses well within the linear range, it is possible to plot the response to a particular contrast grating as a function of spatial position and obtain the same result as plotting sensitivity versus spatial position. Such a plot is shown in Figure 25.3, and the data points are compared to a sine wave. The excellent agreement between the curve and

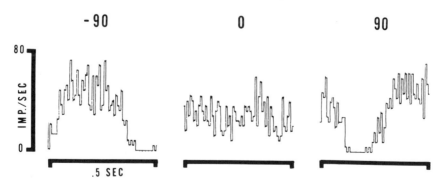

Figure 25.1. Averaged response histograms of an eel X cell at three positions of a contrast-reversal grating. The numbers above each record are the relative position or spatial phase of the grating in degrees. Note the positive response at −90°, negative response at 90°, and lack of response at 0°—the null position. The grating was modulated at 2 Hz so the duration of the record (.5 sec) represents a full temporal cycle of the stimulus. The stimulus contrast was .1 and the spatial frequency was 1.3 cycles mm^{-1}. [Redrawn from R.M. Shapley & J. Gordon, The eel retina: Ganglion cell classes and spatial mechanisms. *Journal of General Physiology,* 1978, *71,* 139–155.]

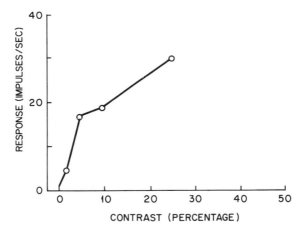

Figure 25.2. Average response amplitude of an eel X cell to increasing contrasts of a contrast-reversal grating. The grating was positioned for maximum response. The responses were Fourier analyzed and the amplitude of the fundamental component is shown. The temporal modulation rate was 2 Hz. [Redrawn from R.M. Shapley & J. Gordon, The eel retina: Ganglion cell classes and spatial mechanisms. *Journal of General Physiology*, 1978, *71*, 139–155.]

the points demonstrates that the sensitivity to the sinusoidal grating is a sinusoidal function of position. This result taken together with the sinusoidal time course of responses to sinusoidal temporal modulation is strong evidence for linear spatial summation. These cells behave very similarly to the X ganglion cells of the cat retina.

Using drifting gratings of different frequencies, we measured the spatial sensitiv-

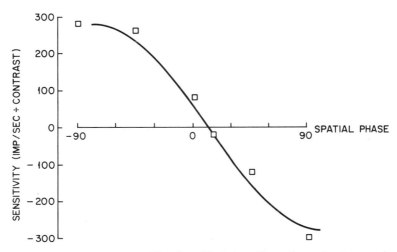

Figure 25.3. Sensitivity of an eel X cell to different positions of a contrast-reversal grating. The data points (□) are sensitivity in impulses per second divided by contrast. The solid curve is a best-fitting sine wave. Only one-half of a cycle is shown since the other half is simply the mirror image of this one. [Redrawn from R.M. Shapley & J. Gordon, The eel retina: Ganglion cell classes and spatial mechanisms. *Journal of General Physiology*, 1978, *71*, 139–155.]

ity of these eel and frog X cells. Again, because we were working in the linear range, response amplitude was a measure of sensitivity. Most of the cells we studied responded best to a particular spatial frequency and showed a decrease in sensitivity both to high- and low-frequency gratings. This result is shown in Figure 25.4 in which the sensitivities of two eel X cells are plotted as a function of spatial frequency. Such a curve is the cells' spatial frequency sensitivity (SFS). The reason for the high- and low-spatial frequency decline (Figure 25.4, ★) has been attributed by Enroth-Cugell and Robson (1966) to the cell's receptive field characteristics. The high-frequency decline occurs because the period of the grating becomes smaller than the size of the receptive field center. When this happens the total amount of light in the field center is the same at all times even though the bars moving through the field change the distribution of light within the center. Since the cell sums signals linearly, the total amount of light determines the response. If this is constant, then the response is constant, and so the cell does not resolve the grating. This leads to an insensitivity to high spatial frequencies.

The low-frequency decline is due to an area surrounding the central field that produces responses opposite in sign to the center. Low-frequency gratings are approximately equivalent to diffuse light in which the center and surround are stimulated simultaneously. Since their responses are of opposite sign and the responses sum, the result is a decline in sensitivity to low-frequency spatial stimuli. The peak of the sensitivity function (Figure 25.4, ★) corresponds to a grating in which one bar of a grating (one-half of a cycle) approximately fills the center of the cell's receptive field.

The receptive field profile shown in Figure 25.5 was determined with a sinusoidally modulated bar. It is for the same cell whose SFS is shown in Figure 25.4. It has a central response area which is on and flanking areas which are off. The size of

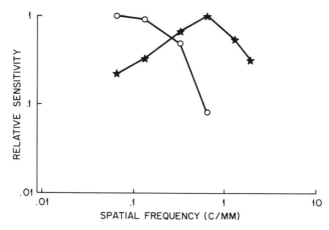

Figure 25.4. Relative sensitivity of two eel X cells to drifting sinusoidal gratings of different spatial frequency. The ★s represent an on-center, off surround cell, whereas the open circles represent an off cell with no surround. The gratings were moving at a rate of 2 Hz. [Redrawn from R.M. Shapley & J. Gordon, The eel retina: Ganglion cell classes and spatial mechanisms. *Journal of General Physiology*, 1978, *71*, 139–155.]

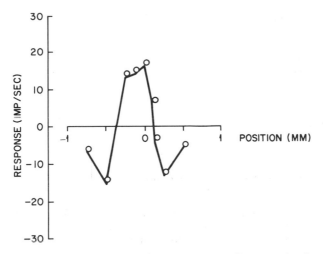

Figure 25.5. Receptive field profile of an eel on-center, off surround cell mapped with a narrow bar. The bar was sinusoidally modulated above and below the mean background level at 1 Hz and a contrast of .25. The width of the bar was .3 mm on the retina. [Redrawn from R.M. Shapley & J. Gordon, The eel retina: Ganglion cell classes and spatial mechanisms. *Journal of General Physiology,* 1978, *71,* 139–155.]

the central area is about .5 mm, which corresponds to the peak of the SFS at slightly less than 1 cycle mm^{-1} or a half cycle (one bar) of slightly more than .5 mm. Thus the shape of the SFS is well predicted by a concentric receptive field organization in which the signals within the receptive field center sum linearly as do the signals between the center and surround of the receptive field. This is basically the same as the linear model proposed by Rodieck (1965) for the cat retina (solid lines, Figure 25.13).

Some eel and frog cells that responded at light offset only (off cells) did not have any apparent surround mechanism. Consistent with this was the finding of no low-frequency decline in their SFSs (Figure 25.4, open circles).

IV. X̄ Cells

Now let us consider another class of ganglion cells that appears in both eel and frog but that does not show linear spatial summation. We will call these cells X̄, since they are neither like the X cells previously described nor are they like the Y cells to be described later. These cells give on–off responses to lights in most parts of their receptive fields. Their responses to a contrast-reversal grating (Figure 25.6) have a dominant fundamental response and small amount of frequency doubling or second harmonic response when the grating is positioned for maximal response amplitude (−90° and +90°). When the grating is positioned at what would be a null for an X cell (0°), there is an almost pure frequency-doubled response. If the spatial frequency of the grating is changed, the response magnitude may change depending on the characteristics of the cell's

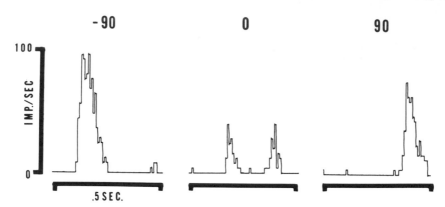

Figure 25.6. Averaged response histograms of an eel $\overline{X}$ cell to three positions of a contrast-reversal grating. The numbers above each record are the spatial phase of the grating in degrees. The grating was modulated at 2 Hz, its contrast was .3, and its spatial frequency was .65 cycle mm^{-1}. [Redrawn from R.M. Shapley and J. Gordon, The eel retina: Ganglion cell classes and spatial mechanisms. *Journal of General Physiology,* 1978, *71,* 139–155.]

SFS. However, as shown in Figure 25.7, the relative magnitudes of the fundamental and second harmonic responses do not change very much as a function of spatial frequency. The second harmonic/first harmonic ratio increases from about .4 at low spatial frequencies to about .8 at high spatial frequencies. The relative amount of second harmonic is considerably larger than that seen in X cells in which the second harmonic was never more than one-tenth of the fundamental. Careful mapping of the receptive fields of the $\overline{X}$ cells showed that, while they had both on and off responses in most areas, the on and off areas were not exactly concentric and were not exactly the same size.

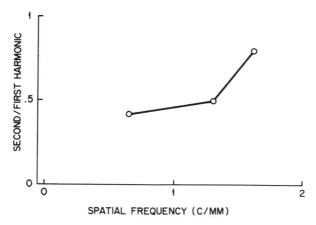

Figure 25.7. Response histograms, like those in Figure 25.6, were Fourier analyzed. The ratio of the second harmonic component divided by the fundamental is plotted as a function of spatial frequency of the stimulus for an eel $\overline{X}$ cell. The temporal modulation of the stimulation was 2 Hz and its contrast was .3.

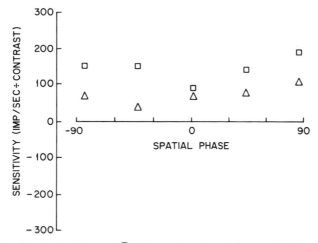

Figure 25.8. Sensitivity of an eel $\bar{X}$ cell as a function of the spatial phase of a contrast-reversal grating. The open squares represent the fundamental component of the responses, while the open triangles represent the second harmonic component of the responses. Both components appear relatively independent of spatial phase. [Redrawn from R.M. Shapley & J. Gordon, The eel retina: Ganglion cell classes and spatial mechanisms. *Journal of General Physiology,* 1978, *71,* 139-155.]

The sensitivity of X cells to contrast-reversal gratings had a sinusoidal dependence on the relative position or phase of the grating (Figure 25.3). No such dependence was found for cells. In fact, as shown in Figure 25.8, the sensitivities of both the fundamental (□) and second harmonic responses (△) of an X cell are relatively independent of the spatial phase of the grating.

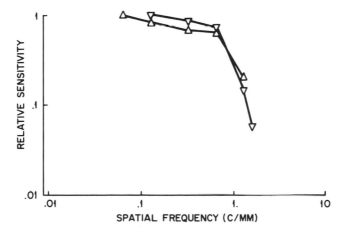

Figure 25.9. Relative sensitivity of two eel $\bar{X}$ cells to drifting sinusoidal gratings of different spatial frequency. The drift rate was 1 (▽) or 2 (△) Hz. Note the lack of a low-frequency decline. [Redrawn from R.M. Shapley and J. Gordon, The eel retina: Ganglion cell classes and spatial mechanisms. *Journal of General Physiology,* 1978, *71,* 139-155.]

The SFS of the eel $\overline{X}$ cells had a high-frequency decline but usually no low-frequency decline (Figure 25.9). This is consistent with the receptive field mapping showing no surround to the on and off areas. Note that some frog $\overline{X}$ cells do show a low-frequency decline although they also have no mappable surround, which is most likely due to the silent surround (inhibiting an excitatory response but producing no ganglion cell response of its own) described by Barlow (1953). Figure 25.10 shows a model consistent with the characteristics of the $\overline{X}$ cells. The on (excitatory) and off (inhibitory) responses sum separately and linearly within themselves. Thus the resolution of the cell is determined by its receptive field size. However, before the on and off processes combine they are half-wave rectified. Therefore, they do not cancel each other and the responses are frequency doubled. If the receptive fields of the on and off mechanisms were exactly concentric then there might actually be a null position. In this case, the nulls within each mechanism would occur in the same place. In fact, some frog $\overline{X}$ cells apparently did have concentric fields and therefore did have null positions for the contrast-reversal gratings. The fact that there is usually no null and that the response waveform varies with spatial phase indicates that the two fields are not exactly lined up with one another. It also suggests that their total sensitivities (perhaps due to different summation areas) are not exactly the same. This is consistent with our receptive field maps previously described.

The $\overline{X}$ nonlinear cells are not similar to the Y nonlinear cells of the cat, to be considered in the next section. Rather they seem more like the on–off W cells of the cat (Stone & Fukuda, 1974). These, like the $\overline{X}$ cells, give local on–off responses and are not sensitive to fine gratings, that is, gratings whose bars are much smaller than the receptive field of the cell.

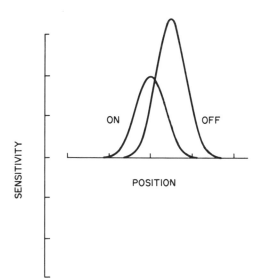

Figure 25.10. Spatial model of an $\overline{X}$ cell receptive field. The spatial extent of the on and off areas overlap, but they are not concentric, and they do not have the same sensitivity. Stimulation of the on area produces on excitation while stimulation of the off area produces off excitation. Since the responses from each area are half-wave rectified they do not cancel each other when both areas are stimulated simultaneously. [Redrawn from R.M. Shapley & J. Gordon, The eel retina: Ganglion cell classes and spatial mechanisms. *Journal of General Physiology,* 1978, *71,* 139–155.]

V. Y Cells

Finally, let us consider a group of ganglion cells found in the frog retina but not in the eel retina. These cells were either locally on–off to stimulation anywhere in the field or yielded off responses everywhere, were off to diffuse light, and had small local on regions within the larger off receptive field. The responses to a low-spatial frequency contrast-reversal grating (Figure 25.11, top) were always frequency doubled to every stimulus position, but there were positions in which one of the components was larger; that is, there was apparently some fundamental component in addition to the second harmonic response. When the spatial frequency was increased, however, both response components had approximately the same magnitude regardless of stimulus spatial phase (Figure 25.11, bottom). Fourier analysis of the responses allowed quantitative separation of first and second harmonics and a plot of the second harmonic/first harmonic ratio for different spatial frequencies is shown in Figure 25.12. As spatial frequency increases, the second harmonic takes over and completely dominates the response. At high spatial frequencies the second harmonic is five times larger than the fundamental. This behavior is very much like that of Y-type cat ganglion cells (Hochstein & Shapley, 1976a, 1976b).

The frog Y cells are also like those of the cat in other important ways. For example, the sensitivity of these cells to high spatial frequency drifting gratings cannot be predicted by the receptive field size of the cell. Rather, the cells resolve gratings that are much finer than the receptive field center, implying that the recep-

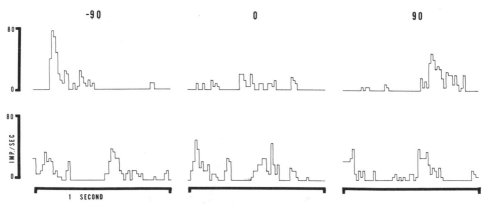

Figure 25.11. Averaged response histograms of a frog Y cell to three positions and two spatial frequencies of a contrast-reversal grating. The numbers above the records are the spatial phase of the grating in degrees. The upper set of records are for a low spatial frequency (.7 cycle mm^{-1}) at .125 contrast while the lower set of records are for a high spatial frequency (4.2 cycles mm^{-1}) at .5 contrast. The temporal modulation rate was 1 Hz. The upper responses are of the fundamental temporal frequency and are responsive to spatial phase. The lower responses show frequency doubling and are phase insensitive.

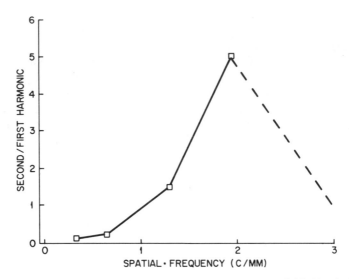

Figure 25.12. Ratio of the second harmonic response component divided by the fundamental plotted as a function of spatial frequency for a frog Y cell. These were determined in the same way as those in Figure 25.7. This ratio increases steeply with increasing spatial frequency (□). The dashed line is an extrapolation back to the ratio of 1 that would be expected when the spatial frequency of the grating becomes very high so that both harmonics are in the noise.

tive field is made up of subfields or subunits. Some features of the receptive field model used by Hochstein and Shapley (1976b) to explain this finding in the cat (Figure 25.13) are applicable to the frog data as well. In this model there is a linear field that sums signals from within its entire area and produces the fundamental response. Thus a low-frequency grating is a good stimulus for the fundamental

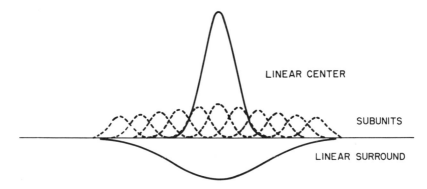

Figure 25.13. Spatial model of a Y-cell receptive field. There is a linear center and surround (solid curve) as in an X cell. In addition there are fine nonlinear rectifying subunits (dashed curves) that overlap the linear center and surround. [Redrawn from Hochstein & Shapley (1976b).]

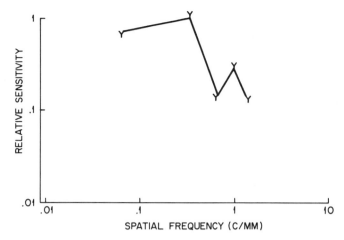

Figure 25.14.   Relative sensitivity of a frog Y cell as a function of the spatial frequency of a drifting sinusoidal grating. The drift rate was 1 Hz. There is a small but consistent low-frequency decline.

response, and there will be a null position for the fundamental response. The second harmonic response, however, is produced by small rectifying subunits. They are much smaller than the total receptive field and so resolve fine gratings. Thus, the second harmonic component of the response remains large when the spatial frequency of the grating is increased and the fundamental response decreases.

The SFS of a frog Y cell is shown in Figure 25.14. There is a weak low-frequency cutoff which, like that in cat Y cells, is very sensitive to the temporal modulation of the stimulus. In the frog it is greater if the temporal modulation of the stimulus is decreased. The secondary peak at high frequencies is also seen in the cat (Hochstein & Shapley, 1976b), although the reason for it is not known.

Some of the frog Y cells, as mentioned, responded to diffuse light primarily at its offset. In fact, in a number of these apparent ''off'' cells there was no on component at all to slow temporal modulation of the stimulus. An experiment on such a cell using a slowly modulated contrast-reversal grating gave a null and no-frequency doubling; that is, the cell appeared to be a linear X cell even though at higher temporal frequencies the behavior was Y-like. Thus the second harmonic component had a low temporal frequency cutoff while the fundamental did not.

VI. On–Off Responses

It is apparent that there are two somewhat different types of mechanisms that can generate frequency-doubled or on–off responses. Both mechanisms can result in local on–off responses, and on–off responses to diffuse light. The fundamental difference between them concerns the size and number of rectifying subunits that make up their receptive fields. In the $\overline{X}$ or W-like cells there is one large on area and one large off area. Each area sums within itself and the rectified output is transmitted to the ganglion cell. In the Y-like cells there are many little overlapping subunits, each summing within its little area, and the rectified outputs of all of them are transmitted to the ganglion cell.

It is now thought that the retinal elements in the distal retina, including the receptors, horizontal cells, and bipolar cells, are basically linear (e.g., Toyoda, 1974). It is presumed, therefore, that the X cells and the linear portion of X and Y cells are derived from input involving direct bipolar transmission. Many amacrine cells, however, are quite nonlinear and in fact are the first retinal elements showing frequency doubling. It is possible then that the rectifying elements in $\overline{X}$ and Y cells are provided by amacrine cells. The many types and sizes of amacrines may explain the differences in the characteristics of the rectifying elements between $\overline{X}$ and Y cells.

VII. Ganglion Cell Classification

We think that the techniques used in our experiments provide a way to suggest and examine models of functional connectivity of retinal neurons. The three distinct classes we described, and which appear similar to cat cells, differ from one another in terms of the way in which they sum signals within their receptive fields. Thus they give some insights into retinal wiring, which we have considered. We thought it reasonable to try to relate these classes to the older classification schemes that have been used for frog ganglion cells (Hartline, 1938, 1940a, 1940b; Maturana, Lettvin, McCulloch, & Pitts, 1960; Reuter, 1969; Keating & Gaze, 1970).

Our sample of cells is still rather small but it has become clear that there is no one-to-one correspondence between our division of the cells and the earlier divisions. Most of our X cells would fit into classes one and two of Maturana *et al.* (1960). However, we mentioned some X cells with just off responses and no surrounds that would fit Hartline's off classes and Maturana's Class 4. Our $\overline{X}$ cells either responded to full field lights with an off response, or with an on–off response and various weightings of on and off components. Thus they could be from Hartline's on–off class (Maturana's Class 3) or Hartline's off class (Maturana's Class 4). We should note that Hartline was always extremely careful to point out that his classes were not discrete but rather were points along a continuum.

Finally, our frog Y cells came either from cells with local and full field on–off responses, or from cells with full field off responses and local on areas within the off field. Thus, they too come from the on–off, off continuum, but in terms of construction of their receptive fields they are quite different from the $\overline{X}$ cells. The problems associated with the various classification schemes have been previously discussed in detail with particular reference to frog ganglion cells (Gordon & Hood, 1976, pp. 29–86). Similar issues arise in classifying retinal ganglion cells in the cat (Hochstein & Shapley, 1976a). We think that our way of studying these cells allows us not only to categorize them into distinct classes but also to develop testable models for the way in which the retina is organized.

ACKNOWLEDGMENT

Computer time was provided, in part, by the City University of New York University Computer Center.

REFERENCES

Adrian, E.D., & Matthews, R. The discharge of impulses in the optic nerve and its relation to the electric changes in the retina. *Journal of Physiology,* 1927, *63,* 378–414. (a)

Adrian, E.D., & Matthews, R. The process involved in retinal excitation. *Journal of Physiology,* 1927, *64,* 279–301. (b)

Adrian, E.D., & Matthews, R. The interaction of retinal neurones. *Journal of Physiology,* 1928, *65,* 273–298.

Barlow, H.B. Summation and inhibition in the frog's retina. *Journal of Physiology,* 1953, *119,* 69–88.

Beatty, D.D. Visual pigments of the American eel *Anguilla rostrata. Vision Research,* 1975, *15,* 771–776.

Carlisle, D.B., & Denton, E.J. On the metamorphosis of the visual pigments of *Anguilla anguilla* (L.). *Journal of the Marine Biological Association of the United Kingdom,* 1959, *38,* 97–102.

Enroth-Cugell, C., & Robson, J.G. The contrast sensitivity of the retinal ganglion cells of the cat. *Journal of Physiology,* 1966, *187,* 517–552.

Gordon, J., & Graham, N. Early light and dark adaptation in frog on–off retinal ganglion cells. *Vision Research,* 1973, *13,* 647–659.

Gordon, J., & Hood, D.C. The anatomy and physiology of the frog retina. In K.V. Fite (Ed.), *The amphibian visual system: A multidisciplinary approach.* New York: Academic Press, 1976.

Hartline, H.K. The response of single optic nerve fibers in the vertebrate eye to illumination of the retina. *American Journal of Physiology,* 1938, *121,* 400–415.

Hartline, H.K. The receptive fields of optic nerve fibers. *American Journal of Physiology,* 1940, *130,* 690–699. (a)

Hartline, H.K. The effects of spatial summation in the retina on the excitation of the fibers of the optic nerve. *American Journal of Physiology,* 1940, *130,* 700–711. (b)

Hochstein, S., & Shapley, R.M. Quantitative analysis of retinal ganglion cell classifications. *Journal of Physiology,* 1976, *262,* 237–264. (a)

Hochstein, S., & Shapley, R.M. Linear and nonlinear spatial subunits in Y cat retinal ganglion cells. *Journal of Physiology,* 1976, *262,* 265–284. (b)

Keating, M.J., & Gaze, R.M. Observations on the surround properties of the receptive fields of frog retinal ganglion cells. *Quarterly Journal of Experimental Physiology,* 1970, *55,* 129–140.

Maturana, H.R., Lettvin, J.Y., McCulloch, W.S., & Pitts, W.H. Anatomy and physiology of vision in the frog, *Rana pipiens. Journal of General Physiology,* 1960, *43* (Supplement), 125–175.

Reuter, T. Visual pigments and ganglion cell activity in the retinae of tadpoles and adult frogs *(Rana temporaria). Acta Zoologica Fennica,* 1969, *122,* 1–64.

Rodieck, R.W. Quantitative analysis of cat retinal ganglion cell response to visual stimuli. *Vision Research,* 1965, *5,* 583–610.

Shapley, R.M., & Gordon, J. The eel retina: Ganglion cell classes and spatial mechanisms. *Journal of General Physiology,* 1978, *71,* 139–155.

Stone, J., & Fukuda, Y. Properties of cat retinal ganglion cells. A comparison of W-cells with X- and Y-cells. *Journal of Neurophysiology,* 1974, *37,* 722–748.

Toyoda, J. Frequency characteristics of retinal neurons in the carp. *Journal of General Physiology,* 1974, *63,* 214–234.

26. Subjective Contours, Visual Acuity, and Line Contrast

R. H. Day and M. K. Jory

I. Introduction

Visually perceived edges and borders are usually correlated with changes in the rate of change over space of such stimulus properties as luminance, hue, and texture density. However, contours are occasionally perceived in the absence of any discontinuities in the stimulus surface, that is, in regions that are physically uniform. These apparent edges, variously called subjective, cognitive, quasi-perceptual, illusory, or anomalous contours, were first noted by Schumann (1904), and later studied by Prandtl (1927), Ehrenstein (1941), and Kanizsa (1955). Subjective contours, as we shall call them here, have recently attracted a great deal of attention and speculation as to their origin (Coren, 1972; Gregory, 1972).

During the course of a series of experiments concerned with the basis of subjective contours it occurred to us that these effects might derive from two brightness phenomena that can be observed in line patterns. We call these assimilation and dissimilation of brightness. Assimilation of brightness, first reported by von Bezold (1874) and Rood (1879), and independently and extensively investigated by Helson and his associates (Helson, 1943; Helson & Joy, 1962; Helson & Rohles, 1959), is essentially a loss or suppression of brightness contrast between lines and interspaces lying more or less side by side. Dissimilation of brightness, a term we have coined, was first described by Ehrenstein (1941) and is essentially an enhancement of brightness contrast occurring mainly, as far as we have observed, in gaps between lines lying end to end. For convenience we refer to these two effects together as "line contrast" to distinguish them from simultaneous brightness contrast. Assimilation is opposite in sign to simultaneous contrast and dissimilation the same. However, in bracketing assimilation and dissimilation of brightness together we do not wish to imply that they are opponent processes or even necessarily related, as we

331

originally thought. Nor do we wish to suggest that dissimilation and simultaneous contrast are unrelated.

Our reasoning was as follows. If the brightness of a white region is reduced through assimilation and that of an adjoining region is enhanced by dissimilation, then a subjective contour would be expected to occur between the two regions. Informal observation and a preliminary experiment strongly supported this view; subjective contours seemed to represent an apparent discontinuity between assimilated and dissimilated areas. We then argued that assimilation and dissimilation of brightness should markedly affect the visibility of fine detail. A white interspace between two parallel dark lines should have a higher threshold than a strip formed of gaps in black lines lying end to end. Furthermore, a dark element in a light region between black lines should be more difficult to detect than when seen alone in a plain field of the same luminance.

Here we are primarily concerned with reporting two experiments showing that assimilation and dissimilation of brightness have a marked effect on visual acuity. We wish also to suggest that the detection of small elements enclosed within dark lines, the enclosing contour effect (Craik & Zangwill, 1939; Youniss & Calvin, 1961), is due to assimilation of brightness. As far as we know, involvement of these two brightness effects in visual resolution of detail has not been recognized so far, although the outcome of some earlier experiments can be so interpreted. Before turning to the experiments themselves it is necessary briefly to describe and demonstrate assimilation and dissimilation of brightness and to show their role in the formation of subjective contours.

II. Assimilation and Dissimilation of Brightness

Assimilation and dissimilation of brightness can be observed in Figure 26.1A in which parallel black and white lines on a uniform gray surround are interrupted by gaps that form a narrow strip across the pattern. The gray interspaces between the black parallels on the right appear darker than the gray ground surrounding the pattern and those between the white lines on the left lighter than the ground. It is as if the difference in brightness between the black and white lines and their gray interspaces has been suppressed. Contrariwise, the narrow strip at right angles to the black lines appears lighter than the gray surround and that at right angles to the white lines appears darker. Perceptually the difference in brightness between the strip and the black and white lines is enhanced. We have called this enhancement effect dissimilation of brightness.

In his early demonstration, von Bezold (1874) superimposed black and white arabesques on blue or red grounds. In these patterns, reproduced by Burnham (1953) and Evans (1948), the blue and red areas overlaid by white arabesques are notably lighter than those overlaid by black. Assimilation was later described by Newhall (1942) and Helson (1943). Parametric studies have been reported by Burnham (1953), Helson and Rohles (1959), and Helson and Joy (1962). Dissimilation

Figure 26.1. Examples of assimilation and dissimilation of brightness. Assimilation, which is a suppression of differences in brightness, occurs as apparent darkening and lightening of interspaces, respectively, between black and white lines in (A) and as apparent darkening of interspaces between the parallel, radiating, and concentric lines in (B–D), respectively. Dissimilation is an enhancement of brightness differences and occurs as apparent darkening and lightening, respectively, in the horizontal strip formed by the ends of black and white lines in (A) and as apparent lightening in the strip, ring, and cross of (B–D), respectively.

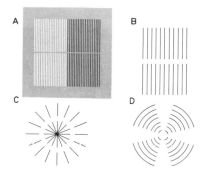

of brightness at the termination of lines occurs in patterns used by Ehrenstein (1941, 1954), Jung and Spillman (1970), and Spillman, Fuld, and Gerrits (1976). It is described specifically by Frisby and Clatworthy (1975) and Kennedy (1975). Spillman *et al.* (1976) and Kennedy (1975) also commented on the subjective contours formed along line ends.

Further instances of assimilation and dissimilation of brightness are shown in Figure 26.1B–D. In each case it can be observed that the brightness of white regions enclosed between lines has undergone assimilation to the black and is less than that of the white ground of the same luminance. Contrariwise, the brightness of the regions that cut transversely across the patterns with edges marked by the ends of lines is dissimilated from the black and is noticeably greater than that of the area surrounding the figures.

The possibility that assimilation or dissimilation of brightness is due to "mixing" of small adjacent regions of different luminance either as a result of voluntary eye movements or their below- or near-threshold angular subtense ("mosaic mixture") is unlikely. Both effects occur when the separation between the elements is too great for mixing through eye movement and both occur during very brief exposures (Burnham, 1953; Helson & Rohles, 1959; Jung, 1973; Spillman *et al.,* 1976).

Casual inspection of the patterns shown in Figure 26.1 suggests that dissimilation of brightness occurs in spaces or gaps between the ends of lines. Evidence for this was obtained when small cross-lines or "feet" were added to the ends of lines. The effect of these orthogonal cross-lines was to change the definition of the space by line ends to that by short line edges. The change and its effects on brightness in the gap can be observed clearly by comparing the upper and lower patterns in Figure 26.2A. In the upper pattern, enhancement of brightness relative to the surround of the figure occurs in the vertical gap defined by the ends of lines forming a grating. Addition of the short cross-lines so that the gap is now enclosed by two parallel dashed lines results in elimination of brightness enhancement. A similar change of brightness occurs in Figure 26.2B.

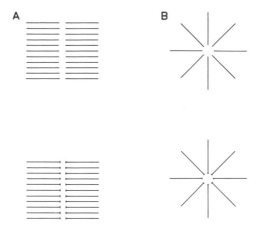

Figure 26.2. Elimination of dissimilation with the addition of short cross-lines to the ends of horizontal lines in (A) and radiating lines in (B).

III. Subjective Contours

We argued that if opposed changes in brightness occur between two contiguous regions of uniform luminance as a result of brightness assimilation in line interspaces in one region and dissimilation of gaps between them in another adjacent to it, then a visible contour may be expected to occur between the two regions. That this is so can be observed in Figure 26.1. In Figure 26.1B subjective contours can be observed along the edges of the horizontal strip separating the regions of decreased and increased brightness. Similar contours can be seen forming the edges of the annulus in Figure 26.1C and the cross in Figure 26.1D. The subjective contours along the edges of the horizontal strip on the left and right of Figure 26.1A show that they occur when assimilation results in increased brightness and dissimilation in decreased brightness, and vice versa.

The central feature of our proposal is that subjective contours are secondary outcomes of the changes in brightness. Changes in brightness occur also as a result of simultaneous contrast between larger areas of different luminance. It is to be

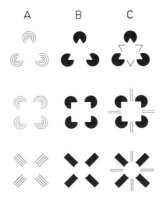

Figure 26.3. Subjective contours attributable to (A) assimilation and dissimilation of brightness ("line contrast") in line figures; (B) simultaneous brightness contrast in figures with larger elements; and (C) both assimilation and dissimilation of brightness and simultaneous brightness contrast. The upper figure in group (C) is the Kanizsa figure.

expected, therefore, that if differences in brightness between adjacent regions of uniform luminance result from simultaneous contrast, then subjective contours should also occur. Examples of subjective contours attributable to assimilation and dissimilation of brightness, simultaneous brightness contrast, and a combination of both effects are shown in Figure 26.3. It can be noted that in these terms the subjective contours in the well-known Kanizsa figure (Kanizsa, 1955) are probably due to a combination of the two classes of brightness effect.

We have obtained evidence for the role of brightness differences in the formation of subjective contours in an experiment in which observers compared the brightnesses of adjacent regions both with the surround of the same luminance and with each other.

IV. Resolution of Detail in Line Patterns

Riggs (1965) has pointed out that experiments in which the physical contrast of a test element is varied can be classed as studies either of the relation of visual acuity to contrast or of brightness discrimination. Such experiments represent a region of overlap between the two visual functions. Results from a number of investigations (Aubert, 1865; Cobb & Moss, 1927; Lythgoe, 1932) show that acuity for detail is maximal for the highest degree of physical contrast between test element and background. We reasoned, therefore, that if through assimilation the brightness difference, that is, apparent contrast, between lines and interspaces arranged side by side were reduced, then their resolution threshold would be increased, that is, acuity would be poorer. In addition, if as a result of dissimilation of brightness apparent contrast were enhanced then the threshold would be decreased. We have tested this in two experiments, the first exploratory and open to some criticism of procedure, and the second more formal and rigorous.

In the first experiment 10 paid undergraduate subjects indicated when vertical, white target gaps at the centers of three patterns (shown in Figure 26.4) were just visible as the patterns approached or receded. The patterns were centered in a circular aperture 20 cm in diameter in a screen that moved backward and forward on tracks. The target gap in each pattern was .2 mm wide. Each subject underwent four balanced trials with each pattern, two approaching and two receding. The task throughout was to indicate when the target gap was just visible.

We expected that the threshold for Figure 26.4A would be low as a result of high contrast between the assimilated white area separating the horizontal lines and the dissimilated area separating the ends of the lines. We also expected that the threshold for the resolution of Figure 26.4B would be relatively high because of assimilation of the white of the target gap between the black lines. Finally, we expected that the cross-lines bounding the target gap in Figure 26.4C would result in reduced contrast, as previously pointed out, and, therefore, in a higher threshold.

The mean distances for resolution of the target together with resolution thresholds in terms of angular subtense are shown in Table 26.1. It can be seen that the

EXPERIMENT I   EXPERIMENT II

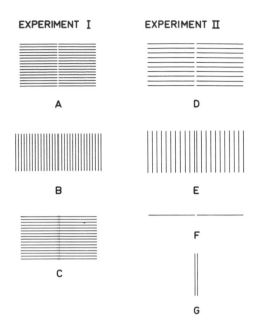

Figure 26.4. Stimulus patterns with vertical target gaps used in Experiments I (A–C) and II (D–G). For purposes of clarity in reproduction the central gaps are twice the size relative to figure widths than they were in the original patterns.

threshold for the gap in Figure 26.4A was about five to six times lower than for those in Figure 26.4B and C. Statistical tests have shown that there is a clearly significant difference between the threshold measures for the pattern in Figure 26.4A and those in Figure 26.4B and C, but no difference between the two latter patterns. In short, the expectations based on apparent contrast due to assimilation and dissimilation of brightness were realized.

The purpose of the second experiment was twofold, to check the results of the first experiment under better controlled conditions and to establish whether the effects of line contrast operate with patterns consisting merely of two lines. Viewing distance (1.3 m), exposure time (2 sec), and field luminance (95 cd m^{-2}) were controlled by presenting the stimulus patterns in a tachistoscope. This time we used a double random staircase procedure to establish thresholds for patterns similar to those shown in Figure 26.4D–G, two essentially the same as those used earlier and two consisting merely of a pair of lines. The patterns were accurate reductions on matte surfaces of much larger, carefully prepared originals. The central, vertical target gaps varied in width from 11 sec to 1 min 33 sec in 10-sec steps. The lines were 21 sec wide and 2 min 52 sec apart. A group of 12 paid undergraduate subjects participated under the four conditions represented in Figure 26.4. It was expected that, as in the first experiment, the threshold for Figure 26.4D in which both assimilation and dissimilation of brightness increased contrast would be lower than in Figure 26.4E in which assimilation reduced it. In Figure 26.4F and G, only dissimilation and assimilation occurred, respectively, so that the threshold for the former was expected to be less than for the latter, but not to the same extent as that between Figure 26.4D and E.

TABLE 26.1

Mean Distances and Visual Angles for Resolution of Target Gaps in the Patterns
Used in Experiments I (Figure 26.4, A–C) and II (Figure 26.4, D–G)[a]

	Pattern			
	A	B	C	
Experiment I				
Mean resolution distance (m)	3.41	.68	.55	
SD	.53	.11	.16	
Mean resolution angle (sec)	11.88	60.84	74.88	
	D	E	F	G
Experiment II				
Mean resolution angle (sec)	15.58	41.67	34.58	46.50
SD	6.98	12.34	14.14	12.26

[a] Standard deviations (SD) of distances are shown for Experiment I and of angles for
Experiment II.

Mean resolution thresholds are shown in Table 26.1. It can be seen that the
expectations in terms of contrast due to assimilation and dissimilation were realized.
The threshold for the pattern represented in Figure 26.4D was less than that represented in Figure 26.4E and that in Figure 26.4F less than that in Figure 26.4G, but
that the difference between the latter pair was less than that between the former pair.
The differences are statistically reliable. Note also that the difference in resolution
threshold between the stimulus patterns shown in Figure 26.4D and E was less than
that between those shown in Figure 26.4A and B. Whereas in the first experiment
the thresholds differed by a factor of about 5, in the second experiment it was about 3.

V. The Enclosing Contour Effect

If the brightness difference between two black lines lying side by side and a white
region between is diminished by assimilation of brightness, it would be expected
that apparent contrast between the white region and a small figure such as a black
dot would also be reduced. In consequence the threshold for detecting the dot would
be expected to rise. That a rise does occur under these conditions was shown in
experiments by Craik and Zangwill (1939), who established the threshold for small
figures and points enclosed between straight lines and within an irregular outline.
Threshold rises occurred also when a point was located near straight lines. Later, in
independent experiments, Youniss and Calvin (1961) showed that the time taken to
recognize tachistoscopically presented nonsense syllables enclosed within a circle or
triangle was greater than when they were presented without an enclosing contour.
Vernon (1961) pointed out the essential similarity between the outcomes of these
experiments and those from Craik and Zangwill's experiments.

VI. Discussion

The data presented here show that the two classes of line contrast, assimilation and dissimilation of brightness, are involved in the generation of subjective contours, in the visibility of real contours and detail, and in the enclosing contour effect. In regard to visual acuity, it seems to us that the relatively high threshold for the resolution of the space between parallels—the minimum separable—is due in part to assimilation of brightness and consequent contrast loss.

A further point needs to be made about the role of line contrast in the generation of subjective contours. The formation of these contours in regions such as the corners of the triangle and square in Figure 26.3A is, as pointed out, probably due to assimilation of brightness between the concentric lines and dissimilation of brightness in the gaps between their ends. Thus the subjective contour occurs between the region of suppressed and enhanced brightness. However, the contour also extends across the break between the corners to complete the triangle and square. It is as if the enhanced brightness in the corners of the figures has filled the total triangular or square areas. Such spreading of contrast effects bears a close similarity to the Craik–O'Brien effect (Cornsweet, 1970). Thus it is necessary to distinguish between *formation* of subjective contours through assimilation and dissimilation of brightness and *completion* of contours due to spreading of enhanced brightness within the defined region.

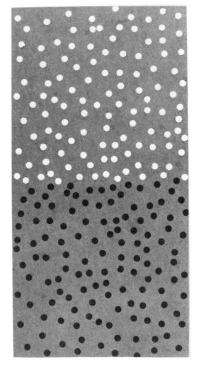

Figure 26.5. Example of assimilation of brightness in a pattern of irregularly arranged spots. The gray between the white spots appears lighter than that between the dark spots. A similar pattern was first shown to the senior author by D. M. Mackay of the University of Keele.

Both assimilation and dissimilation have been known for a long time. We wish to reemphasize, however, that in bracketing the two effects together under the heading of line contrast we do not intend to imply either an opponent or any other form of relationship between them. As far as we have observed dissimilation of brightness is confined to gaps between line ends. Assimilation of brightness seems to occur in patterns in which elements, including lines, are regularly or irregularly distributed. This can be observed in Figure 26.5 in a pattern consisting of black and white spots on a gray field, which was shown recently to one of us by D. M. Mackay of the University of Keele. The range of conditions under which both effects occur has yet to be explored in detail.

We wish to make another point in conclusion. The relationship between dissimilation of brightness and classic (simultaneous) brightness contrast is an issue for further enquiry. It is conceivable that the two are identical and that the former is merely a special case of the latter, occurring in a gap between two relatively long lines. There is much more yet to be discovered and to be theorized.

REFERENCES

Aubert, H. *Physiologie der Netzhaut*. Bredau: Morgenstern, 1865.

Burnham, R. W. Bezold's colour mixture effect. *American Journal of Psychology*, 1953, *66*, 377–385.

Cobb, P. W., & Moss, F. K. The relation between extent and contrast in the liminal stimulus for vision. *Journal of Experimental Psychology*, 1927, *10*, 350–364.

Coren, S. Subjective contour and apparent depth. *Psychological Review*, 1972, *79*, 359–367.

Cornsweet, T. N. *Visual perception*. New York: Academic Press, 1970.

Craik, K. J. W., & Zangwill, O. L. Observations relating to the threshold of a small figure within the contour of a closed-line figure. *British Journal of Psychology*, 1939, *30*, 139–150.

Ehrenstein, W. Uber Abwandlungen der L. Hermannschen Helligkeit-serscheinung. *Zeitschrifte für Psychologie*, 1941, *150*, 83–91.

Ehrenstein, W. *Probleme der ganzheitspsychologischen Wahrnehmungslehre* (3rd ed.). Leipzig: J. A. Barth, 1954.

Evans, R. M. *An introduction to color*. New York: Wiley, 1948.

Frisby, J. P., & Clatworthy, J. L. Illusory contours: Curious cases of simultaneous brightness contrast? *Perception*, 1975, *4*, 349–357.

Gregory, R. L. Cognitive contours. *Nature*, 1972, *238*, 51–52.

Helson, H. Some factors and implications of colour constancy. *Journal of the Optical Society of America*, 1943, *33*, 555–567.

Helson, H., & Joy, V. L. Domains of lightness assimilation and contrast. *Psychologische Beitrage*, 1962, *6*, 405–415.

Helson, H., & Rohles, F. H. A quantitative study of the reversal of classical lightness contrast. *American Journal of Psychology*, 1959, *72*, 530–538.

Jung, R., & Spillman, L. Receptive field estimation and perceptual integration in human vision. In F. A. Young & D. B. Lindsley (Eds.), *Early experience and visual information processing*. Washington, D.C.: National Academy of Sciences, 1970.

Kanizsa, G. Marzini quasi-percettivi in campi con stimolazione omogenea. *Rivista di Psicologia*, 1955, *49*, 7–30.

Kennedy, J. M. Depth at an edge, coplanarity, slant depth, change in direction and change in brightness in the production of subjective contours. *Italian Journal of Psychology*, 1975, *2*, 107–123.

Lythgoe, R. J. The measurement of visual acuity. *Medical Research Council Special Reports,* Series 173. London: H. M. Stationery Office, 1932.

Newhall, S. M. The reversal of simultaneous brightness contrast. *Journal of Experimental Psychology,* 1942, *31,* 393–409.

Prandtl, A. Uber gleischsinnige Induktion unde die Lichtverteilung in gitterartingen Mustern. *Zeitschrifte für Sinnesphysiologie,* 1927, *58,* 263–307.

Riggs, L. A. Visual acuity. In C. H. Graham (Ed.), *Vision and visual perception.* New York: Wiley, 1965.

Rood, O. N. *Modern chromatics.* London: Kegan Paul, 1879.

Schumann, F. Einige Beobachtungen ueber die Zusammenfassung von Gesichtseindrucken zu Einheiten. *Psychologische Studien,* 1904, *1,* 1–32.

Spillman, L., Fuld, K., & Gerrits, H. J. M. Brightness contrast in the Ehrenstein illusion. *Vision Research,* 1976, *16,* 713–719.

Vernon, M. D. Comment on "the enclosing contour effect." *Perceptual and Motor Skills,* 1961, *13,* 334.

von Bezold, W. *Die Farbenlehre,* 1874. [*The theory of colour*] (S. R. Koehler, trans.). Boston: L. Prang, 1876.

Youniss, J., & Calvin, A. D. The enclosing contour effect. *Perceptual and Motor Skills,* 1961, *13,* 75–81.

27. Effects of Fixational Eye Movements on Contrast Sensitivity

Ülker Tulunay-Keesey

I. Introduction

It has been known for over a century that the eye exhibits small, continual movements during fixation. Lorrin Riggs and his associates (Ratliff & Riggs, 1950) were able to measure these movements with great precision by making use of a contact lens which the observer wore and which followed the movements of the eye with fidelity. A small plane-surface mirror was embedded on the temporal side of this lens. A collimated beam of light was reflected from the mirror and focused on a strip of moving film. Because the contact lens mirror was placed in a parallel beam of light, only the rotational movements of the eye caused a displacement of the beam without contamination due to translational movements of the head. The rotational movements of the head were minimized by the use of a bite board and a head rest. Both the horizontal and the vertical movements of the eye could be recorded.

Ratliff and Riggs distinguished three broad categories of movement: tremors, drifts, and saccades. The tremor motion was described as being very small, rarely exceeding 20 sec of arc in amplitude, but quite fast, with a frequency of between 30 and 70 Hz. Drifts were characterized as the gradual shifting of the direction of gaze; their mean amplitude was measured to be 5 min of arc, and rate of occurrence between 1 and 5 times per sec. The saccades, which were also irregular, had a mean amplitude of 5 min of arc, but occasionally a saccade of 20 min of arc occurred; their duration did not exceed 200 msec. This categorization has been verified with minor variations (see Ditchburn, 1973).

The motions of the eyeball cause displacements of the image on the retina, but amplitude of eye motion and image displacement do not correspond exactly, since the center of rotation and the nodal point of the eyeball are not the same. The correspondence is close enough, however, to permit calculation of extent of image motion from the measured rotations of the eyeball. It is certain, for example, that

341

when fixation is relaxed, a given point of the retinal image cannot remain on a single receptor for more than a few hundredths of a second.

One of the problems investigated during the early 1950s was the effect of eye movements during natural fixation on acuity. Ratliff (1952) measured these movements during brief, 75-msec presentations of grating targets. He found that correct identification of targets correlated better with periods during which the smaller amount of eye motion took place. The conclusion was that motions of the retinal image that result from the eye movements did not enhance visual acuity.

A better way of studying effects of eye motion on vision would be to hold the retinal image motionless while allowing the eyeball to move. In this way the image could be viewed for longer periods of time and psychophysical measures of visual function obtained with and without image motion could be compared directly.

The trick was to move the retinal image as much as the eye moved. To achieve this the eye movement recording system was modified so that the beam reflecting from the contact lens mirror was focused on a screen (Figure 27.1). The beam carried the image of a target. This target on the screen moved in proportion to the movements of the eye through twice the angular extent as the rotation of the eyeball. Viewing was done through a pathway that was twice the distance from the eye to the screen. Measured through this longer pathway at the point where the eye was situated, the motion of the image on the screen was halved, that is, it was the same as the rotation of the eye, and the retinal image remained stationary with respect to the receptors.

One of the startling phenomena associated with viewing a target whose image is stable on the retina is that the spatial detail is perceived sharply at first, but after a few seconds of viewing, all contrast within the image fades and the target appears uniform despite the physical distribution of light. Some of the early work done in Riggs' laboratory indicates that the function of the motion of the retinal image is to maintain vision, and not necessarily to improve visual acuity (Riggs, Ratliff,

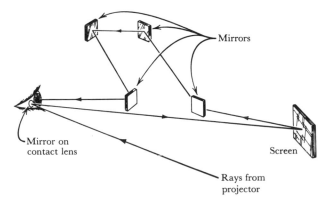

Figure 27.1. A method for producing a stationary image on the retina even though the eye itself is not stationary. [From F. Ratliff, *Mach bands: Quantitative studies on neural networks in the retina.* Copyright 1965 by Holden-Day, Inc.]

Cornsweet, & Cornsweet, 1953; for summaries of work with stabilized images see Ditchburn, 1973; Yarbus, 1967).

The preceding summarizes the essential features of the two types of image stabilization apparatus I have used, the optical and the electronic systems, and also some of the questions constituting the basis of some of my research.

With regard to the construction and calibration of the apparatus, I refer the reader to Riggs and Tulunay (1959), Riggs and Schick (1968), Jones, Webster, and Keesey (1972), and Jones and Keesey (1975). These two pieces of equipment referred to previously compensate for both the vertical and horizontal components of eye movements, although in the case of the electronic stabilization system only 71% compensation is achieved for the vertical component. This drawback is overcome by using targets containing luminance variations only along the horizontal dimension, such as vertically oriented gratings.

Some of my research utilizing image stabilization concentrated on two questions. One was directed to the role of image motion in maintenance of vision, and the other was concerned with the contribution of image motion to contrast sensitivity. The following is a summary of my research addressed to these questions, as well as of the supporting evidence from other laboratories.

II. Motions of the Retinal Image and Maintained Visibility of Targets

The disappearance of the stabilized image, regardless of its contrast level, emphasized the single most important function of image motion, that of maintaining the visibility of targets. Therefore the relative importance of the three different components of eye movements became a question of interest. This question was examined by moving the stabilized image in a controlled fashion with different amplitude and frequencies, or by varying temporally the contrast of the stabilized image in order to subject a given retinal location to known amounts of luminance change. Work done in various laboratories with a variety of targets, such as Mach bands, bipartite fields, and dark or bright bars, shows that large and slow movements of the image with an amplitude of about 1 min or arc and frequencies in the range of from 1 to 3 Hz maintain the best visibility of the stabilized target. Similarly, temporal modulation of the contrast of a stabilized target with rates of about 1–4 Hz is optimal. Rates about 15 Hz, regardless of the contrast, yield a visibility level that is not different from the level obtained when the bar is steady (Figure 27.2). These results indicate that visibility is not prolonged by those changes of luminance resulting from tremor motion under normal viewing conditions, while slow changes of luminance, resulting from the drift component of normal eye movements, are beneficial for prolonged visibility (Riggs & Tulunay, 1959; Keesey & Riggs, 1962; Krauskopf, 1957; Ditchburn, Fender, & Mayne, 1959; Keesey, 1969, 1973).

The role of the saccades in maintaining visibility has not been clearly defined in

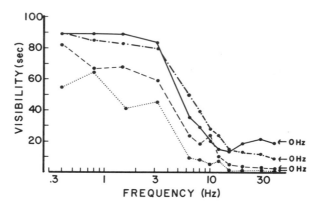

Figure 27.2. Visibility of a bar as a function of sine wave flicker frequency for selected contrast ratios: .06 (dotted line); .25 (dashes); 1 (dash–dot); and 10 (solid line). Each point is an average of 10 judgments. Visibility of bar when it was steady (0 Hz) is indicated by arrows along appropriate contrast lines. Stabilized viewing. [From Keesey (1973).]

the studies mentioned. However, the general trend of results (e.g., Gerrits, 1970) lends credence to the contention that continuous visibility of targets can be supported without the saccadic component of eye movement. The possibility will be discussed that abrupt changes in luminance determine sensitivity rather than continued visibility of above-threshold targets.

III. Role of Image Motion in Visual Sensitivity

The classic measures of acuity have long been used as indications of the sensitivity of the visual system. Usually the target is of high contrast and a critical dimension; for example, the width of a line, a vernier displacement, is varied until the observer can just see it. The measures of acuity are considerably smaller than may be expected on the basis of the size of the individual receptors. For example, a dark line of .5 sec of arc in width is easily detectable under favorable conditions, yet the single cone in the center of the fovea is many times larger, about 20 sec of arc.

One of the principal mechanisms suggested for the discrimination of fine patterns by the relatively coarse receptor layer depends on eye motion (Marshall & Talbot, 1942). Target scanning is said to promote stimulation of those receptors falling under the luminance gradient. This suggestion implies an improvement of acuity as a function of an increase in exposure duration because of the resulting increase in the amount of image motion. However, experiments wherein the target image was stabilized provided data to the contrary. Acuity did improve as a function of the duration of exposure of the target but was neither enhanced nor impaired by image movements that were present during inspection period. It was suggested that acuity is based on the discrimination of the spatial pattern of illumination, regardless of any temporal changes of intensity over the receptors caused by small movements of the image (Keesey, 1960).

The sensitivity of the visual system can also be assessed by determining the threshold contrast of given size objects. A convenient stimulus for this type of measure is repetitive light and dark bars whose luminance along the horizontal dimension is distributed sinusoidally. Contrast is expressed as the ratio of the difference between the brightest and the dimmest part of the image to the sum of the brightest and the dimmest parts. One of the advantages of this type of stimulus is that the mean luminance does not change as a function of contrast or spatial frequency; therefore, the adaptation level of the retina remains constant.

There is general agreement that the human visual system is most sensitive to spatial frequencies between 2 and 4 cycles deg^{-1}. Sensitivity is attenuated for the lower and higher frequencies. There is also general agreement that sensitivity to low frequencies, as opposed to high frequencies, can be manipulated by the temporal aspects of the stimulus, such as flicker and exposure duration. Therefore, it is reasonable to expect that the movement of the retinal image contributes to sensitivity at low spatial frequencies.

We measured spatial contrast sensitivity with the normally moving and the stabilized retinal image of sine-wave gratings (Tulunay-Keesey & Jones, 1976). Exposure duration of the target was varied from 6 msec to 4 sec. Between exposures of the target, the field was evenly illuminated at the same level as the space-average luminance of the target. The results (Figure 27.3) indicated that sensitivity increased

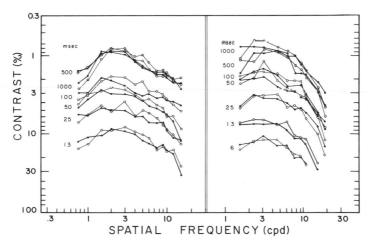

Figure 27.3. Threshold contrast (%) necessary to see gratings is plotted for spatial frequencies ranging from .75 to 15 cycles deg^{-1} (RMJ, left panel) and 1.5 to 18 cycles deg^{-1} (UTK, right panel). Both axes are in log scale. Percentage of contrast decreases upward. Exposure durations range from 6 to 1000 msec. The data for the duration of 250 msec are omitted for UTK; exposures of 6 and 250 msec were not used for RMJ. The closed symbols designate the unstabilized, the open symbols the stabilized viewing conditions. [From Tulunay-Keesey & Jones (1976).]

rapidly for any given frequency as a function of exposure duration up to about 50 msec. The rate of increase approached zero as the exposure was lengthened to durations longer than 1 sec (not shown). Exposure duration was also the primary determiner of the shape of the contrast sensitivity curve; low-frequency attenuation developed within 50 to 100 msec and was substantial for the longer durations of 500 msec or longer. For example, the slope of the curve relating log threshold to log spatial frequency up to 3 cycles deg^{-1} increased from .2 for target durations of 13 msec to .7 for the 1-sec exposures. Image stabilization sometimes yielded the more attenuated curves, which indicated that for low spatial frequencies lack of image motion could serve to decrease sensitivity while for the middle-range frequencies of 2 to 7 cycles deg^{-1} it could increase sensitivity. But point by point comparison of normal and stabilized threshold contrasts for each spatial frequency for a given exposure duration did not yield differences at accepted levels of statistical significance. It appeared, therefore, that image motion was of secondary, if any, importance in determining sensitivity to contrast of low spatial frequencies.

The effect of image motion became apparent, however, when the target was presented for indefinite durations and the observer was asked to adjust the contrast to threshold. The stabilized thresholds were found to be about .2 log unit higher than the unstabilized thresholds over most of the frequency range used in this experiment (Figure 27.4).

The important difference between the two methods of threshold acquisition was in the mode of target onset. For the staircase method, the grating was flashed on with a sudden onset, and judgment was made soon after onset, under either stabilized or unstabilized conditions. On the other hand, contrast changed gradually during the method of adjustment. A threshold setting was difficult to make under the stabilized conditions, for even a brief inspection of a low-contrast target led to rapid

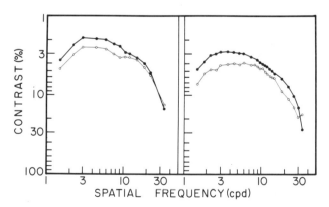

Figure 27.4. Threshold contrast (%) for detecting gratings of spatial frequencies ranging between 1.5 and 30 cycles deg^{-1}. Left panel, RMJ. Right panel, UTK. Percentage of contrast decreases upward. Both axes are in log scale. Exposure duration is indefinite, thresholds are obtained by the method of adjustment. Open symbols are for the stabilized, closed symbols for the unstabilized conditions. [From Tulunay-Keesey & Jones (1976).]

disappearance and a further increase of contrast had to be made to find a new level of visibility. The question arises whether fading of the image and decrease of sensitivity are synonymous. The data resulting from both methods taken together indicate that absence of image motion induces fading and lower contrast sensitivity, but considerable image motion occurring during long exposures of a target, up to 4 sec in our experiments, with sharp onset and offset does not determine sensitivity. A strong possibility exists that transients resulting from sharp onset of the target mask any effect of transients induced by image motion. Therefore we attempted to assess the relative contribution of transients induced either by image motion or the onset of the target. We chose an exposure of a duration within which disappearance would easily take place, and presented the target either with a sharp onset of approximately 10 msec or a gradual onset of 2.5 sec. The steady plateau was 10 sec for the former condition and 7.5 sec for the latter. The targets were viewed under both stabilized and normal conditions. The staircase method was used for securing thresholds. Figure 27.5 gives an index of the effect of image motion alone, which can be found by comparing two curves obtained with the gradual onset under normal and stabilized conditions. The data suggest that the presence of image motion increases sensitivity to frequencies lower than 3 cycles deg^{-1} by about .2 log unit. A comparison of two contrast sensitivity curves obtained under stabilized conditions, one with gradual onset, the other with sharp onset, presumably gives an indication of the effect of onset transients alone. As Figure 27.6 indicates, onset transients increase low-frequency sensitivity by a larger amount than transients generated by image motion. It would appear that onset transients affect contrast sensitivity more than do transients resulting from normal image motion occurring during fixation.

It should be noted that elimination of either image motion or onset transients does not have the effect of changing the slope of the contrast sensitivity curve. Among the variables we have examined, length of exposure seemed to be the one manipulating the amount of low-frequency attenuation.

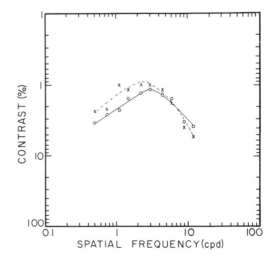

Figure 27.5. Threshold contrast for gratings of spatial frequencies ranging between .5 and 12 cycles deg^{-1}. Percentage of contrast decreases upward. Both axes in log scale. Stimulus onset and offset gradual, with 2.5-sec rise and decay ramp. Plateau of steady contrast of 7.5 sec. Crosses indicate normal, open circles stabilized viewing. Subject UTK.

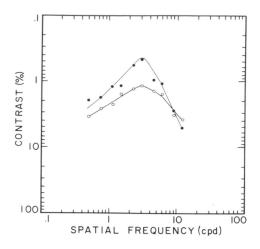

Figure 27.6. Threshold contrast for gratings of spatial frequencies ranging between .5 and 12 cycles deg^{-1}. Percentage of contrast decreases upward. Both axes are in log scale. Stabilized viewing: closed circles, sudden onset and offset, 10-sec duration; open circles, ramp onset and offset, with 2.5-sec rise and decay time. Plateau of steady contrast of 7.5 sec. Subject UTK.

IV. Conclusion

In summary, it appears that contrast sensitivity (and as a special case, acuity) is dependent mainly on events that develop in time. They may be related to an increase in efficiency of light and the development of neural interactions. Attenuation to low-frequency sensitivity may well be the result of two opposing mechanisms acting asynchronously such as the excitatory and inhibitory mechanisms found within receptive fields of vertebrate ganglion cells. Because the shape of the curve does not depend on the presence or absence of image motion, it is suggested that temporal changes brought about by the motion of a gradient of light on the retina do not interfere with the timing of this type of spatial neural interaction. However, temporal changes to some degree set the level of sensitivity of the mechanism.

Another theoretical framework within which these results can be interpreted assumes that there are channels in the visual system that are tuned to specific spatial frequencies. These channels have different sensitivities that presumably produce the contrast sensitivity curve (Campbell & Robson, 1968). There also is a substantial amount of data (Keesey, 1972; Keesey & Jones, 1972; and see Kulikowski & Tolhurst, 1973) indicating that there are two mechanisms, one specialized for transient, and the other for mediating sustained information. The same data suggest that low spatial frequencies may be detected by the transient, the higher frequencies by the sustained spatial mechanism. The physiological analogues of these mechanisms are, of course, the transient and sustained cells found at all levels in the vertebrate visual system.

The sharp onset of the grating pattern can be regarded as a temporal waveform containing high temporal frequency components of large amplitude. It is expected, then, that the visibility of low spatial frequencies would be aided by such temporal stimulation. Our results confirm this expectation and also indicate that the threshold lowering effect, however small, of image motion may be mediated by a similar transient mechanism.

A classic measure of the sensitivity of the visual system is increment threshold. Westheimer (1965, 1967) showed that the area as well as the luminance of the background upon which incremental light is superimposed determines threshold. For example, in the fovea, increment threshold for a small 2 min of arc spot superimposed on a constant luminance background increases (desensitization) as the background is enlarged up to 6 or 7 min or arc. The threshold decreases (sensitization) as the background diameter is increased up to 10 to 15 min of arc, and reaches a steady level upon further enlargements of the background. The increase and

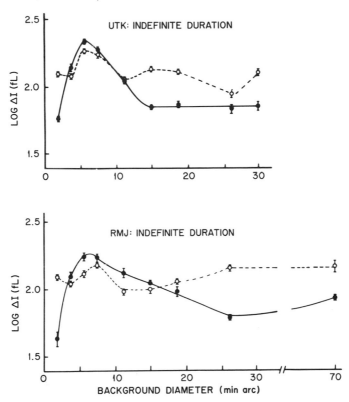

Figure 27.7. Increment thresholds for a tiny test spot of 1.8 min of arc superimposed on backgrounds ranging from 1.8 to 30 min arc in diameter. The adapting background of 10 mL was presented continuously. Closed circles and solid lines show the data obtained under normal (unstabilized) viewing conditions. Open circles and dashed lines are for stabilized viewing. Each data point represents the geometric mean of 10 threshold intensities; two extreme values of 12 judgments have been excluded. Vertical bars show 1 SE. Threshold was the same under either normal or stabilized viewing. [From Tulunay-Keesey & Vassilev (1974).]

decrease in the psychophysical threshold are generally ascribed to summation of excitation and inhibition, respectively.

We examined the increment threshold under stabilized conditions and confirmed that size-dependent change is indeed a basic property of human vision; that is, thresholds taken on stabilized and unstabilized, normally moving backgrounds show an increase and decrease at comparable diameters (Figure 27.7) (Tulunay-Keesey & Vassilev, 1974; Tulunay-Keesey & Jones, 1977). However, the following differences between stabilized and nonstabilized thresholds are to be noted: (a) Thresholds taken on backgrounds of 5–6 min of arc are higher by about .1 to .2 log unit when the background moves normally on the retina than when it is stabilized. On the other hand, moving backgrounds of diameters exceeding 10 min of arc consistently yield lower thresholds. (b) Decrease of threshold (sensitization) is independent of the delay between the onset of the background and the test flash under unstabilized viewing conditions. However, stabilized viewing yields a sensitization effect that is dependent on the temporal relation between onset of background and test flash. For example, under stabilized conditions, when the delay is 100 msec, a large sensitization effect is obtained of a magnitude equal to the one produced with normal, unstabilized viewing. With longer delays of 200 and 400 msec the effect is smaller and dissipates when the delay is longer (Figure 27.8).

If sensitization is indeed a reflection of inhibition, our results suggest that inhibition develops within 100 msec. The persistence of sensitization during image

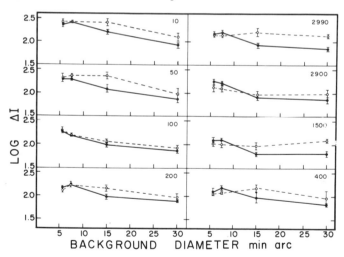

Figure 27.8. Increment threshold (Δ*I*) as a function of background diameter of 5, 7, 15, and 30 min arc. Incremental flash was a 1.8-min arc, 10-msec spot superimposed on a background of varying diameter and a constant luminance of 3 mL. Background was on for 3 sec and off for 3 sec. Each pair of curves represents one delay between the onset of the background and the test flash. Each point is an average of 10 judgments, and the vertical lines indicate the standard error. Open circles and dashed lines represent increment threshold taken on stabilized backgrounds; the closed circles and solid lines on unstabilized backgrounds. Subject UTK. [From Tulunay-Keesey & Jones (1977).]

movement and the attainment of lower thresholds through the use of large moving backgrounds suggest that edge movement of the background image perpetuates the effectiveness of the inhibitory mechanism and regulates the activity measured in its center.

These experiments and those with gratings lead us to conclude that image motion has a role in regulating contrast sensitivity. The mechanism by which this is done is not clear. If we accept that regulation is achieved by movement of the edge within the inhibitory surround of receptive fields, we then must ask how this can be achieved in the case of a repetitive low-frequency pattern of, say, 1 cycle deg^{-1}, which covers many overlapping receptive fields of different sizes and sensitivities in the fovea. If we accept [as suggested by some of our earlier results and those of Kulikowski and Tolhurst (1973)] that there are two systems, one specialized for detecting temporal and the other spatial contrast, then we may pose the question of whether edge motion defines the temporal mechanism.

We hope questions such as these help us formulate future experiments enabling us to propose a coherent hypothesis for the role of image motion in contrast sensitivity.

ACKNOWLEDGMENTS

This chapter is a summary of work that continues, in essence, experiments Lorrin Riggs and I started when I was a graduate student. I have had the valuable assistance of Mr. R.M. Jones and Ms. B.J. Bruhn in carrying out various phases of the work.

REFERENCES

Campbell, F.W., & Robson, J.G. Application of Fourier analysis to the visibility of gratings. *Journal of Physiology,* 1968, *197,* 551–566.

Ditchburn, R.W. *Eye movements and visual perception.* Oxford: Clarendon Press, 1973.

Ditchburn, R.W., Fender, D.H., & Mayne, S. Vision with controlled movements of the retinal image. *Journal of Physiology,* 1959, *145,* 98–108.

Gerrits, H.J.M., & Vendrik, A.J.H. Artificial movements of a stabilized image. *Vision Research,* 1970, *10,* 1443–1456.

Jones, R.M., & Keesey, U.T. Accuracy of image stabilization by an optical electronic feedback system. *Vision Research,* 1975, *15,* 57–61.

Jones, R., Webster, J., & Keesey, U.T. An active feedback system for stabilizing visual images. *IEEE Transactions of Bio-medical Engineering,* 1972, *19,* 29–33.

Keesey, U.T. Effects of involuntary eye movements on visual acuity. *Journal of the Optical Society of America,* 1960, *50,* 769–774.

Keesey, U.T. Visibility of a stabilized target as a function of frequency and amplitude of luminance modulation. *Journal of the Optical Society of America,* 1969, *59,* 604–610.

Keesey, U.T. Flicker and pattern detection: A comparison of thresholds. *Journal of the Optical Society of America,* 1972, *62,* 446–448.

Keesey, U.T. Stabilized target visibility as a function of contrast and flicker frequency. *Vision Research,* 1973, *13,* 1367–1373.

Keesey, U.T., & Jones, R.M. Flicker and pattern detection: A comparison of thresholds. II. *Journal of the Optical Society of America,* 1972, *62,* 1395.

Keesey, U.T., & Riggs, L.A. Visibility of Mach bands with imposed motions of the retinal image. *Journal of the Optical Society of America,* 1962, *52,* 719-720.

Krauskopf, J. Effect of retinal image motion on the contrast thresholds for maintained vision. *Journal of the Optical Society of America,* 1957, *47,* 740-744.

Kulikowski, J.J., & Tolhurst, D. Psychophysical evidence for sustained and transient detectors in human vision. *Journal of Physiology,* 1973, *232,* 149-162.

Marshall, W.H., & Talbot, S.A. Recent evidence for neural mechanisms in vision leading to a general theory of sensory activity. *Biological Symposia,* 1942, *7,* 117-164.

Ratliff, F. The role of physiological nystagmus in monocular acuity. *Journal of Experimental Psychology,* 1952, *43,* 163-172.

Ratliff, F. *Mach bands: Quantitative studies on neural networks in the retina.* San Francisco: Holden-Day, 1965.

Ratliff, F., & Riggs, L.A. Involuntary motions of the eye during monocular fixation. *Journal of Experimental Psychology,* 1950, *40,* 687-701.

Riggs, L.A., Ratliff, F., Cornsweet, J.C., & Cornsweet, T.N. The disappearance of steadily fixated visual test objects. *Journal of the Optical Society of America,* 1953, *43,* 495-501.

Riggs, L.A., & Schick, A.M.L. Accuracy of retinal image stabilization achieved with a plane mirror on a tightly fitting contact lens. *Vision Research,* 1968, *8,* 159-169.

Riggs, L.A., & Tulunay, U. Visual effects of varying the extent of compensation for eye movements. *Journal of the Optical Society of America,* 1959, *49,* 741-745.

Tulunay-Keesey, U., & Jones, R.M. The effect of micromovements of the eye and exposure duration on contrast sensitivity. *Vision Research,* 1976, *16,* 481-488.

Tulunay-Keesey, U., & Jones, R.M. Spatial sensitization as a function of delay. *Vision Research,* 1977, *17,* 1191-1199.

Tulunay-Keesey, U., & Vassilev, A. Foveal spatial sensitization with stabilized vision. *Vision Research,* 1974, *14,* 101-105.

Westheimer, G. Spatial interactions in the human retina during scotopic vision. *Journal of Physiology,* 1965, *181,* 881-894.

Westheimer, G. Spatial interaction in human cone vision. *Journal of Physiology,* 1967, *190,* 139-154.

Yarbus, A.L. *Eye movements and vision,* L.A. Riggs (Ed.). New York: Plenum Press, 1967.

28. Saccadic Eye Movements and the Perception of a Clear and Continuous Visual World[1]

Frances C. Volkmann and Robert K. Moore

In 1905 Raymond Dodge introduced a paper entitled "The Illusion of Clear Vision during Eye Movement" by referring to an even earlier paper (Dodge, 1900) which maintained that under normal viewing conditions vision is absent during saccadic eye movements (Dodge, 1905):

> The evidence was clear enough. The only really surprising fact was that it should have needed expression at all. It would seem as though rapidly recurring moments of practical blindness to events in the environment ought to need no detailed proof. That the matter did require proof and that this was received with some scepticism created a new problem in psychological optics, viz., the cause of the illusion of continuous clear vision during eye movements of the simple reaction type [p. 193].

In this chapter we will discuss some research related to the question of why the phenomenal world remains *clear* as we glance from one object to another. We will then offer some preliminary data and speculations concerned with the question of why the phenomenal world remains *continuous* over long periods of saccadic eye movements and fixational pauses.

I. Saccadic Suppression and Visual Clarity

A. The Phenomenon of Saccadic Suppression

The early investigators contended that the reason the phenomenal world remains clear and stable as we look about is that some sort of impairment of vision occurs for

[1]This research was supported by Grants GB-41103 (BNS74-01135) and BNS76-01450 from the National Science Foundation to Frances C. Volkmann and Lorrin A. Riggs, and was conducted primarily at Smith College.

the smeared images that are swept across the retina during saccades (Dodge, 1900, 1905; Holt, 1903; Woodworth, 1906). Quantitative experiments in the 1960s (for reviews see Matin, 1974; Volkmann, 1976; Cumming, 1978), some from the Riggs laboratory (Volkmann, 1962; Volkmann, Schick, & Riggs, 1968; Lederberg, 1970), showed that although the eye is not completely "blind" during saccades, visual performance on a variety of discriminations is significantly worse during saccades than it is during fixation. This decrement in performance, now called saccadic suppression, occurs even when care is taken to minimize image smear and otherwise to equate the stimuli reaching the eye in the two conditions.

A number of mechanisms have been proposed to account for saccadic suppression, among them (a) a centrally originating neural suppression, (b) an impairment produced in normal viewing by image smear on the moving retina, (c) shearing forces in the retina, and (d) visual masking effects resulting from spatial and temporal interactions on the retina as we look about in a contoured environment (see Matin, 1974; Brooks & Fuchs, 1975; Breitmeyer & Ganz, 1976). Although we interpret the experimental literature as showing that neural suppression combines with optical effects (which vary with viewing conditions) to produce visual impairment during saccades (Riggs, Merton, & Morton, 1974; Volkmann, Riggs, Moore, & White, in press; Volkmann, Riggs, White, & Moore, in press; Moore, Volkmann, & Riggs, in preparation), this interpretation is of secondary importance today. Here we wish to discuss the effects of saccadic suppression rather than its causes.

B. The Time Course of Saccadic Suppression

To favor the clear vision that can occur in normal viewing only during steady fixation, it would be advantageous to an organism for saccadic suppression to occur with a time course that is at least as long as the saccade itself. Early quantitative work showed that this is generally the case (Latour, 1962; Volkmann et al., 1968). Typically, the probability of detection of a pattern of added brightness flashed against a steady light background begins to decrease when the flash precedes saccade onset by about 50 msec, reaches a minimum when the flash comes during the saccade, and returns slowly to the value for steady fixation over a period of 100 msec or longer. More recently, we have extended the analysis to the time course of changes in contrast sensitivity to sinusoidal test gratings presented in brief exposures in various temporal relations to saccades (Volkmann, Riggs, White, & Moore, in press).

The experimental apparatus and technique have been described elsewhere (Volkmann, Riggs, White, & Moore, in preparation). Briefly, the observer sat in a uniformly illuminated Ganzfeld and viewed monocularly, through a window in the Ganzfeld, a 9.5° square fixation field containing two sets of fixation marks located 6° apart. On signal from the experimenter, the observer executed a horizontal saccade from between one set of fixation marks to the other, and on another signal about 1–2 sec later, executed a second saccade back to between the first marks. A horizontally oriented sinusoidal grating replaced the fixation field in a 10-msec exposure at a predetermined time before, during, or after one saccade of the pair. A blank field replaced the fixation field, also in a 10-msec exposure, in the same temporal relation to the other saccade of the pair. The space-average luminance of the grating and of the uniform field was equal to that of the fixation field and the Ganzfeld. Although these are photopic conditions, the entire visual field was such that effects of contour masking and retinal image smear were minimized. The observer was required to make a temporal forced-choice judgment of which saccade within the pair was accompanied by exposure of the grating.

Figure 28.1 shows the time course of the saccadic suppression of contrast sensitivity obtained with this experimental arrangement, based on the combined data of three observers, at four values of spatial frequency. These are relative sensitivity functions; contrast threshold for the fixating eye at each spatial frequency was taken to be zero. Plotted points indicate 75% correct contrast thresholds derived from linear regression lines fitted to psychophysical performance data at each of eight temporal relationships. Each point represents the midpoint of a 100-msec interval, though samples were taken every 50 msec on a sliding scale to counteract the effects of small numbers of observations in some of the time bins.

Two features of these curves are of interest here: (a) Their general shape shows that the saccadic suppression of contrast sensitivity follows roughly the same time course as do the discriminations investigated previously; and (b) they seem to show considerable oscillation in sensitivity after the saccade, and in some cases do not return to fixating eye threshold in the range of times investigated. In this respect the curves also resemble earlier data, and previous investigators have speculated about the existence and possible sources of such oscillations in sensitivity and their implications for the recovery of clear vision (Latour, 1966; Volkmann *et al.*, 1968).

Figure 28.1. Relative contrast sensitivity as a function of the temporal relation between stimulus and saccade. Data pooled from three observers are shown for four spatial frequencies. Points are interpolated from regressions and plotted relative to the sensitivity for the fixating eye. For further details see text.

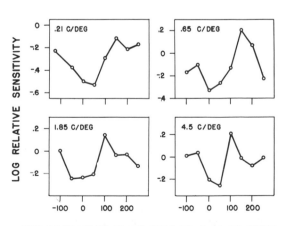

TIME OF STIMULUS IN RELATION TO SACCADE ONSET

C. The Fine Structure of Visual Recovery
   following Saccades

Data such as those shown in Figure 28.1 emphasized the need for a careful, fine-grained analysis of visual sensitivity to stimuli presented at precisely specified times up to several hundred milliseconds after saccades. Such an analysis is shown in two different ways in Figure 28.2.

Using a constant stimulus method of stimulus presentation and a temporal forced-choice response, contrast sensitivity functions were obtained for a .65 cycle deg^{-1} horizontal test grating. A 5-msec exposure of the grating or of a blank field was triggered by each saccade to arrive at 1 of 20 predetermined times after saccade onset. Four values of contrast were presented 48 times each to obtain each of the 20 contrast threshold values. All of the functions were obtained concurrently. The observers were informed that the stimuli would arrive at various times during or after saccades, but were not given information by which to predict the precise time of occurrence of any given stimulus.

The curves of Figure 28.2A show the recovery from saccadic suppression of contrast sensitivity at each of the 20 times of stimulus occurrence for two observers. The horizontal dashed line on each graph indicates contrast threshold as found in separately conducted trials with steady fixation. The curves for both observers show

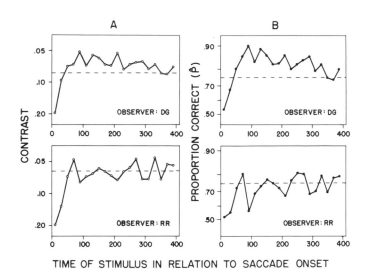

Figure 28.2. (A) Contrast sensitivity as a function of the temporal relation between stimulus and saccade. Data are shown for two observers, DG and RR. Plotted points are contrast thresholds interpolated from regressions; the dashed line is the contrast threshold determined for the fixating eye. (B) Estimated proportion of correct responses as a function of the temporal relation between stimulus and saccade. Plotted points are estimated for the same two observers and from the same data as in (A) and interpolated at the contrast determined to be the contrast threshold for the fixating eye. The dashed line is the 75% expected performance at that contrast.

a rapid initial rise of sensitivity from the low point during the saccade. In fact, within 50 msec after the onset of the saccade (the duration of which is about 30 msec) contrast threshold has already reached the fixating eye level. For Observer DG, sensitivity appears to exceed that of the fixating eye by a small amount during the next 300 msec. The data for RR do not show this effect, however.

Thresholds of both observers appear to oscillate as a function of time of stimulation after the saccade, and there is some evidence of periodicity: For Observer DG, the high points at 90, 210, and 330 msec suggest a period of approximately 120 msec. The same period, but out of phase, is suggested by the low points at 110, 230, and 350 msec. For Observer RR a period of approximately 100 msec is suggested by the high points at 70, 170, 270, and 370 msec, and again out of phase with these, the low points at 90, 190, and 290 msec. This periodicity is similar to that of *alpha* activity typically seen in the human electroencephalogram; Lindsley (1952) has speculated that such activity may be of importance in saccadic suppression.

The curves of Figure 28.2B were constructed in an attempt to make clear the probability of detection of gratings of a particular contrast at various intervals of time following the saccade. Points on these curves are estimates of the proportion of correct choices; they were obtained by interpolation from the same raw data used to construct the contrast sensitivity functions in Figure 28.2A. The particular contrast chosen for this manipulation of the data is that at which the same observer had been correct 75% of the time under conditions of steady fixation. It may be seen from the curves in Figure 28.2B that correct identification rises from the chance level of 50% to values as high as or even higher than the 75% threshold value obtained for the fixating eye. These curves also make even more evident the fluctuations that take place throughout an otherwise steady trend of recovery. These oscillations are not as large, however, as those reported by Latour (1966), to occur preceding saccades. For Observer DG, these oscillations are superposed on a longer period during which sensitivity exceeds that of the fixating eye and only gradually decreases to fixating eye level. For RR, on the other hand, the oscillations are superposed on a very gradual trend toward the total recovery of sensitivity after the saccade.

D. Implications for a Clear Visual World

This analysis of the temporal fine structure of contrast sensitivity indicates that substantial recovery from saccadic suppression is relatively rapid, although in our experiments suppression always outlasts the saccade. Moreover, recovery is accomplished without large oscillations in sensitivity that might operate to decrease the phenomenal clarity of stimuli viewed at the conclusion of a saccade.

We view these data as showing *minimum* values of suppression, in terms of both magnitude and duration, since they were obtained in an experimental situation that minimized the potential contributions of contour masking, retinal smear, large shifts in luminance, and changes in accommodation (Volkmann, Riggs, Moore, & White, in press). Under more usual conditions of viewing, both the magnitude and time course of suppression would be expected to be larger, and maximum sensitivity would indeed be reserved for the stationary objects of regard which rest on the fovea well after the end of a saccade.

II. Time Distortions around Saccades and the Perception of Visual Continuity

The time course of saccadic suppression is important to understanding our "illusion" of clear vision at all times, since the normally blurred stimuli that arrive during saccades are not seen. However, it does little to explain our perception of continuous vision through periods of interruption which may last as long as 150 msec around each saccade. We have begun some preliminary work aimed at the question of why the perceptual world remains not only clear but also continuous throughout the saccades we make in normal visual exploration.

A. The Perception of Time of Occurrence of Stimuli in Relation to Ballistic Motor Events: Preliminary Findings

During the latter part of the experiment previously described (Section I, C), an observer remarked that although the instructions had indicated that stimuli would be presented "during or after" saccades, she was convinced that almost all of the stimuli had in fact been presented during saccades. We decided to pursue this remark by presenting grating stimuli at various times after saccades and by asking observers to judge whether a given stimulus arrived during or after a saccade. We used horizontal gratings at above-threshold values of contrast, presented in 5-msec exposures. The left-hand graphs of Figure 28.3 show the results for two observers for several values of grating contrast ranging from only slightly above threshold (.10–.15) to highly visible (.40). The data are clear in showing a prolonged period of time after the saccade throughout which the observer perceives the stimulus as having arrived during the saccade. A predominance of these "during" judgments occurred until 250–280 msec after saccade onset, indicating that the stimulus must arrive, on the average, more than 200 msec after the *completion* of the saccade before it is discriminated as having come after it. These data also show that the timing of a stimulus, relative to a saccade, is not perceived any more accurately for a high-contrast stimulus than for a low-contrast stimulus.

These results raised a number of questions that we have only begun to explore: How dependent are they on the psychophysical procedure used? Are they specific to saccades and visual stimuli, or do these long delays occur in conjunction with other motor tasks and with stimuli in other sensory modalities?

The right-hand graphs of Figure 28.3 show some additional preliminary results. At the top right are plots of the discrimination of the time of occurrence of a 5-msec tone burst in relation to a saccade, and at the bottom right is plotted the same discrimination applied to a 5-msec interruption of light occurring at various times

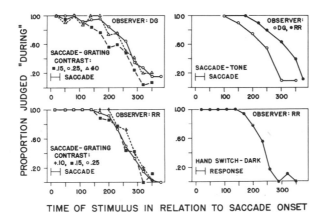

TIME OF STIMULUS IN RELATION TO SACCADE ONSET

Figure 28.3. Proportions of stimuli judged by the observer to have occurred during the saccade. Curves on left are for 5-msec exposures of a grating at the designated levels of contrast. At top right are curves for a 5-msec auditory stimulus. At bottom right are one observer's judgments of the time of interruption of a steady light; here, the motor response is not a saccade but a quick sliding motion imparted to an electric hand switch. Note that in all cases the actual duration of the motor response is less than 35 msec, whereas the affected interval of time extends to about 300 msec after the beginning of the motor response.

after the onset of a manual response, namely, the movement of a hand switch from one side to the other. It is evident that the long period of time after the response, throughout which the stimulus is judged as occurring during the response, is not specific to saccades or to visual stimuli.

There are many directions in which we may pursue the implications of these preliminary findings. Physiologically, the discrimination requires a comparison of the relative times of occurrence of two central events: one associated with a sensory stimulus, and the other with a peripheral motor event. The critical central representation of this motor event may result from proprioceptive feedback, but would seem more likely to result from a corollary discharge accompanying the efferent signal. In the case of eye movements, this is presumably the signal to the extraocular muscles to execute a saccade (Sperry, 1950; von Holst, 1954). Electrophysiology may eventually reveal the location, the time course, and the duration of this event. An example of a cortical response with somewhat similar time course and duration is provided by Mountcastle (1975, compare Figures 16 and 17 with our Figure 28.4).

The present findings may also be related to information processing and timing, selective attention, and motor control mechanisms (for reviews, see Keele, 1973; Marteniuk, 1976; Stelmach, 1976; Welford, 1976). To take an example from the early literature: Certain aspects of this task are reminiscent of the "complication experiment," and the related phenomenon of prior entry (see Boring, 1950, pp. 142–147; Sternberg & Knoll, 1973). Although the magnitudes of the differences in times of prior entry are small, it is possible that our much longer intervals may be composed in part of temporal distortions due to such an attentional phenomenon.

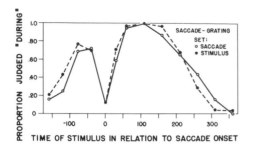

Figure 28.4. Proportion of stimuli judged to have occurred during a saccade. Solid line: Observer set to pay close attention to the stimulus. Broken line: Observer set to pay close attention to the saccade.

To evaluate this possibility, we conducted an experiment in which two sets of instructions were used, one in which the observer concentrated as completely as possible on the *saccade* on each trial, the other in which she concentrated on the *stimulus exposure*. In addition, the grating was presented *before* as well as *during* and *after* saccades, and the observer judged the time of occurrence of the stimulus relative to each saccade using the three categories of *before, during,* or *after*.

Figure 28.4 shows the results. This observer, RR, was highly trained, although she was not familiar with the aim or results of our experiments; she had served in this apparatus for over 50,000 saccades. Nevertheless, instructions to attend selectively did not alter the results. The data for stimuli arriving after the saccade replicate the earlier results using a two-category judgment and a more restricted range of stimuli. The data for stimuli arriving before the saccade may be interpreted tentatively as showing two separate events:

1. Stimuli arriving as early as 80 msec before saccade onset are discriminated 70–80% of the time as having occurred during the saccade. A smooth, bell-shaped envelope might well describe the proportion of "during" responses from approximately 200 msec before saccade onset to 350 msec after it.
2. Superposed on this smooth envelope is an abrupt change in the discrimination between about 20 msec prior to saccade onset and 20 msec after it (thus including most of the duration of the saccade).

Stimuli that arrived during this brief interval were discriminated as having "preceded" the saccade. We suspect that this may be a secondary effect, specific to the conditions of our experiment. One consideration here is the subject's anticipation of each event, since the experimenter used signals from a blinking electronic metronome to achieve an almost perfectly repeated timing of the "ready" and "go" signals to the observer to execute a saccade. The drop in the curve may mark the intrusion of the anticipated go signal. We are currently undertaking experiments to eliminate the possibility of anticipation of such rhythmic signals.

B. Implications for the Relation between Distortions of Time and Saccadic Suppression

The preliminary data presented here (Section II) indicate that certain stimuli occurring as long as 250 msec after a brief ballistic response, and from about 100 msec before it, are judged to have arrived during the response. Although this effect appears not to be specific to saccades, it may be important to the saccadic system. Not only do stimuli arriving in temporal proximity to saccades seem to arrive during them, but the time interval over which this effect operates is sufficient to encompass the duration of the impairment in vision also occurring in relation to saccades (i.e., saccadic suppression). Under conditions of normal viewing, clear vision can only be generated during the fixational pauses that occur between saccades, and not during the saccades themselves. The temporal illusion that we have described may have the effect that the interval of the saccade, in which the retinal image must be smeared and degraded, is "filled in" by the prolonged period of clear vision that is in fact generated before and after the saccade but is experienced as accompanying it. "Continuous clear vision" is the biologically fortunate result.

ACKNOWLEDGMENTS

We acknowledge with appreciation the contributions of Lorrin A. Riggs, who participated in these experiments as a co-principal investigator, of Jerrilynn Peters, Research Assistant on the project, of Dani P. Giannone and Ruth I. Richardsen, who served as observers, of Maria E. Benet and Delores M. Mei, who helped with data collection, and of John Volkmann, who contributed many ideas and criticisms to the manuscript.

REFERENCES

Boring, E. G. *A history of experimental psychology* (2nd ed.). New York: Appleton-Century-Crofts, 1950.

Breitmeyer, B. G., & Ganz, L. Implications of sustained and transient channels for theories of visual pattern masking, saccadic suppression, and information processing. *Psychological Review*, 1976, *83*, 1–36.

Brooks, B. A., & Fuchs, A. F. Influence of stimulus parameters on visual sensitivity during saccadic eye movement. *Vision Research*, 1975, *15*, 1389–1398.

Cumming, G. D. Eye movements and visual perception. In E. C. Carterette, & M. Friedman (Eds.), *Handbook of perception* (Vol. 8). New York: Academic Press, 1978.

Dodge, R. Visual perception during eye movement. *Psychological Review*, 1900, *7*, 454–465.

Dodge, R. The illusion of clear vision during eye movement. *Psychological Bulletin*, 1905, *2*, 193–99.

Holt, E. B. Eye-movement and central anaesthesia. I. The problem of anaesthesia during eye-movement. *Psychological Monographs*, 1903, *4* (17), 3–46.

Keele, S. W. *Attention and human performance*. Pacific Palisades, California: Goodyear, 1973.

Latour, P. L. Visual threshold during eye movements. *Vision Research*, 1962, *2*, 261–262.

Latour, P. L. Cortical control of eye movements. Unpublished doctoral thesis, Institute for Perception RVO-TNO, Soesterberg, The Netherlands, 1966.

Lederberg, V. Color recognition during voluntary saccades. *Journal of the Optical Society of America*, 1970, *60*, 835–842.

Lindsley, D. B. Psychological phenomena and the electroencephalogram. *Electroencephalography and Clinical Neurophysiology*, 1952, *4*, 443–456.

Marteniuk, R. G. *Information processing in motor skills*. New York: Holt, Rinehart, and Winston, 1976.

Matin, E. Saccadic suppression: A review and an analysis. *Psychological Bulletin*, 1974, *81*, 899–917.

Moore, R. K., Volkmann, F. C., & Riggs, L. A. *Relative contribution to saccadic suppression of retinal image smear*. In preparation.

Mountcastle, V. B. *The world around us: Neural command functions for selective attention*. The F. O. Schmitt Lecture in Neuroscience, 1975, Neurosciences Research Program. Cambridge, Massachusetts: MIT Press.

Riggs, L. A., Merton, P. A., & Morton, H. B. Suppression of visual phosphenes during saccadic eye movements. *Vision Research,* 1974, *14,* 997–1010.

Sperry, R. W. Neural basis of the spontaneous optokinetic response produced by visual inversion. *Journal of Comparative and Physiological Psychology,* 1950, *43,* 482–489.

Stelmach, G. E. (Ed.), *Motor control*. New York: Academic Press, 1976.

Sternberg, S., & Knoll, R. L. The perception of temporal order: Fundamental issues and a general model. In S. Kornblum (Ed.), *Attention and performance IV*. New York: Academic Press, 1973.

Volkmann, F. C. Vision during voluntary saccadic eye movements. *Journal of the Optical Society of America,* 1962, *52,* 571–578.

Volkmann, F. C. Saccadic suppression: A brief review. In R. A. Monty & J. W. Senders (Eds.), *Eye movements and psychological processes*. Hillsdale, New Jersey: Lawrence Erlbaum, 1976.

Volkmann, F. C., Riggs, L. A., Moore, R. K., & White, K. D. Central and peripheral determinants of saccadic suppression. In J. W. Senders, D. F. Fisher, & R. A. Monty (Eds.), *Eye movements and the higher psychological functions*. Hillsdale, New Jersey: Lawrence Erlbaum, 1976.

Volkmann, F. C., Riggs, L. A., Moore, R. K., & White, K. D. Central and peripheral determinants of saccadic suppression. In J. W. Senders, D. F. Fisher, & R. A. Monty (Eds.), *Eye movements and the higher psychological functions*. Hillsdale, New Jersey: Lawrence Erlbaum, in press.

Volkmann, F. C., Riggs, L. A., White, K. D., & Moore, R. K. Contrast sensitivity during saccadic eye movements. *Vision Research,* in press.

Volkmann, F. C., Schick, A. M. L., & Riggs, L. A. Time course of visual inhibition during voluntary saccades. *Journal of the Optical Society of America.* 1968, *58,* 562–569.

von Holst, E. Relations between the central nervous system and the peripheral organs. *British Journal of Animal Behaviour,* 1954, *2,* 89–94.

Welford, A. T. *Skilled performance: Perceptual and motor skills*. Glenview, Illinois: Scott, Foresman, 1976.

Woodworth, R. S. Vision and localization during eye movements. *Psychological Bulletin,* 1906, *3,* 68–70.

29. Potentials That Precede Small Saccades[1]

John C. Armington

There has been considerable speculation regarding the importance of microsaccadic eye movements for vision, but despite much research, their role still remains uncertain. A good many experiments have been done to see whether microsaccades can be related to any specific visual function, but they have been largely unsuccessful. For example, stabilized image experiments show that saccades as well as other forms of eye movement are not needed to maintain visual acuity (Keesey, 1960). Saccades are not essential to prevent stabilized visual fields from fading (Steinman, Haddad, Skavenski, & Wyman, 1973). Saccades are not the only means of restoring the position of the eye when it has slipped off the target. They do not help the eye when counting objects in the visual field (Kowler & Steinman, 1977). In fact, it has been suggested that small saccades may have a slight adverse effect on vision (Steinman *et al.,* 1973). In spite of all of these negative findings regarding the necessity of small saccadic eye movements for *specific* visual activities, their intimate relation to the visual process must still be acknowledged. It is clear that they produce significant electrophysiological response activity in the retina and in the brain (Armington & Bloom, 1974). It may also be significant that an elaborate neural system is involved in their production (Robinson, 1964; Fuchs, 1976, pp. 39–53). This chapter is concerned with small electrophysiological potentials that precede small saccadic movements.

I. Experimental Method

A union of well-known and relatively simple techniques is used for recording. The needed apparatus consist of an eye movement recording system, an elec-

[1]This research was supported by Public Health Service Grant EY 00568.

trophysiological recording system, a computer, and a display that presents fixation stimuli to the subject (Armington, 1972). The general procedure is to use saccadic eye movements for triggering a computer that is programmed to average electroencephalographic potentials. For most of the present work saccades were produced as the subject shifted his gaze from one to another of a pair of fixation points that were presented by a Maxwellian view stimulator. A mirror mounted on a snugly fitting contact lens was the essential element of the optical lever and photoelectric system used for recording saccades. The signal it provided was sent to analogue computer circuitry that provided the computer with a synchronization pulse whenever a saccade of specified direction and amplitude occurred. The electrophysiological potentials were picked up and amplified with conventional electroencephalographic equipment prior to averaging.

II. Examples of Recordings

The features of the recordings are identified in Figure 29.1. The upper tracing arises from the eye movement system. It shows that an averaged saccadic eye movement has shifted the eye horizontally to the right at point A. The middle tracing shows the averaged activity appearing at the same time as the saccade between electrodes attached to the vertex and to the joined earlobes. An upward deflection, denoting negativity of the vertex electrode, begins well before the saccade and is labeled with a B. It gives way to a positive change at point C and then to a more rapid positive spike at point D. The latter potential peaks just as the saccade

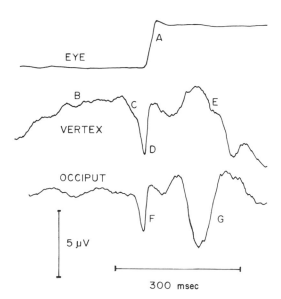

Figure 29.1. Schema of the potentials that accompany saccadic eye movement.

begins. Response activity, having a complex waveform, follows the saccade, and it is marked with an E. The bottom tracing was obtained simultaneously from electrodes on the occipital midline and the ears. It shows a sharp negative spike at F that is apparently the same as seen in the vertex recording. Response activity also follows the saccade with this electrode placement, and it is identified with letter G.

Recordings of the sort shown in Figure 29.1 may be obtained in association with saccades whose amplitudes range well below 1° of visual arc, but their features seem to be the same as those that have been reported for larger saccades (Becker, Hoehne, Iwase, & Kornhuber, 1972). The slow negative potential, B, has been associated with "readiness" (Becker, Hoehne, Iwase, & Kornhuber, 1973) and "contingent negative variation" (McAdam & Seales, 1969). It is prominent in some subjects but not others. In the present case it was found when the saccades were made in step with an auditory or tactile pacing signal. It was not found when the saccades were self-paced without any external signal.

The positive potential that precedes small saccades also compares with similar activity that precedes larger movements. The early, gradually descending part of this complex, C, has been given the descriptive name of premotor positivity (Becker et al., 1972). Although it is seen only at the vertex in Figure 29.1, later figures in the present chapter show that this waveform can appear when the electrode is in the occipital region. The sharp positive spike, D and F, in the middle and bottom recordings is the most well defined of the premotion potentials. Its similarity with the occipital and vertex electrode placements indicates that it would not be seen if recordings were taken between electrodes at these two sites (Riggs, Merton, & Morton, 1974). There is speculation that the positive spike is related to specific functions. It has been called the "rectus" potential, a term which relates it to the action of the extraocular muscles (Riggs et al., 1974; Becker et al., 1972), and in another context, it has been suggested to be an electrophysiological sign of the first phases of correlary discharge (Kurtzberg & Vaughan, 1977).

The response potentials shown in Figure 29.1 have been described rather thoroughly elsewhere (Armington & Bloom, 1974). Their properties seem to be the same as those of responses recorded by conventional methods of visual stimulation. Thus, the present discussion will be limited to potentials that precede microsaccades, and particular attention will be given to the positive spike.

The recordings that are produced with saccade triggering exhibit the variability that is characteristic of all electroencephalography. To meet this problem, the strategy illustrated in Figure 29.2 has been adopted. The left half of the figure shows averaged recordings from an electrode on the midline about 3 cm anterior to the inion with reference to the joined earlobes. Recording was performed while the subject made self-paced saccadic eye movements between two fixation points spaced at a visual angle of 27 min. Averages of the saccades that provided the trigger signal are shown to the right. The columns, from top to bottom, show six averaged recordings obtained during six viewing periods, each of which lasted 10 min. Grand averages based on all six sessions, and thus on an hour's total recording

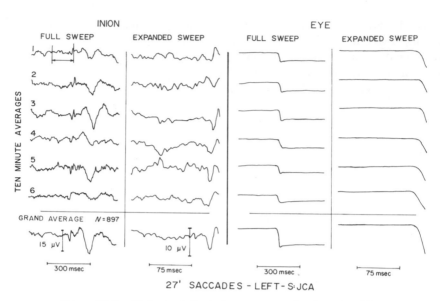

Figure 29.2. Methods of displaying and averaging the potentials.

time, are shown at the bottom of each column. The columns marked "Full Sweep" show the entire epoch that was sampled. To permit a more detailed examination of the potentials in the immediate vicinity of saccadic onset, a section of the records has been expanded and displayed to the right. The interval that has been expanded in this case is indicated by the double arrow in the tracing at the upper left-hand corner. The positive spike is seen clearly at the right end of the expanded recordings from the inion, and the onset of the corresponding average saccade is seen in the eye movement recording.

The saccades in Figure 29.2 are similar, but not identical, for all the experimental trials. Their regularity indicates that the averaging process is well synchronized. Nevertheless, the time relations between saccades and the positive spikes may be examined with best accuracy by looking at tracings from single averages rather than grand totals. Examples are shown in Figure 29.3 for two subjects on an expanded scale that stretches beyond the duration of the saccades. In this case, the saccades were made between fixation points that were spaced by 81 min of visual angle. These and many other recordings show that the peak of the positive spike is nearly coincident with the beginning of the saccade. The spike starts well before the saccade, but its onset is more difficult to fix exactly. In some cases, for example, the vertex recording from JCA with right saccades, an abrupt onset is seen about 10 msec ahead of any movement; in other cases, perhaps because the spike is confounded with premotor positivity, the onset is more gradual and extends 40 msec or more in front of the saccade. In all cases, the spike terminates while the saccade is still well under way.

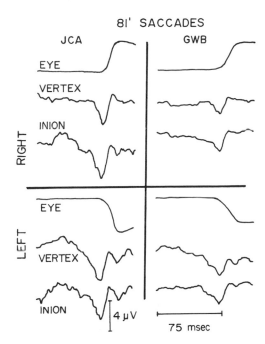

Figure 29.3. A display to show the temporal relations between the saccades and the positive potentials.

III. Amplitude of Movement

An important question is whether any relation exists between the features of these potentials and the amplitudes of the saccades that accompany them. This has been investigated with self-paced saccades. Jumps were made between pairs of fixation points that were spaced at differing intervals. Examples of grand average recordings obtained from the inion of one subject are shown in Figure 29.4 for right and for left saccades. An increase in activity with amplitude of eye movement is clearly evident. The positive spike becomes larger. Also, the onset of positivity is evident earlier with relatively large (81 min of arc) saccades than with small.

Amplitude measurements of the positive potential were made from the base line at the start of the recordings. The total deflection was measured. No attempt was made to distinguish the spike from premotion positivity. These measures are plotted against saccade amplitude in Figure 29.5. The data are based on grand averages from both right and left movements and are shown for two subjects. A regular growth in response amplitude with movement amplitude is evident, but the relation is not a linear one. The response levels off at about 10 μV. In fact, the potentials described in the literature for saccades that extend to many degrees of visual angle (Becker *et al.*, 1972; Kurtzberg & Vaughan, 1977) are not much larger than those found here. This nonlinearity will need to be taken into account when future attempts are made to establish the physiological origins of these positive signals.

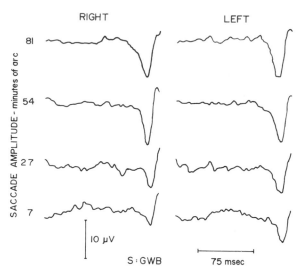

Figure 29.4.   Potentials obtained to right and left saccades of several amplitudes. The recording electrode is placed on the midline about 3 cm anterior to the inion.

IV. Direction of Movement

The recordings described so far were all obtained with the electrodes on the two ears joined together as a so-called reference. There is always uncertainty regarding the inactivity of such placements, however. In the present case, an interaction was found between the direction of eye movement, the choice of reference condition,

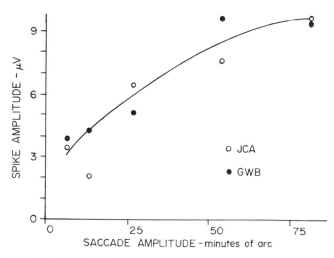

Figure 29.5.   Change in the size of the positive spike with saccadic amplitude.

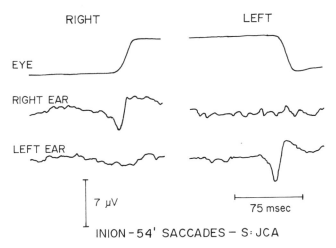

INION - 54' SACCADES - S: JCA

Figure 29.6. Potentials accompanying right and left movement and referred to the two ears independently.

and the amplitude of the positive spike. This is illustrated in Figure 29.6 where recordings from an electrode on the occipital midline are referred to each of the two ears separately. When the subject made saccades to the right, a large potential appeared between the placements on the right ear and the occipital position. Conversely, a large potential was seen with the left ear placement when saccades were made to the left. The recordings in this figure are for a single 10-min viewing period. However, a number of recordings have been performed with several subjects with electrodes on the vertex and with saccades of several amplitudes. Usually, some potential is obtained at both sides of the head, but the larger potential is always seen on the side toward which the eye is moved. These directional characteristics disappear entirely when the ears are joined together as a common reference.

All the results described so far pertain to horizontal saccades. Positive activity

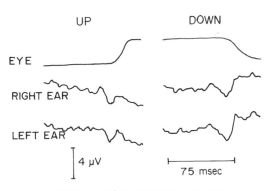

Figure 29.7. Potentials accompanying vertical saccades.

VERTEX - 8I' SACCADES - S:JCA

also accompanies vertical movement. An example showing the potentials obtained with up and down movements is presented in Figure 29.7. The scalp electrode was on the vertex and was referred to the two ears separately. A positive spike similar to that seen with horizontal movements is apparent for both directions of movement regardless of which ear is used as a reference. The positive potential is of the same order of magnitude as that found with horizontal movement. The figure shows samples from a single 10-min period of recording, but grand averages were taken from six such periods. Although no examples are shown, but as is true of all of these recordings, the positive spike stood out more clearly when the grand average was taken.

V. Fixation Saccades

The concern up to this point has been with saccades that were executed between pairs of fixation points. Small fixation saccades may occur when the subject tries to hold his eye on a single point, and these also are accompanied by antecedent potentials. Occipital examples are show in Figure 29.8. This figure shows grand totals from six viewing periods with an expanded sweep. Results are presented for two subjects and, in each case, the recording of the average saccade is superimposed on the electroencephalographic recording. Both subjects show positive activity close to saccade onset, but the difference between the two is striking. The positive spike is quite small in the data of GWB, in relation to both that of subject JCA and his own result with two closely spaced fixation points. A reason for this result is that GWB's fixation saccades are smaller than those of JCA. Thus, the average saccade has a less distinct onset. Since the computer could be less accurately synchronized with GWB's small saccades, small blurring of the recordings was the outcome. Nonethe-

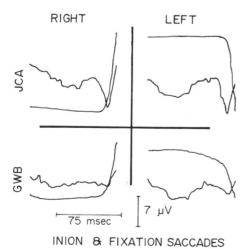

INION & FIXATION SACCADES

Figure 29.8. Potentials accompanying fixation saccades.

less, the results do make it clear that a positive potential does appear in conjunction with fixation saccades.

VI. Discussion

The data presented here indicate that the potentials that accompany small saccadic eye movements, including fixation saccades, are essentially similar to those seen with large eye movements. Although simple in waveform, their behavior is most likely more complex. Many questions arise regarding their nature, the extent to which they represent neural, muscular, and ocular activity, their relation to alpha waves in the electroencephalogram, and their significance for visual function. The experiments outlined here do not provide final answers to these questions, but they certainly have a bearing upon them. Future systematic study of the mass action potentials that antecede small saccades will yield information of considerable value.

ACKNOWLEDGMENTS

Portions of this research were conducted in collaboration with Matthias Korth, Vance Zemon, and Gary Barnes. Technical assistance was rendered by Laurel Rose and Rose White.

REFERENCES

Armington, J. C. Using the Lab-8 for experimentation with the human visual system. *Behavior Research Methods & Instrumentation,* 1972, *4,* 61–63.

Armington, J. C., & Bloom, M. B. Relations between the amplitudes of spontaneous saccades and visual responses. *Journal of the Optical Society of America,* 1974, *64,* 1263–1271.

Becker, W., Hoehne, O., Iwase, K., & Kornhuber, H. H. Bereitschaftspotential, prämotorische Positivierung und andere Hirnpotentiale bei sakkadischen Augenbewegungen. *Vision Research,* 1972, *12,* 421–436.

Becker, W., Hoehne, O., Iwase, K., & Kornhuber, H. H. Cerebral and ocular muscle potentials preceding voluntary eye movements in man. In W. C. McCallum & J. R. Knott (Eds.), *Event-related slow potentials of the brain. Electroencephalography and Clinical Neurophysiology,* 1973, *33,* 94–104 (suppl.).

Fuchs, A. F. The neurophysiology of saccades. In R. A. Monty & J. W. Senders (Eds.), *Eye movements and psychological processes.* Hillsdale, New Jersey: Erlbaum, 1976.

Keesey, U. Tulunay. Effects of eye movements on visual acuity. *Journal of the Optical Society of America,* 1960, *50,* 769–774.

Kowler, E., & Steinman, R. M. The role of small saccades in counting. *Vision Research,* 1977, *17,* 141–146.

Kurtzberg, P., & Vaughan, H. G., Jr. Electrophysiological observations on the visuomotor system and visual neurosensorium. In J. E. Desmedt (Ed.), *Visual evoked potentials in man: New developments.* Oxford: Clarendon, 1977. Pp. 314–331.

McAdam, D. W., & Seales, D. M. Bereitschaftspotential enhancement with increased level of motivation. *Electroencephalography and Clinical Neurophysiology,* 1969, *27,* 73–75.

Riggs, L. A., Merton, P. A., & Morton, H. B. Suppression of visual phosphenes during saccadic eye movements. *Vision Research,* 1974, *14,* 997–1011.

Robinson, D. A. The mechanics of human saccadic eye movement. *Journal of Physiology,* 1964, *174,* 245–264.

Steinman, R. M. Haddad, G. M., Skavenski, A. A., & Wyman, D. Miniature eye movement. *Science,* 1973, *181,* 810–819.

30. A Spatial Interference Effect with Stereoscopic Visual Acuity and the Tuning of Depth-Sensitive Channels

Thomas W. Butler

I. Introduction

Westheimer and his associates have been interested for some time in a number of different visual acuity tasks that Westheimer has called the "hyperacuities." A number of tasks are included in this class, including the whole family of vernier-type tasks, as well as sensitivity to differences in the tilt of short lines and sensitivity to small differences in depth. The one feature these judgments have in common is that they are all performed with a higher degree of accuracy than would be expected from the sharpness of the human eye's optics or the fineness of the retinal mosaic. The implication is that this hyperaccurate performance is probably due to some sort of neural sharpening of the signal from the eyes.

Spatial interference with an acuity of this type was reported by Westheimer and Hauske (1975), who put flanking lines around a vernier acuity pattern. The flanking lines were parallel to the vernier target, but caused an increase in the vernier offset threshold when they were a particular distance from the pattern. Two characteristics of the results were counterintuitive: First, one would expect a flanking line of this type to act as a comparison stimulus for the subject and to improve his performance rather than degrade it, as actually happened. Second, the interference effect was not monotonically related to the distance of the flanks from the target. When the flanks were so close that the line-spread functions of their images overlapped with that of the target line, performance was hindered, as one would expect. When the two flanks were moved away, performance improved temporarily, but larger distances between the target and the flanks produced another increase of threshold. This interference was maximal at about 2 min of arc stimulus-to-flank distance, too far away for physical optical factors to account for it. At yet greater separations, the interference lessened and was usually absent by the time the flanks were 4–6 min of arc away. Experiments that examined the effects of onset asynchrony between the

373

target and flanks and the effects of dichoptic presentation (that is, presentation of the target to one eye and the flanks to the other) all suggest that this interference has a neural basis and probably occurs at a cortical level.

Similar interference effects were demonstrated for line tilt thresholds by Westheimer, Shimamura, and McKee (1976). The threshold amount of tilt necessary for a subject to discriminate between a line tipped to the right and one tipped to the left was affected in much the same way by flanking lines, though some differences specific to the task did surface. The experiments discussed here tested for similar effects in the stereo domain.

The fundamental stimulus in all these experiments was composed of two vertical lines 10 min of arc long. One line was directly above the other, and their endpoints were separated by a 3 min of arc gap. Its appearance was similar to that of a traditional vernier pattern. The lines were drawn on two display oscilloscopes by a PDP-11 computer. The lights from the two oscilloscopes were polarized in opposite directions, and the two images were superimposed with a pellicle mirror. Subjects viewed the combined images through Polaroid analyzers from a distance of 2.5 m. The impression of depth was produced by displacing the top line of each pair by equal small amounts in opposite directions on the two oscilloscopes. In this way retinal disparity was introduced, but the position of the top line in the fused image remained aligned with the bottom test line. The lower test line always appeared in the same depth as the fixation plane, and the upper test line appeared at seven discrete positions in depth. The middle position was the same depth as the lower test line, and three positions in front and three positions in back were used, spaced at equal intervals in depth. The computer randomly presented one of these stimuli for 200 msec every 3 sec, and the subject responded after each presentation whether the top line had appeared in front of or behind the lower line. Immediate feedback was given for incorrect responses. The resulting data were fit with a psychometric function by the method of probits (see Finney, 1952).

One subject who was extremely practiced showed retinal disparity thresholds of about 6 sec of arc with this stimulus. The other, more typical subject showed thresholds of about 17 sec of arc. This value is typical for stereo presentations of this short duration (Ogle & Weil, 1958).

A. The Initial Finding

In the first experiment I was simply interested in the existence of a spatial interference effect of the type described earlier. The same pattern was used as in the control condition, but with four flanking lines 6 min of arc long symmetrically placed around the stimulus, as in Figure 30.1. All of the flanks appeared in the same depth as the lower test line, while the top test line moved in depth just as before. Figure 30.1 shows the stereo threshold values that were obtained for a range of stimulus-to-flank distances. It is clear that the interference for which we tested was present, with maximum interference occurring at about 2–2.5 min of arc stimulus-

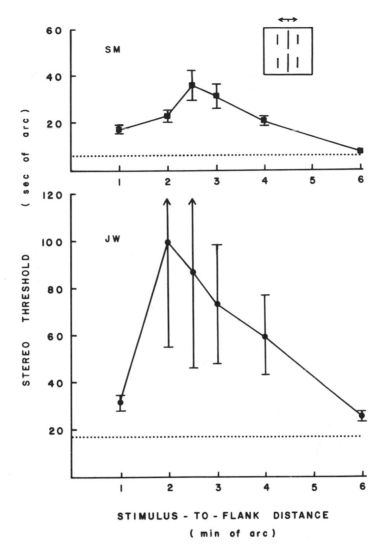

Figure 30.1. Stereo thresholds when the stimulus configuration shown in the inset was used with a range of stimulus-to-flank distances. The thresholds were elevated most at distances of 2–2.5 sec of arc. The dashed line indicates threshold for the control condition with no flanking lines present. All flanks remained in the same depth as the fixation plane, as did the lower test line, while the upper test line moved in depth. One stimulus was presented for 200 msec every 3 sec. In between presentations fixation was maintained with a fixation pattern of four dots placed around the location of the target in a rectangle subtending 47 min × 38 min arc. The fixation pattern was not present during the presentations.

to-flank distance. Each subject showed about a sixfold threshold increase at that distance.

All of the values plotted on these graphs are the result of a probit analysis of at least 300 responses per point. Error bars indicate the size of ±1 SE. Their absence indicates the error was too small to plot.

B. Subsequent Experiments

Additional experiments were performed to determine which of the stimulus components were necessary for the interference to appear.

In Experiment 2 the stimulus was the same as in Experiment 1, except that the flanks around the upper test line changed their position in depth with that test line instead of remaining at the same depth as the lower test line and its flanks. As shown in Figure 30.2, no interference occurs in this condition. If anything, the thresholds may be lower over the first 4 min of arc of stimulus-to-flank distances. This suggests that the top three lines were all seen as a unit and that the task was essentially the same as the control condition, but with more structured targets.

In Experiment 3 the stimulus was again the same as in Experiment 1, except that this time the flanks around the lower test line were omitted. The flanks around the upper line still remained at the same depth as the lower test line. The data in Figure 30.3 show that this condition is clearly sufficient to produce the interference effect. Interference produced with this condition is at least as large as that found in Experiment 1.

Data from one subject in Experiment 4 (Figure 30.4) show that this is not true when only the flanks around the lower test line are present. In this condition no interference occurs.

A fifth experiment placed a single flanking line on the right side of the upper test line. Once again, the flank remained at the same depth as the lower test line. This condition also produced no interference, as shown in Figure 30.5. Subjects reported that after one or two trials they could simply "look around" this single flanking line and ignore it totally.

It appears that the necessary condition for producing this interference is to have two flanking lines stationary in depth that surround a test line appearing at different depths.

Mitchell and O'Hagan (1972) have also described an interference effect with stereoscopic acuity, but it is probably not the same one that is described here. They found that monocularly presented interfering stimuli elevated stereo thresholds, but their interfering stimuli were much larger than those used in the present study, and they were placed an order of magnitude farther from the stereo target than those used here (Mitchell & O'Hagan, 1972). The nonmonotonic nature of the present effect and the small spatial area over which it occurs suggest that it is not the same as other stereoscopic interference effects that have been described (e.g., Richards, 1972).

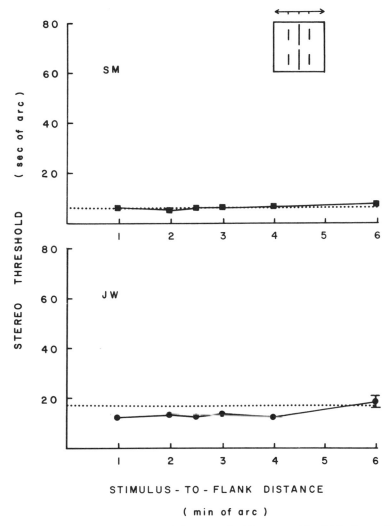

Figure 30.2. When the flanks around the upper test line moved in depth along with it, no interference of the type shown in Figure 30.1 seemed to be present.

II. Depth Tuning of Processing Channels

While it is probably premature to speculate about the neural substrate of this effect, it may still be exploited in order to study a number of characteristics of stereoscopic vision that are not easily examined otherwise. One general course of investigation being pursued in our laboratory that makes use of this tool is an examination of the depth tuning of channels responsible for fine stereoscopic acuity.

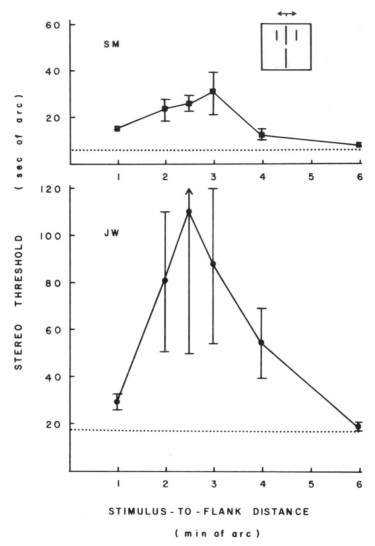

Figure 30.3. Omitting the flanks around the lower test line did not affect the interference effect. Flanks around the upper test line remained stationary in the plane of fixation.

These depth-tuning experiments used stimuli similar to those already described, but with some differences. The same two vertical test lines are present as before, and interfering stimuli are placed around the top stimulus line. The interfering stimuli, though, are not vertical lines as before, but are a sort of louver pattern composed of four short horizontal lines on each side of the test line, as shown in Figure 30.6. For the data presented here, these louver lines were 3 min of arc long, and their near endpoints were a mean distance of 2.5 min of arc away from the test line.

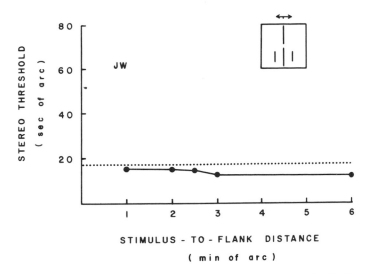

Figure 30.4.   Omitting the flanks around the upper test line, while leaving flanks around the lower test line, eliminated the interference effect.

Depth tuning was measured by placing the interfering louvers at different station-ary depth positions relative to the lower test line, and by examining their interfering effectiveness at these different locations in depth. The upper test line moved in depth just as before. Subjects were tested with the interfering louvers behind, in front of, and at the same depth as the lower test line. The resulting stereo thresholds are shown in Figure 30.6. The threshold elevations were largest when the louvers appeared in the same plane as the rest of the target, and they decreased very quickly when the louvers moved away from the target in depth. Three subjects were used. The two subjects whose results are shown in the lower panels of Figure 30.6 viewed the targets for 500 msec instead of the usual 200 msec because they had difficulty in fusing the stimulus appropriately at the shorter duration. The use of a 500-msec presentation made the task easier for them, and apparently did not disrupt the effect since their results are qualitatively the same as those of Subject SM.

The striking feature about all of the curves is the narrowness of their tuning. The tuning curve for Subject SM has a half-bandwidth of only 24 sec of arc of retinal disparity, which is very narrow indeed. At the 2.5-m viewing distance used here, this translates to just slightly more than 1 cm in real depth. Therefore when the louvers were moved more than the equivalent of 5 mm in front of or behind the stereo target, their interfering effect dropped to less than half of its peak value. The tuning of the other two subjects' curves is wider, with half-bandwidths of approximately 36 sec of arc and 1 min 10 sec of arc, respectively; but even these values are strikingly narrow. This finding has at least one implication for stereo processing: In the plane of fixation, the channels through which stereo information is processed must either be very narrow, or, if wide, the channels must overlap to a great extent with their peaks quite close together.

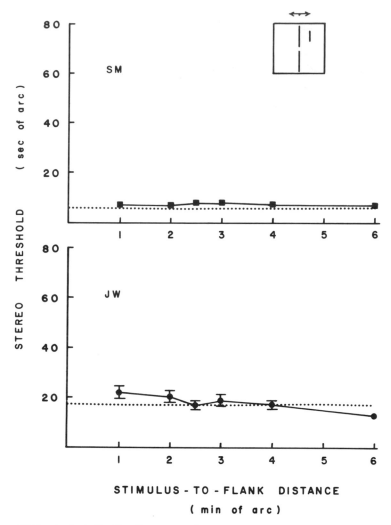

Figure 30.5. A single flanking line next to the upper test line was not sufficient to produce interference. This flank was stationary in the fixation plane.

This finding indicates a much tighter tuning than that which would be inferred on the basis of the results of Blakemore and Hague (1972). They adapted subjects to gratings of a given spatial frequency and then measured the contrast thresholds of binocular gratings of the same frequency. These gratings were presented at a range of retinal disparity values. Although they did find differential adaptation for gratings of different disparities, the bandwidth of the effect appeared to be much larger than that found in the present study. Contrast thresholds for gratings differing in retinal disparity from the adapting grating by as much as 6 min of arc were elevated by as

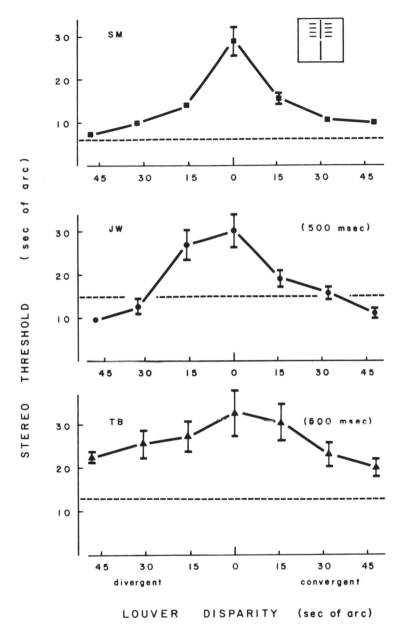

Figure 30.6. To study depth tuning, subjects made stero judgments with the flanking lines around the upper test line replaced with a louver pattern (see inset). Flanking louvers were stationary in depth, but appeared at different positions in depth relative to the fixation plane. The abscissas represent the positions of the louvers in depth relative to the fixation plane. Interference was maximal when the louvers were in the same depth as the target, and decreased rapidly when the louvers were removed from that plane.

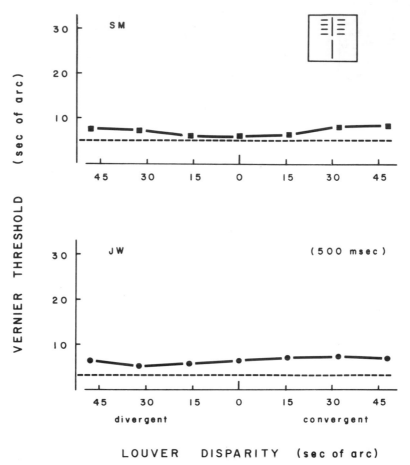

Figure 30.7. A vernier analogue of the experiment in Figure 30.6. Subjects made vernier judgments with the same configuration of interfering louvers as in Figure 30.6. The louvers did not change in their capacity to interfere when they appeared in different depths as they did with stereo judgments.

much as a factor of 2. This finding would not necessarily indicate the fine tuning that is implied by the present results.

A control experiment provides evidence that the interference on which this result is based is truly interference with stereo processing, and not simply the result of a monocular interference effect of the type described by Westheimer and Hauske (1975). This control was necessary because, as Walls (1943) proposed, stereo acuity may be the result of additional processing of vernier-type information from the two eyes. Walls noted that both tasks are based on the precise relative localization of objects, and that the essential difference between stereo and vernier tasks is that in stereo acuity the relative localization information from two different sources is processed and compared. Whether this serial scheme of stereopsis is valid is still not certain, though a number of investigators, including Berry (1948) from the laboratory at Brown University, have examined the relationship between the two acuities. If the proposal is valid, then a disruption of processing at either level would impair stereo acuity.

To test for the effects of interference at the level of monocular processing, a vernier analogue of the previous experiment was performed. The stimulus was the same as in the "tuning" experiment, except that the upper test line was displaced laterally instead of in depth. The louver lines still appeared in different depths, just as before. The subject's task was to determine whether the upper test line was to the right or to the left of the lower test line in each presentation. Vernier thresholds for two subjects in which the louvers appeared at a number of different depths are shown in Figure 30.7. It is clear that these vernier thresholds are not affected by the interfering louvers in the same way that stereo thresholds were affected. A fairly uniform, small threshold elevation is shown in the vernier data across the whole range of louver depths, with no peak interference effect occurring when the louvers appeared in the same depth as the vernier target. This suggests that the interference shown in the stereo depth-tuning experiment is a phenomenon occurring in the stereo domain, and that the tuning curves shown in Figure 30.6 represent the depth tuning of a mechanism that processes stereo information. The fact that it is possible to interfere with stereo acuity without affecting vernier acuity also suggests that the processing of vernier and stereo information may indeed be more separate than Walls would have us believe (Walls, 1943).

ACKNOWLEDGMENTS

The experiments reported here were conducted in the laboratory of Dr. Gerald Westheimer where the author holds Postdoctoral Fellowship EY 05136-02 from the National Institutes of Health. Dr. Westheimer's encouragement and support are gratefully acknowledged.

REFERENCES

Berry, R.N. Quantitative relations among vernier, real depth, and stereoscopic depth acuities. *Journal of Experimental Psychology,* 1948, *38,* 708–721.

Blakemore, C., & Hague, B. Evidence for disparity detecting neurones in the human visual system. *Journal of Physiology (London),* 1972, *225,* 437–455.

Finney, D.J. *Probit analysis* (2nd ed.). Cambridge: University Press, 1952.

Mitchell, D.E., & O'Hagan, S. Accuracy of stereoscopic localization of small line segments that differ in size and orientation for the two eyes. *Vision Research,* 1972, *12,* 437–454.

Ogle, K.N., & Weil, M.P. Stereoscopic vision and the duration of the stimulus. *Archives of Ophthalmology,* 1958, *59,* 4–17.

Richards, W. Disparity masking. *Vision Research,* 1972, *12,* 1113–1124.

Walls, G.L. Factors in human resolution. *Journal of the Optical Society of America,* 1943, *33,* 487–505.

Westheimer, G., & Hauske, G. Temporal and spatial interference with vernier acuity. *Vision Research,* 1975, *15,* 1137–1141.

Westheimer, G., Shimamura, K., & McKee, S.M. Interference with line-orientation sensitivity. *Journal of the Optical Society of America,* 1976, *66,* 332–338.

31. Assessment of Visual Acuity in Infants[1]

Velma Dobson and Davida Y. Teller

Over the past 20 years, three techniques—optokinetic nystagmus (OKN), preferential looking (PL), and the visually evoked cortical potential (VECP)—have been developed to test visual acuity in infants. The three techniques use different types of stimuli, score acuity differently, and may well tap acuity information at different levels of the visual system. Therefore, there is no reason why they should give exactly the same acuity values. However, in adults and animals, under some circumstances, OKN and the VECP give acuity values similar to those found behaviorally in a psychophysical task or with a Snellen chart (Berkley & Watkins, 1971, 1973; Campbell & Maffei, 1970; Regan & Richards, 1971; Reinecke & Cogan, 1958; Voipio, 1961, Wolin & Dillman, 1964) It is therefore of interest to compare the infant results found using different techniques.

This chapter will summarize the results of OKN, PL, and VECP studies of visual acuity in infants and show that acuity values obtained with the VECP are typically higher than those measured with PL or OKN. We will then discuss the possibility that differences in acuity results across techniques may be due largely to differences in scoring. Finally, we will report an experiment we carried out to see whether part of the acuity difference could be due to differences in the stimuli used to test acuity.

I. Optokinetic Nystagmus

In the OKN procedure the stimulus is typically a moving square-wave grating that subtends part or all the infant's visual field. The grating may be moved across a canopy above the infant, or it may rotate in front of the infant on a hand-held drum.

[1]This research was supported in part by National Institutes of Health Postdoctoral Fellowship EY 01523 to Velma Dobson, and Grant BNS 76-01503 from the National Science Foundation.

385

The movement of the stripes elicits pursuit eye movements, which follow the stripes until the eye reaches the edge of the orbit, at which point a saccade is made and the pursuit movements begin again.

Figure 31.1 summarizes acuity data obtained with OKN from various laboratories. The data of Enoch and Rabinowicz (1976) are from one infant and indicate the smallest stripe width eliciting OKN eye movements in that infant. The data of Gorman, Cogan, and Gellis (1957, 1959), Dayton, Jones, Aiu, Rawson, Steele, and Rose (1964), and Fantz, Ordy, and Udelf (1962) are based on five or more subjects at each age. In these studies, acuity is estimated as the stripe width on which 75% or more of infants tested showed OKN. With the exception of one point from the subject tested by Enoch and Rabinowicz, there is agreement to within 1 octave across studies at each age. Stripe resolution increases from about 20 min of arc in the newborn to 5 min of arc by 6 months.

II. Preferential Looking

In the PL procedure, the infant is shown two stimuli simultaneously—typically an acuity grating and a homogeneous field of equal space average luminance. If the infant stares at one stimulus more than the other or responds differentially to the two stimuli in any way, it follows that the infant can discriminate the grating from the homogeneous field.

A schematic drawing of a PL stimulus arrangement is shown in Figure 31.2.

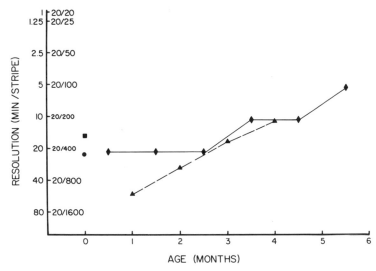

Figure 31.1. Visual resolution in infants, as measured with OKN. Minimum stripe width resolved (in minutes of visual angle and approximate Snellen equivalent) is plotted as a function of age. (●) Gorman *et al.* (1957, 1959); (◆) Fantz *et al.* (1962); (■) Dayton *et al.* (1964); (▲) Enoch and Rabinowicz (1976).

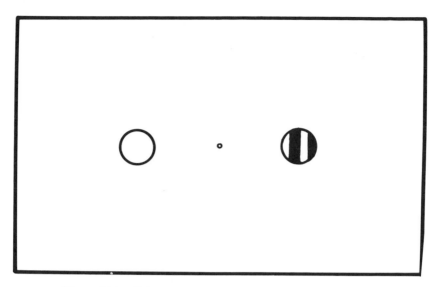

Figure 31.2.   Schematic diagram of a PL stimulus arrangement.

Here, the infant is shown a stimulus field with a square-wave grating located to one side of center and a blank gray field of equal space-average luminance located to the other side. A peephole in the center of the screen allows an observer to watch the infant. In the traditional version of the PL procedure (Fantz et al., 1962), the observer is required to record some aspect of the infant's behavior, for example, direction of first fixation or duration of fixation of each stimulus. In the forced-choice preferential looking (FPL) technique (Teller, Morse, Borton, & Regal, 1974), the observer (who is blind as to the location of the grating pattern) is required to judge, on the basis of the infant's looking behavior, whether the grating is on the left or the right.

Figure 31.3 shows representative results of studies that have used the traditional PL technique or the FPL modification to measure acuity in infants. In general, there is considerable agreement among the results of the various studies even though the data come from different laboratories and from different variations of the PL procedure. Acuity increases from about 20 min of arc at 1 month to about 5 min of arc at 6 months. At each age between 2 and 6 months, the data fall within about a 1-octave range.

In these studies, stimuli were either stationary square-wave gratings (Allen, 1978; Fantz et al., 1962; Held, in press; Teller et al., 1974) or sine-wave gratings (Atkinson & Braddick, 1977; Atkinson, Braddick, & Moar, 1977a; Banks & Salapatek, 1978). The criterion for scoring acuity was typically rather strict. Fantz et al. (1962) estimated acuity as the minimum stripe width that 75% or more of the infants of a particular age fixated longer than they fixated the homogeneous gray field. Teller et al. (1974), Allen (1978), and Held et al. (in press) estimated acuity as the stripe width that produced 75% correct by the observer in the FPL procedure.

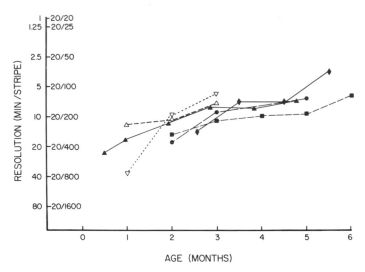

Figure 31.3. Visual resolution in infants, as measured with preferential looking (PL). Axes as in Figure 31.1. (◆) Fantz *et al.* (1962); (●) Teller *et al.* (1974); (■) Held (in press); (▲) Allen (1978); (△) Banks and Salapatek (1978); (▽) Atkinson and Braddick (1977), and Atkinson *et al.* (1977a).

Finally, the acuity values shown for Banks and Salapatek (1978), Atkinson and Braddick (1977), and Atkinson *et al.* (1977a) are the high-frequency cutoffs estimated from their measurements of contrast sensitivity functions in infants from 1 to 3 months of age. Contrast threshold was estimated by Banks and Salapatek as the (interpolated) contrast on which the infant's first fixation away from midline was in the direction of the grating on 75% of the trials. Atkinson and Braddick, and Atkinson *et al.*, on the other hand, used the FPL procedure and estimated contrast threshold as the stripe width that produced 70% correct by the observer. Thus, in all the PL studies, the scoring rule adopted was such that it was necessary for the observer to get a rather high percentage correct or for a large percentage of infants to show preferential fixation before a particular stripe width was taken as an estimate of visual resolution.

III. Visually Evoked Cortical Potential

In the VECP procedure, electrodes are taped on the scalp over the occipital pole, and the VECP is recorded to a checkerboard or grating stimulus pattern. Since the VECP is a response elicited by a *change* in the stimulus, stimuli are by necessity temporally modulated, either by flashing the pattern on and off, by phase-alternating elements of the pattern, or by alternating the pattern with a field of the same space-average luminance.

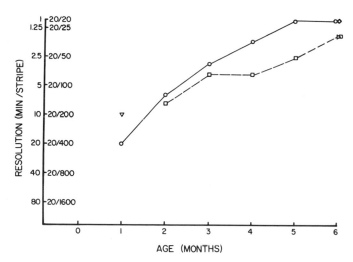

Figure 31.4. Visual resolution in infants, as measured with the VECP. Axes as in Figure 31.1 (○) Marg *et al.* (1976); (◇) Sokol and Dobson (1976); (□) Sokol (1978); (△) Harris *et al.* (1976); (▽) Harter *et al.* (1977).

Figure 31.4 shows the results of studies using the VECP to estimate acuity in infants. In general, acuity results of the various studies agree to within an octave at each age. Stimulus configuration varied considerably among studies. Harter, Deaton, and Odom (1977) used flashed checkerboards; Marg, Freeman, Peltzman, and Goldstein (1976) used square-wave gratings alternated with a homogeneous field of equal space-average luminance; Harris, Atkinson, and Braddick (1976) used phase-alternated sine-wave gratings, and Sokol (1978) and Sokol and Dobson (1976) used phase-alternated checkerboards.

As it happens, the criterion for scoring acuity was in each case a generous one. Marg *et al.* (1976) estimated acuity as the smallest stripe width that would produce a VECP detectably different from that produced in response to a defocused 30 cycles deg^{-1} grating. Sokol (1978) plotted amplitude of the steady-state VECP as a function of check size and extrapolated to estimate the smallest check size that would elicit a VECP. Harter *et al.* (1977) used a similar technique, except that acuity was extrapolated from a plot of the amplitude of the most positive component occurring between 320 and 400 msec after the flash (termed P4) versus check size. Sokol and Dobson concluded that 6-month-old infants show 20/20 acuity on the basis of the similarity of adult and 6-month amplitude versus check size functions. Finally, the acuity estimate of Harris *et al.* (1976) is based on the cutoff frequency of a contrast sensitivity function obtained for one infant. In their study, contrast threshold was estimated by extrapolating to zero on a plot of steady-state VECP versus log contrast.

IV. Comparison of Acuity Results across Techniques

Thus far, we have seen that within each technique—OKN, PL, and VECP—there is considerable agreement concerning the manner in which acuity develops between birth and 6 months of age. Figure 31.5 presents a comparison of some typical results across techniques. In general, all three techniques show that acuity increases over the first 6 months. However, especially at the older ages, the VECP values are on the average about 1.5 octaves better than those found with OKN or PL. We will now attempt to answer the question of why VECP acuity values are so much better than values obtained with OKN and PL.

A. Level at Which Acuity Information Is Tapped

One obvious difference between the techniques is that they tap acuity information at different levels of the visual system. Thus, information recorded in the VECP may not be available at the levels tapped by PL and OKN.

B. Influence of Scoring

A second factor that may contribute to the difference in acuity among techniques is the difference in criteria used to estimate acuity in each technique. In VECP

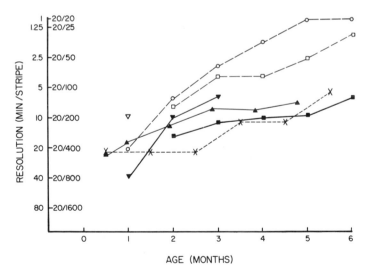

Figure 31.5. Representative results of OKN, PL, and VECP measurements of visual resolution in infants. Axes as in Figure 31.1. In general, PL and OKN results show estimates of resolution 1 to 2 octaves poorer than those obtained with the VECP. (X) Fantz *et al.* (1962), OKN; (▲) Allen (1978), FPL; (■) Held *et al.* (in press), FPL; (▼) Atkinson and Braddick (1977), and Atkinson *et al.* (1977a), FPL; (□) Sokol (1978), VECP; (○) Marg *et al.* (1976), VECP; (▽) Harter *et al.* (1977), VECP.

estimates of acuity, the criterion has traditionally been rather generous, for example, extrapolation to zero on a plot of amplitude versus check size. The PL and OKN criteria, on the other hand, are usually less generous, for example, 75% correct by an observer or 75% of infants showing preferential fixation or OKN. If the data from PL and OKN testing were replotted using more generous scoring criteria, an improvement in acuity values would be expected.

The effect of replotting the data using more generous criteria is illustrated in Figure 31.6 for FPL data and in Figure 31.7 for OKN data. Figure 31.6 shows the FPL data of Allen (1978) plotted according to criteria of 55, 65, and 75% correct by the observer. Criteria of 65 and 55% improve acuity values by about .5 and 1 octave, respectively. Even higher acuity values would be obtained by extrapolating to 50%, the criterion that may be most comparable to the VECP criterion of extrapolating to zero response amplitude.

Figure 31.7 shows the effect of using a less strict criterion in evaluating OKN data. Closed symbols show data of Figure 31.1 and represent the smallest stripe width eliciting OKN in 75% of infants. Open symbols are the same data replotted to show acuity as the smallest stripe width eliciting OKN in *any* infant in the study. As in the PL results, the use of the more generous criterion for evaluating OKN data improves acuity values by at least 1 octave. Note that the acuity values of Fantz *et al.* (1962) at 3.5, 4.5, and 5.5 months undoubtedly underestimate resolution, since 5-min stripes were the smallest stripe width used and a large percentage of infants at these ages preferred stripes to gray.

Figure 31.8 replots the OKN data of Fantz *et al.* (1962) and the FPL data of Allen

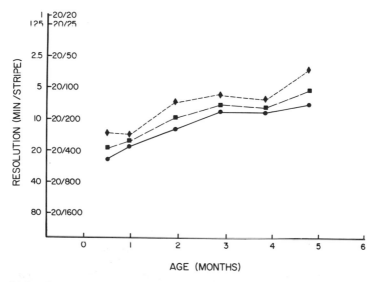

Figure 31.6. Forced-choice preferential looking data of Allen (1978) plotted according to criteria of 55 (◆), 65 (■), and 75% (●) correct by the observer. Use of more generous criteria results in higher estimates of visual resolution. Axes as in Figure 31.1.

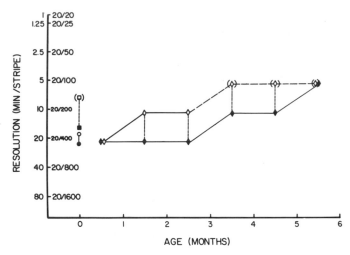

Figure 31.7. Optokinetic nystagmus estimates of visual resolution, plotted to show the in-crease in acuity occurring when resolution is estimated as the smallest stripe width eliciting OKN in any infant in the study (open symbols) rather than as the stripe width on which 75% of infants showed OKN (closed symbols). Symbols enclosed in parentheses are the smallest stripe width used in the study and may underestimate acuity. Axes as in Figure 31.1. (○,●) Gorman *et al.* (1957, 1959); (◇,◆) Fantz *et al.* (1962); (□,■) Dayton *et al.* (1964).

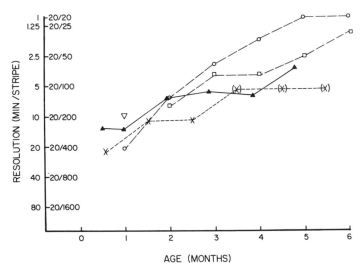

Figure 31.8. Representative results of OKN, PL, and VECP measurements of visual resolu-tion in infants. The VECP data as in Figure 31.5. The PL and OKN data replotted according to more generous criteria of Figures 31.6 and 31.7, respectively. Use of more generous criteria in scoring PL and OKN data greatly reduces differences in OKN, PL, and VECP estimates of resolution. Axes as in Figure 31.1 (X) Fantz *et al.* (1962), OKN; (▲) Allen (1978), FPL; (□) Sokol (1978), VECP; (○) Marg *et al.* (1976), VECP; (▽) Harter *et al.* (1977), VECP.

(1978) based on more generous criteria for scoring acuity, along with the VECP data of Sokol and Marg. Using what may be more comparable criteria for estimating acuity in the three techniques produces acuity estimates that are more similar across techniques [although the data from Marg *et al.*'s (1976) subjects in months 4 and 5 still stand as considerably higher acuity values than have yet been seen in other labs by *any* technique]. Thus, we propose that the finding of consistently *lower* acuity values with OKN and PL is due largely to the relatively ungenerous criteria typically used to score OKN and PL data.

C. Influence of Stimulus Differences

In addition to differences in scoring between techniques, there are also stimulus differences that may contribute to differences in acuity values. Stimuli in the PL technique are typically stationary gratings, whereas the VECP stimulus is often a temporally modulated checkerboard. It seemed possible to us that the use of more spatially complex and/or temporally modulated stimuli might induce the infants to show higher PL acuity than they show with stationary stripes.

To investigate this possibility, we used a variety of stimulus configurations to test acuity in a group of 2-month-old infants with the FPL procedure (Dobson, Teller, & Belgum, in press). Each infant's acuity was estimated using both checkerboard patterns and square-wave gratings. For some subjects, the checks were phase-alternated at 10 alternations per second, while for other subjects the checks remained stationary. Gratings remained stationary for all subjects. Our goal was to see whether using a more complex stimulus (a stationary checkerboard) or a temporally modulated stimulus (a phase-alternated checkerboard) would produce PL acuity values approaching acuity values found with the VECP.

Stimuli were generated on two cathode ray tubes (CRTs), one to the left and one to the right of the infant. The CRT faces were embedded in a green plastic screen approximately equal in hue and luminance to the scope faces. On any one trial, one CRT face displayed a homogeneous field and the other CRT face showed either a grating or a checkerboard pattern equal in space-average luminance to the homogeneous field. Testing was carried out with the FPL procedure in which the observer's task is to judge the location of the patterned stimulus on the basis of the infant's behavior.

The results for one infant are shown in Figure 31.9. For both checks and stripes, the observer's percentage correct ranges from near chance (50%), for stimuli too small to produce differential fixation by the infant, to near 100% for large stimuli that the infant clearly discriminated from the homogeneous field. Acuity was estimated as the stripe or check width that would produce a score of 75%, as indicated by the arrows below the abscissa. For this infant, there was virtually no difference in acuity for phase-alternated checks and stationary stripes.

Figure 31.10 shows a summary of the data of all our subjects. The solid diagonal line represents the set of locations in which an infant's data point would be expected to fall if the infant's acuity values for checks and stripes were equal. If checker-

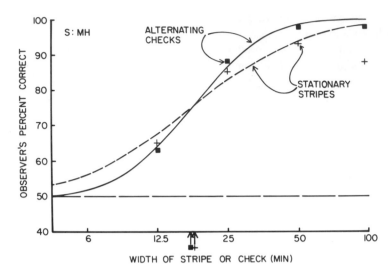

Figure 31.9. Observer's percentage correct versus stripe or check width for one infant. (+) Vertical gratings; (■) phase-alternated checks. Solid and dashed curves indicate cumulative normal ogives that were computer fit to data for checks and stripes, respectively. Arrows below abscissa indicate stripe or check width corresponding to 75% correct on each computer-fit ogive. For this subject, resolution of checks and stripes was similar.

boards lead to higher acuity values than do stripes, the data points would fall above the solid diagonal line. In the extreme, if the whole 1.5-octave difference previously found between PL and VECP acuity were due to temporal modulation of the stimulus or to the use of a more complex pattern in the VECP procedure, we would expect the data to cluster along the dashed diagonal line.

The data shown in Figure 31.10 tend to cluster along the solid diagonal line rather than above it. Thus, since the acuity values of subjects tested with stationary checkerboards and phase-alternated checkerboards are very similar to their acuity values for stationary gratings, we conclude that neither temporal modulation nor the increased complexity of the checkerboard pattern significantly affects PL acuity estimates.

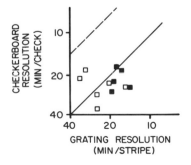

Figure 31.10. Comparison of visual resolution for checkerboard and grating stimuli within individual infants. The solid line indicates the locus of equal acuity for the two stimulus conditions being compared. Points above (below) this line indicate finer acuity for checks (stripes). The dashed diagonal line indicates acuity for checks which is 1.5 octaves better than acuity for stripes. (■) Data of subjects tested with phase-alternated checks and stationary gratings. (□) Data of subjects tested with stationary checks and stationary gratings.

Recently, Atkinson, Braddick, and Moar (1977b) have also found that temporal variation of a stimulus does not affect acuity as measured with the FPL procedure. They tested infants at 1, 2, and 3 months of age and showed that for each infant, similar acuity values were obtained with stationary gratings and gratings drifting at a rate of 3 Hz. Thus, the data from both laboratories are in good agreement and indicate that stimulus differences are probably not a major cause of acuity differences found with the PL and VECP procedures.

V. Summary

Optokinetic nystagmus, preferential looking, and the visually evoked cortical potential have been successfully used to measure acuity in infants less than 6 months of age. The results of all three techniques indicate an improvement in acuity over the 6-month period. When comparable scoring criteria are used to estimate acuity, the combined results of the three procedures indicate that acuity increases from about 20/300 in the newborn period to close to 20/20 by 6 months. Each technique has its own particular advantages and disadvantages, for example, the PL technique is relatively inexpensive but lengthy, the VECP is quick but requires expensive equipment. Since each technique may tap different pathways, we foresee advantages to the further development of all three techniques, both for the laboratory study of infant visual development and for clinical assessment of acuity in infants.

ACKNOWLEDGMENTS

We thank Jane Allen, Janette Atkinson, Richard Held, Martin Banks, and Sam Sokol for unpublished data presented here, and Marjorie Zachow for secretarial assistance.

REFERENCES

Allen, J. Visual acuity development in human infants up to 6 months of age. Unpublished doctoral dissertation, University of Washington, 1978.

Atkinson, J., & Braddick, O. Contrast sensitivity in the infant. In H. Sperreise & L. H. van der Tweel (Eds.), *Spatial Contrast*. New York: Elsevier-North Holland, 1977.

Atkinson, J., Braddick, O., & Moar, K. Development of contrast sensitivity over the first three months of life in the human infant. *Vision Research,* 1977, *17,* 1037–1044. (a)

Atkinson, J., Braddick, O., & Moar, K. Contrast sensitivity of the human infant for moving and static patterns. *Vision Research,* 1977, *17,* 1045–1047. (b)

Banks, M. S., & Salapatek, P. Acuity and contrast sensitivity in one-, two-, and three-month-old human infants. *Investigative Ophthalmology and Visual Science,* 1978, *17,* 361–365.

Berkley, M., & Watkins, D. W. Visual acuity of the cat estimated from evoked cerebral potentials. *Nature New Biology,* 1971, *234,* 91–92.

Berkley, M., & Watkins, D. W. Grating resolution and refraction in the cat estimated from evoked cerebral potentials. *Vision Research,* 1973, *13,* 403–415.

Campbell, F. W., & Maffei, L. Electrophynological evidence for the existence of orientation and size detectors in the human visual system. *Journal of Physiology,* 1970, *207,* 635–652.

Dayton, G. O., Jones, M. H., Aiu, P., Rawson, R. A., Steele, B., & Rose, M. Developmental study of coordinated eye movements in the human infant. I. Visual acuity in the newborn human: A study based on induced optokinetic nystagmus recorded by electro-oculography. *Archives of Ophthalmology,* 1964, *71,* 865–870.

Dobson, V., Teller, D. Y., & Belgum, J. Visual acuity in human infants assessed with stationary stripes and phase-alternated checkerboards. *Vision Research,* in press.

Enoch, J. M., & Rabinowicz, I. M. Early surgery and visual correction of an infant born with unilateral eye lens opacity. *Documenta Ophthalmologica,* 1976, *41,* 371–382.

Fantz, R. L., Ordy, J. M., & Udelf, M. S. Maturation of pattern vision in infants during the first six months. *Journal of Comparative and Physiological Psychology,* 1962, *55,* 907–917.

Gorman, J. J., Cogan, D. G., & Gellis, S. S. An apparatus for grading the visual acuity on the basis of optokinetic nystagmus. *Pediatrics,* 1957, *19,* 1088–1092.

Gorman, J. J., Cogan, D. G., & Gellis, S. S. A device for testing visual acuity in infants. *The Sight-Saving Review,* 1959, *29,* 80–84.

Harris, L., Atkinson, J., & Braddick O. Visual contrast sensitivity of a 6-month-old infant measured by the evoked potential. *Nature,* 1976, *264,* 570–571.

Harter, M. R., Deaton, F. K., & Odom, J. V. Maturation of evoked potentials and visual preference in 6–45 day old infants: Effects of check size, visual acuity, and refractive error. *EEG and Clinical Neurophysiology,* 1977, *42,* 595–607.

Held, R. Development of visual acuity in normal and astigmatic infants. In S. Cool (Ed.), *Vision 1977 Symposium.* New York: Springer-Verlag, in press.

Marg, E., Freeman, D. N., Peltzman, P., & Goldstein, P. J. Visual acuity development in human infants: Evoked potential measurements. *Investigative Ophthalmology,* 1976, *15,* 150–153.

Regan, D., & Richards, W. Independence of evoked potentials and apparent size. *Vision Research,* 1971, *11,* 679–684.

Reinecke, R. D., & Cogan, D. C. Standardization of objective visual acuity measurements. *Archives of Ophthalmology,* 1958, *60,* 418–421.

Sokol, S. Measurement of infant visual acuity from pattern reversal evoked potentials. *Vision Research,* 1978, *18,* 33–39.

Sokol, S., & Dobson, V. Pattern reversal visually evoked potentials in infants. *Investigative Ophthalmology,* 1976, *15,* 58–62.

Teller, D. Y., Morse, R., Borton, R., & Regal, D. Visual acuity for vertical and diagonal gratings in human infants. *Vision Research,* 1974, *14,* 1433–1439.

Voipio, H. Objective measurement of visual acuity by arresting optokinetic nystagmus without change in illumination. *Acta Ophthalmologica,* 1961 (Suppl. 66), 1–70.

Wolin, L. R., & Dillman, A. Objective measurement of visual acuity. *Archives of Ophthalmology,* 1964, *71,* 822–826.

32. Spatial Summation in Motion Perception

Santo Salvatore

The contrast and comparison of real and apparent motion have received much attention in the vision literature. Apparent movement was first thought of as a "peculiar class of optical deceptions" or errors of judgment. Later its basic sensory character was recognized and it was suggested that a complete theory of motion should encompass real and apparent movement. Given the proper spatial and temporal sequences motion is ascribed to stationary stimuli. Perception, or interpretation of environmental stimuli, necessarily relies on sensory receptors and their attached neural circuits.

I. A Prototype for Movement

The general class of apparent movement produced by the sequential flashing of stationary stimuli has been dubbed beta with phi being the special case wherein the movement appears disembodied from the objects producing it. Ordinarily the movement progresses from the first to the second stimulus in the sequence. However, if the second stimulus is much brighter than the first there is a secondary reversal movement from the brighter to the dimmer stimulus—called delta.

Gamma movement is the perceived radial movement outward from the fixation point when the level of illumination is suddenly raised. The whole field may be involved, as when turning on a light bulb in a dark room or when a restricted target is involved.

Bartley (1941, 1958) thought of gamma as the prototype of all movement since it produces the necessary retinal conditions for the movement experience. Real movement of a target provides continuous displacement of the image and therefore successive stimulation of the photoreceptors in the retinal mosaic. Bartley analyzed the photic radiation of a delimited stimulus and found it adequate for the purpose

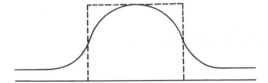

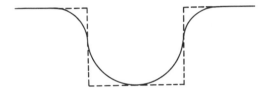

Figure 32.1. Target (---) and retinal (——) luminance gradients. Top: Positive contrast. Target is brighter than background. Bottom: Negative contrast. Target is darker than background.

(Figure 32.1). When the target is first presented the center of the image receives most radiation. Since the latent period of the neurons is inversely related to stimulation intensity the receptors at center will respond or fire before those radial to it. Such a retinal sequence is quite similar to that produced by the traverse of an image of a moving target.

It was suggested to Bartley that since the gamma effect could be produced by a dark target on light ground as well as a bright target on dark ground that the effect was centrally rather than peripherally mediated. Bartley, however, was acquainted with Hartline's (1938) work defining "on" and "off" fibers in the visual pathway and so maintained that a peripheral mechanism is sufficient. With a dark target the off fibers at the center of the image will fire before those radial to it and therefore produce the gamma effect.

II. Real Motion: Directly Perceived or Inferred

Real motion is defined by the conditions of a stationary eye and a moving target. The implication is of the movement of a segment of the retinal image over a relatively stationary retina. The criterion for the absolute threshold of motion is the subjective appearance or disappearance of movement. It is defined as the rate of travel at which movement becomes just perceptible; this is the direct perception of motion such as may be seen when looking at the sweep second hand of a watch. The inferred perception of motion occurs at slower rates of movement such as may be deduced from the change in position of the minute hand of a watch at two different times; with the inferred criterion threshold rates decrease with increased observation time.

Thus, when motion is real there may be more than one avenue for its apprehension. This corresponds to the historical controversy of whether the apprehension of movement is a sensation or a perception—whether the apprehension is mediated by motion receptors or acuity receptors. James (1950) stated that in the inferred case the perception of motion is derived from knowledge that the starting and ending points of the stimulus are separate positions in space. The matter has been very well put by von Kries (1925):

> Psychologically speaking, an indirect perception of motion involves both the idea of an interval of time and that of two places. While it is true that these conditions are always fulfilled in a physical sense, we find that in the case of more rapid motions the impression is a more immediate one. A judgment of spatial displacement does not necessarily have to be made in direct motion. . . [p. 270].

Restating, we can say that there is more than one property or feature analyzer involved in the integration of motion. Possibly the discrimination of a series of positions in space though not in sufficiently rapid succession to stimulate a motion analyzer may activate a secondary mechanism that integrates successive positions into a continuous motion percept—an impletion similar to that of apparent movement.

III. References in the Visual Field

The subjective report of "immediately perceived movement" varies not only with the rate of stimulus movement but also with the location of the moving stimulus in the field (Brown, 1931a, 1931b). Therefore the transition point from inferred to direct perception of motion is dependent on the rate of motion and the inhomogeneity of the field. The same rate of movement perceived in motion directly in an inhomogeneous field will be inferred as having moved in a homogeneous field when its change in position, relative to the observer, is great. The rate of movement, if increased sufficiently, will also yield a direct perception of motion in the homogeneous field.

Without visual references judgment is egocentric in that it is based on the angular displacement of the object relative to the observer's line of sight and threshold is large. With visual references judgment is based on the angular displacement of one environmental object relative to another and threshold is small. The latter type of situation has been summarized by Gibson (1968), who considered the possibility that the essential data in the perception of motion are in the changes of the configuration of contours and boundaries generated by the moving object. As the stimulus moves it occludes the background at the leading edge and reveals the background at the trailing edge. So with references present motion perception may be reduced to visual acuity or changing form.

Aubert (1886) determined the foveal absolute threshold for motion directly perceived to be 1 min of arc sec^{-1}. He added that the point at which phenomenal
movement arises becomes 10–20 min of arc sec^{-1} when the stimulus object is
screened so that reference points provided by the experimenter's apparatus are not
visible. Obviously, the presence of reference points in the visual field, whether
intentional or incidental, reduces the motion threshold. In Ganzfelds, most easily
obtained by the absence of light, Aubert's results have been confirmed. Brown and
Conklin (1954), using such a condition, found the absolute threshold of motion as
the discrimination of the direction of movement to be 9–18 min of arc sec^{-1}. With
similar conditions Fox and Lyman (1970) found that percentage of correct responses
was 75% when the stimulus angular velocity was 45 min of arc sec^{-1} whereas with
the addition of a circle as frame of reference 100% correct detection was attained
when stimulus velocity was 14 min of arc sec^{-1}.

It has been reported that observers revert to angular displacement relative to the
observer when the nearest reference point is 8–10° from the stimulus of interest, that
is, a local Ganzfeld is developed. However, examination of the literature indicates
that a stimulus field of this size is not large enough to markedly increase the value of
threshold. Furthermore the addition of reference lines to small fields reduces the
threshold little since the boundaries of the field itself are serving as reference points.
For example, Leibowitz (1955) obtained little reduction in threshold by the addition
of vertical reference lines. The stimuli were rectangles moving horizonally in a 3.2°
field. Here the addition of reference lines had no effect on threshold with exposure
time of .25 sec and reduced threshold by a factor of less than 2 at an exposure of
16 sec rather than the factor of 10 reported by Aubert. In small fields occlusion and
disocclusion may occur at the edges of the field and the task is converted by the
observer to the detection of object relative movement.

IV. Form and Motion Thresholds

In keeping with the notion that motion perception is mediated by the same neural
mechanism giving rise to form perception or visual acuity, nineteenth-century researchers attempted to document the equality of form, motion, and displacement
thresholds. The displacement threshold—the distance the stimulus must move in
order to be seen as being in movement—was considered the bridge between form
and motion threshold. If these thresholds were equal then illumination and contrast
data developed on visual acuity would be applicable to motion perception.

For foveal vision, Stratton (1902) found the displacement threshold equal to the
vernier threshold. Others, however, found the displacement threshold equal to the
minimum separable and minimum visible measures of visual acuity. Klein (1942)
pointed out that previous investigators had used different targets to determine the
form and motion thresholds, that the comparison will be affected by the visual
acuity measure used, and that the certainty criterion used for the perception of
motion will also influence the motion threshold. The latter point is significant since

observation time is ordinarily a variable in motion perception, whereas visual acuity requires essentially unlimited observation time.

Klein used the same stimulus, a modified Landolt ring in rotary motion, for both thresholds at parafoveal and peripheral locations in the retina. He found that, at photopic illumination levels, the thresholds of motion, form, and displacement are proportional to each other and approximately equal at any given retinal eccentricity. Gordon (1947), utilizing Klein's equipment, found that the three thresholds were also equal at a scotopic level of illumination though maximum sensitivity shifted to the near periphery.

Though these two studies appear to settle the relationship between these three thresholds it must be concluded that the equation holds true for only a very limited set of conditions. Rotary motion sensitivity varies with the degree of curvature (Brown, 1931b), and McGolgin (1960), comparing rotary and linear motion at 45° retinal eccentricity, found the rotary motion threshold to be nearly three times that of the linear motion threshold. In summary, the displacement threshold may be manipulated over a wide range of values by the judicious selection of observation time, type of target, direction of movement, etc.

A summary of studies examining the absolute threshold of motion as a function of retinal eccentricity is presented in Figure 32.2. The photopic studies of Aubert (1886) and Klein (1942) produce curves similar to that of Wertheim (1894), documenting the reciprocal of visual acuity that corresponds to the threshold of form and that is sometimes known as the minimum angle of resolution. At photopic levels

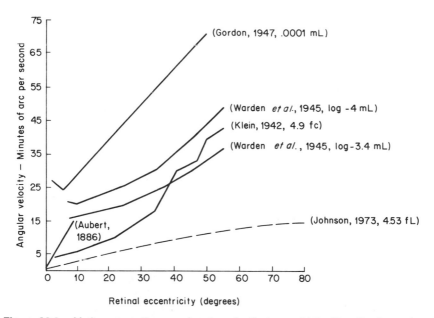

Figure 32.2. Motion perception as a function of retinal eccentricity. Results of experiments reported by the authors shown.

these thresholds are at a minimum in the fovea, vary directly with retinal eccentricities of 20–30°, and then increase more rapidly further in the periphery.

At scotopic conditions these thresholds are elevated in the fovea, reach a minimum at a location 5–10° eccentric to the fovea, and then rise rapidly again in the far periphery.

The generalized shapes of several threshold curves are shown in schematic form in Figure 32.3. The absolute threshold for the detection of light, the minimum angle of resolution, and the absolute thresholds of motion and displacement at scotopic levels of illumination generally conform to curve A. The locus of greatest sensitivity as well as steepness of slope shift with a number of variables. At photopic levels of illumination the several thresholds generally conform to curve B with maximum sensitivity in the fovea.

Referring again to Figure 32.2, note that the most recent study (Johnson, 1973; Johnson & Leibowitz, 1976) produced an atypical threshold motion curve as a function of retinal eccentricity. Threshold is lower for this study at all eccentricities and the curve is negatively accelerated. Approximately 30 years have elapsed between this study and the others in the figure. It is assumed that basic underlying motion sensitivity has not changed and that the difference arises from procedural variables in data collection. Most of the studies in the figure reflect data based on classic psychophysical methods with 100% correct detections whereas Johnson's study utilized an interleaved double staircase method and selected a 50% correct criterion as the threshold measure. Curve C in Figure 32.3 is intended to reflect changes in the threshold curve that may occur when the criterion level is lowered.

V. Stimulus Size as a Factor in Motion Perception

Few studies have varied stimulus size experimentally. Brown's work (1931a, 1931b) is a prominent exception. Brown's transposition effect states that increasing and decreasing either field or stimulus size phenomenally decreases and increases speed, respectively. According to this rule the absolute threshold of motion becomes smaller as either the stimulus size and/or stimulus field is made smaller.

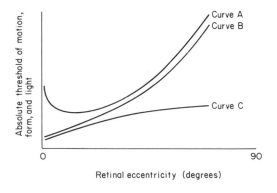

Retinal eccentricity (degrees)

Figure 32.3. Generalized threshold curves for motion, form, and light. Curve A under scotopic conditions. Curve B under photopic conditions. Curve C with lower criterion level.

These results received corroboration by Graham (1968) who varied the length of the moving stimulus—a line subtending a visual angle ranging from 17 to 52 min of arc in a constant stimulus field of 13° diameter. Here increasing line length increased threshold from 3 to 8 min of arc sec^{-1}.

A third study where stimulus size was experimentally varied obtained contrary results. McGolgin (1960) used altimeter hands of several sizes and found that though size had no effect on rotary motion threshold the motion threshold decreased as size increased when the motion was linear. It is noteworthy that these observations were made in the peripheral regions of the retina in a Ganzfeld.

There may be more than one explanation for the apparent increase in speed with a decrease of stimulus size and field size. The smaller the field size the more likely is the stimulus to be maintained in the fovea where vision is most acute. Also the smaller the field the more likely it is for the field outline to act as a reference. A third explanation is stated in terms of Roelof's effect, or asymmetry effect (Sugarman & Cohen, 1968). The subjective median plane is very sensitive to shifts in the visual array. In the case where the stimulus field consists of the total array the median plane is defined by the center of the stimulus field. Stimulus movement away from the median plane will cause field asymmetry that is more noticeable for small rather than large objects and therefore decreases the phenomenal speed of large objects. This applies to foveal but not to peripheral stimuli. A fourth explanation is that of the association of large objects with stationary stimuli.

VI. Motion Analyzers

Recently the alternative hypothesis—that the direct perception of motion is a sensation—has received new support. Electrophysiological work with animals indicates that the apprehension of motion is based on a neural system entirely independent of visual acuity.

Barlow and Levick (1965), recording frequency of firing from the optic nerve of the rabbit, have described cells that respond selectively to the direction of motion. The cell was vigorously excited by a stimulus moving in the preferred direction and inhibited by motion in the reverse or null direction. The response appeared independent of speed of movement or its shape or contrast. Thus the cell detected the feature velocity. This feature detector may be said to be the "true" motion detector since both motion and direction are sensed, thus providing a field vector. Michael (1969), analyzing the inhibitory mechanism underlying the detection of direction, stated that a moving stimulus is not critical. He found that maximum response of the directional mechanism was obtained by flashing stimuli along the preferred axis and that a separation of 20 min of arc between stimuli was able to be tolerated. The cell, therefore, cannot discriminate between continuous motion and change in position. Similarly Grüsser-Cornehls, Grüsser, and Bullock (1963) have described cells in the optic nerve of the frog that detect stroboscopic movement.

At the level of frog movement detectors have been suitably demonstrated by Lettvin, Maturama, Pitts, and McCollough (1961). They have described movement-gated, dark convex boundary detectors in the optic nerve that maintain discharge even after movement has stopped. The discharge, however, is erased by transient dimming or by a shadow passing over the receptive field and will not recur until the boundary moves again. They further describe the following: moving or changing contrast detectors that do not have an enduring response but fire only when the contrast is changing or moving; dimming detectors that respond to dimming of the whole receptive field; and boundary detectors that respond to sharpness of boundary rather than degree of contrast and produce a discharge even when the boundary is brought into the receptive field in total darkness and the light is sub-sequently switched on. These three mechanisms have been identified with Hartline's (1938) on–off, on, and off fibers, respectively.

Signals propagated along the visual pathway are all initiated by transient changes of light on the retinal photoreceptors. One therefore may suspect that under some circumstances any change in stimulation may be regarded as signaling movement. The following, attributed to Gordon Walls (Cornsweet, 1970), illustrates this point: Many birds, when searching for food, assume frozen postures between sharp movements while others are in constant motion while feeding. Walls suggests that the relatively motionless birds do not have involuntary eye movements and maintain a position sufficiently rigid to experience stabilized images. The inhibition then suppresses all retinal signals except those from moving objects and in essence all receptors therefore are converted to moving object detectors.

Though a change in the pattern of light distributed on the retina is necessary for the signaling of movement it is not necessary that the movement feature be pro-cessed at the level of the optic nerve. Generally the lower the organism on the phylogenetic scale the more likely it is to process visual information close to the retina. The spatial and temporal arrangement of the optic nerve impulses must carry all the information about significant aspects of the visual field but it may be decoded at other stations in the brain further along the visual pathway (Riggs, 1965b). At the primate level movement receptors have not been found in the optic nerve. The complex and hypercomplex cells found in the monkey (Hubel & Wiesel, 1962) that are directionally selective to movement through their receptive field are at the cortical level.

VII. The Tentative Model

The present model assumes that underlying retinal structures convert the spatiotemporal distribution of light energy from external sources into neural im-pulses. The absolute threshold of motion is conditioned by the distribution of the pattern of light on the retina. It is further assumed that receptive fields of various types are formed and that the distributed light pattern on a segment of the retina may be analyzed by more than one detector either because the same retinal area is analyzed more than once at any one level of the visual pathway and/or because the retinal segment may receive representation at more than one level in the visual pathway.

Holding to a theory of the proportionality and approximate equality of the form and motion thresholds, as did Klein (1942) and Gordon (1947), then the functions of the absolute threshold of motion across the retina would be of types B and A for photopic and scotopic conditions, respectively. This model assumes identical characteristics for form and motion analyzers. Therefore no shift in sensitivity for motion perception is expected with variations of stimulus size and complexity.

A second theory assumes that the detection of motion is mediated by the same analyzers that decode luminous intensity. With this assumption it would be expected that increasing stimulus size while maintaining stimulus intensity constant would shift the locus of maximum sensitivity peripherally. The peripheral shift would be strong for scotopic and weak for photopic background levels because spatial summation increases with reduction in illumination (Arden & Weale, 1954). This model would predict that an inhomogeneous target would have a higher motion threshold than a homogeneous one with the same diameter.

The present model assumes motion detectors independent of brightness and form analyzers. Units directionally sensitive to motion carry information not useful for brightness or pattern discrimination. At the level of the optic nerve it is expected that several cell types may carry neural information varying with stimulus motion and therefore capable of being decoded. On–off, off, and on units carry impulses whose number and ratio vary with light distribution.

The expected function of the absolute motion threshold across the retina would be predicted to change with change of stimulus features (Figure 32.4). At both levels of illumination it is predicted that the larger target will produce a lower motion threshold because the leading and trailing edges of the larger target will stimulate more receptors whose effects will be summated. The effect should be stronger in the

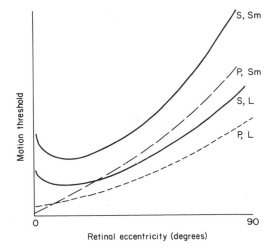

Figure 32.4. Expected results. The expected generalized threshold function for absolute threshold of motion related to background luminance and stimulus size. (P), Photopic; (S), scotopic; (L), large; (Sm), small.

periphery since summation of stimulation continues further into the periphery for the larger target. A complex target is predicted by the model to be more effective than a simple target of equal area and intensity. By virtue of its greater leading and trailing edges the complex target will stimulate more receptors and therefore lower the motion threshold. The greater sensitivity for photopic levels predicted for the small target in the foveal region is based on reports of previous investigators and is not maintained extrafoveally.

A. Method

The subject's visual field was formed by a uniformly backlighted circular screen. The screen was curved to a radius of 24 in. and the subject positioned at the center of curvature. The screen subtended a visual angle of 200° horizontal by 30° vertical. The target always appeared in the center of the screen. The only other inhomogeneity on the screen was a red spot subtending an arc of 15 min at the eye. It served as the fixation point and was varied from 10° to 90° from the target (Figure 32.5). See Salvatore (1974) for a description of equipment and procedural details.

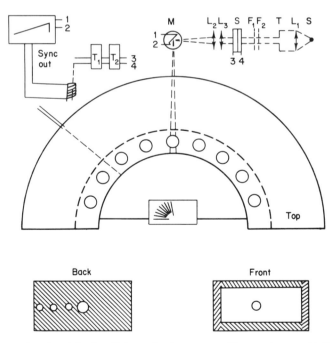

Figure 32.5. The visual display. Schematic of apparatus. The numbers and letters from right to left refer to the following components: S, tungsten light source; L_1, collimating lens; T, target; F_2 and F_1, neutral filters; S, shutter; 3 and 4, electrical shutter connections; L_3 and L_2, focusing lenses; M, movable mirror; 1 and 2, electronic mirror connections; 3 and 4, timer connections to shutter; T_2 and T_1, electronic timers; 1 and 2, electronic connections from function generator to mirror.

With monocular fixation thresholds were determined for the temporal visual field of the right eye. The target was in movement at the onset of the constant 1 sec exposure time. The stimuli were circular spots of light subtending .5 and 2° and a complex target with the same diameter as the large target. The area approximated that of the small target and the perimeter was similar to that of the large target (see Figure 32.6).

All targets were observed at photopic (7 fL) and scotopic (5 × 10⁻⁴ fL) background illumination. The photopic and scotopic targets were 14 and 2×10^{-3} fL, respectively. The stimulus movement was always in the horizontal meridian toward the line of sight.

Four naive volunteers from the university community served as paid subjects. The subject's task was to fixate the red spot and report target movement or stationarity. The method of limits was used with four ascending and descending series for each subject at each eccentricity. The subject was instructed in the use of the direct perception of motion as criterion. The fixation point was not used when observations were made foveally since this would have changed the nature of the experiment. Experiment I obtained information on the two factors of size and eccentricity at each level of illumination. Experiment II obtained information on stimulus complexity at each level of illumination to be compared with the two simple targets.

B. Results and Discussion

The threshold was computed as the average of the ascending and descending series at that particular condition. At scotopic levels (Figure 32.7) the large target

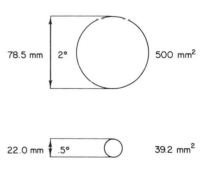

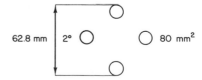

Figure 32.6. The stimuli: Large (top), small (middle), complex (bottom). The area, in square millimeters, is given to the right of each target; the perimeter, in millimeters, is given to the left of each target.

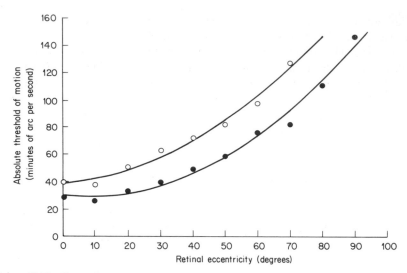

Figure 32.7. Scotopic motion threshold as a function of retinal eccentricity. The parameter is stimulus size. Curves of best fit are for points average of two subjects. Upper curve: .5° stimulus. Lower curve: 2° stimulus.

produced lower motion thresholds at all eccentricities. For both target sizes the curve of best fit was parabolic and maximum sensitivity occurred at 10° eccentric to the line of sight. Analysis of variance shows that both size and eccentricity are significant but the size versus eccentricity interaction is not significant. The difference in sensitivity due to target size is constant across the retina.

At photopic levels of illumination (Figure 32.8) the large target again produced lower motion thresholds at all eccentricities. At photopic levels, however, the curve of best fit for both target sizes was exponential. The threshold was smallest in the foveal region and rose sharply in the periphery. Analysis of variance shows that both size and eccentricity are significant and that the size versus eccentricity interaction is significant. Obviously the effect of target size is minimal at the fovea and increases with eccentricity; the sensitivity differential due to target size becomes larger in the peripheral retina.

We conclude that in the absence of reference points in the visual field absolute motion thresholds across the retina decrease as stimulus size increases. It can be hypothesized that the perception of motion has spatial summation properties similar to those specified by Ricco's law for the perception of light.

In any case spatial summation does occur in the retinal sensory unit or ganglionic receptive field and the summation characteristic holds for the differential threshold of intensity as well as the absolute threshold of detection (Boynton, 1962). The size of the field for which reciprocity holds increases with increasing distance from the fovea. Also, the summation areas are known to vary inversely, with background illumination being largest in complete darkness. Therefore the summation area increases directly with eccentricity and inversely with background luminance

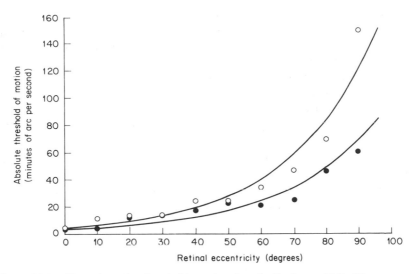

Figure 32.8. Photopic motion threshold as a function of retinal eccentricity. The parameter is stimulus size. Curves of best fit are for points average of two subjects. Upper curve: .5° stimulus. Lower curve: 2° stimulus.

(Teichner & Krebs, 1972). Estimates of receptive field sizes, by electrophysiological recording from optic fibers of the monkey, range from 4 min to 2° of arc with increase of eccentricity from 4° to 56° (Ruch, 1965). Similarly, in the human, summation has been found complete at 20° eccentricity for a 1° field and complete at eccentricity of 35° for a 5.6° field on zero background illumination (Hallet, Marriott, & Rodger, 1962).

The findings of this experiment, that motion thresholds are inversely related to stimulus size across the retina, are entirely consistent with the summation properties previously stated. At scotopic illumination levels receptive fields are large and the stimuli used in the experiment relatively small. Therefore summation may be expected to be complete for both target sizes and the differential sensitivity constant across the retina. At photopic illumination levels receptive fields or summation areas become smaller, particularly in the central retina. Under these conditions the two stimulus sizes used cannot produce differential summation in the central retina since both targets are larger than summation areas. In the periphery receptive fields become larger and provide the opportunity for the flux in the larger target to continue summation. In this case motion sensitivity to the large target at the photopic level increases with eccentricity and provides significant size versus eccentricity interaction.

The greater sensitivity obtained with the large target may be due to its greater luminance since in this case target size and target luminance covary. Or, as an alternative, the greater sensitivity obtained with the large target may be due to the greater retinal area swept by the large target, thus producing a lower threshold on a probabilistic basis.

The replication of the experiment with a complex target explored these possibilities. The complex target (Figure 32.6) has an area similar to that of the small target and a perimeter similar to that of the large target. The complex target has an overall extent equal to that of the large target but delivers one-sixth the radiant flux of the large target to the retina and sweeps a retinal area during movement similar to that of the small target.

At scotopic levels the complex target produces motion thresholds across the retina quite similar to those of the large target. Comparison with the simple targets is provided in Figure 32.9. The curve of best fit is again parabolic and the eccentricity versus complexity interaction is not significant. At photopic levels the complex target produces motion thresholds across the retina similar to those of the large target. Comparison with the simple targets is provided in Figure 32.10. The curve of best fit is again exponential and the eccentricity versus complexity is significant. The interaction is caused by the threshold elevation occurring at the fovea and 10° eccentricity with the complex target.

It is concluded that a reduction of motion threshold is obtainable with the complex target and, since the area of the complex target is similar to that for small target, the reduction is due not to the total radiant flux of the target but to its perimeter. Similarly the lowered threshold is not produced by the retinal area swept but by the edge effect of the perimeter. Thus the summation characteristics apparent in this experiment on motion perception have characteristics distinct from those specified in Ricco's law.

The hypothesis presented here is that the basis for the summation mechanism in motion perception lies in the differential activity of ganglion cell types, i.e., on, off,

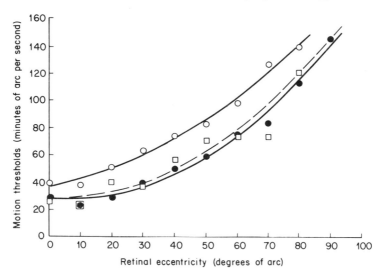

Figure 32.9. Motion thresholds as a function of retinal eccentricity. At scotopic illumination the complex target is compared with small and large targets. Upper curve (○) is for the small target; lower curve (●) is for the large target; broken curve (□) is for the complex target.

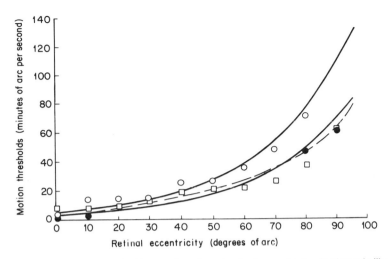

Figure 32.10. Motion thresholds as a function of retinal eccentricity. At photopic illumination the complex target is compared with small and large targets. Upper curve (○) is for the small target; lower curve (●) is for the large target; broken curve (□) is for the complex target.

and on–off. The visual pathway is multistaged and though the patterning of neural impulses occurs at the ganglion cell level the information may not be analyzed or decoded until later stages. The activity of these fibers to moving and stationary stimuli is summarized.

On Receptors. Stimulus onset of both stationary and moving stimuli will increase the frequency of firing and, with continued stimulation, impulse frequency will reduce to the maintained level. However, while at the trailing edge of the moving stimulus the maintained activity will be terminated, the leading edge will activate new receptors. Therefore the overall activity of the on receptor ganglion cell will be greater when the stimulus is moving.

Off Receptors. Stimulus onset inhibits spontaneous activity in the fiber. For the moving stimulus receptors at the trailing edge will fire continuously during its presence whereas for the stationary stimulus they will fire only at stimulus offset.

On–Off Receptors. For the stationary stimulus these receptors will increase impulse frequency at stimulus onset, return to base line during continued stimulation, and again increase at stimulus offset. For the moving stimulus the decrease of firing will not be great with continued stimulation since the leading and trailing edges are activating on and off fibers with continued movement.

The moving stimulus therefore provides more neural activity at the ganglion cell level than a stationary stimulus of like size and intensity. However, the temporal distribution of the neural activity generated by the moving stimulus is distinct from the temporal pattern of the stationary stimulus. Assuming three different fiber types carrying neural information the differentiation of stationary from moving targets can be made in the central nervous system by the patterning of neural activity in the fibers over time.

Further experimentation is required to corroborate the hypothesis of the summation mechanism underlying the perception of motion. Thresholds must be obtained with the parameters of size, diameter, and perimeter of target varied over a wide range of values to ascertain the limits and nature of the receptive fields. The model predicts that increasing the difference between target sizes at photopic levels up to the largest receptive field size of the periphery will increase the eccentricity versus size interaction. This prediction will also hold true at scotopic levels with the proviso that the targets are larger than those used at photopic levels since receptive fields are inversely related to background illumination.

A critical test of the model is an experiment using negative contrast or black targets on a white ground. The model predicts that increasing the negative contrast area or perimeter of the black target will result in lower motion thresholds across the retina. If the prediction holds it will prove Bartley (1941) right: Gamma is the prototype of motion.

The crossover of sensitivity of the two size targets at some point near the fovea at photopic conditions was not obtained. Rather the larger target approached asymptotically the threshold value of the smaller target at zero eccentricity. It is strongly suggested that the crossover did not occur because thresholds were not determined in an inhomogeneous field. The addition of reference points changes the task from the detection of motion to one of visual acuity in the fovea. Since the fovea at photopic conditions is the area of greatest acuity the provision of inhomogeneity facilitates the detection of change in position. Additionally, change of position for small targets in small fields is facilitated by Roelof's effect—detection of field asymmetry.

Shifting of the point of maximum sensitivity to a point further out in the periphery at scotopic conditions also was not obtained. For both target sizes thresholds were at a minimum at 10° eccentricity. Additional stimuli at parafoveal areas possibly would have located the minimum threshold closer to the line of sight. Additionally, threshold in the vicinity of the optic disc was elevated by the decrease of receptor density and the possibility is raised that the threshold values at 10° and 20° eccentricity are higher than would be obtained in other meridians.

It is strongly suspected that the rather high sensitivity obtained in the fovea at scotopic conditions is a gross overestimate. There are multiple reasons for the obtained result. The fixation point was not used at zero eccentricity and the method used to obtain fixation is inexact. Though the subject was locked into the fixation area by a location stimulus a few seconds elapsed before the presentation of the moving target. Within this time small eye movements will relocate the line of regard (Matin, Pearce, Matin, & Kibler, 1966) up to 1°, thereby placing the target on receptors sensitive to low levels of illumination, that is, the rods. The size of the target, .5° and 2°, and its movement, which may travel another .5°, all tend to place the target outside of the intended region—the fovea. Therefore it is likely that the threshold obtained represents that of parafoveal regions rather than zero degrees eccentricity. Additionally, it is possible that the target luminance value of .002 fL may have surpassed the threshold of some cones. For these reasons it appears that the sensitivity value of the scotopic fovea is overestimated by the present experimental findings. Refined control of these parameters may lead to the conclusion that at the fovea motion acuity is zero—as in form acuity.

One more point will be made. It is known that receptive fields become smaller as the fovea is approached and that foveal cones may have singular ganglionic connections. With this model, then, it would be expected that the perception of motion in the fovea at photopic levels is impaired. We noted such impairment in the present experiments. The elevation of threshold at the fovea was more likely to occur with small and complex targets (Figure 32.10). That this effect is not reliable may be due to several overlapping factors. At zero degrees at photopic conditions, as at scotopic conditions, fixation was inexact and the stimulus was likely to strike "motion detectors" of the type previously described. Equally important, though the screen was featureless slight inhomogeneities—such as specks of dust—were present to make relative object movement possible. Also the screen has a specular nature and as the target traverses lenticuli the angle of incident light changes, thereby providing cues to motion. The conclusion is that the type of motion receptors described in this model do not exist in the fovea. Judgment of motion in the fovea occurs as a deduction from change in position. The model predicts that the foveal motion threshold will be elevated when visual structure is removed—as occurs at scotopic conditions.

VIII. Summary

The distinction of motion directly perceived and motion inferred from change in stimulus position has been elaborated. The two modes form the historical controversy of whether motion is a sensation or a perception. The importance of references in the visual field for the motion threshold was pointed out and the implication was drawn that visual references alter the task from motion perception to detection of changing form. Therefore studies conducted in small fields or having other references are not suitable for defining thresholds of motion directly perceived.

A synopsis was given of research attempting to find the equation between displacement threshold and threshold of form. It has been assumed that both form and motion perception are based on the mechanism underlying visual acuity. Electrophysiological work in animals was cited that indicates motion perception is based on a neural system entirely independent of visual acuity. An experiment was conceptualized to test the hypothesis that motion perception is based on mechanisms similar to those underlying the perception of light. It was concluded that the perception of motion directly perceived is not based on visual acuity and that the receptive fields for motion perception have properties distinct from summation areas underlying the perception of light. It is speculated that the integrative mechanism in the perception of motion involves on, off, and on–off receptors at the ganglion cell level which have distinct neural response patterns for stationary and moving objects.

REFERENCES

Arden, G. B., & Weale, R. A. Nervous mechanisms and dark adaptation. *Journal of Physiology (London),* 1954, *125,* 417–426.

Aubert, H. Die bewegungempfindung. *Pfluger Archives,* 1886, *39,* 347–370.

Barlow, H. B., & Levick, W. The mechanism of directionally sensitive units in the rabbit's retina. *Journal of Physiology (London),* 1965, *178,* 477–504.

Bartley, S. H. *Vision. A study of its basis.* New York: D. Van Nostrand Co., 1941.

Bartley, S. H. *The principles of perception.* New York: Harper & Row, 1958.

Boynton, R. M. Spatial vision. In *Annual review of psychology.* Palo Alto, California: Annual Reviews Inc., 1962.

Brown, J. F. The visual perception of velocity. *Psychologische Forschung,* 1931, *14,* 199–232. (a)

Brown, J. F. The thresholds for visual movement. *Psychologische Forschung,* 1931, *14,* 249–268. (b)

Brown, R. H., & Conklin, J. E. The lower threshold of movement as a function of exposure time. *American Journal of Psychology,* 1954, *67,* 104–110.

Cornsweet, T. *Visual perception.* New York: Academic Press, 1970.

Fox, J. N., & Lyman, J. *Structureless field visual perception studies: Applications for automotive and aerospace safety research.* Paper presented at the annual meeting of the Human Factors Society. San Francisco, California, 1970.

Gibson, J. J. What gives rise to the perception of motion? *Psychological Review,* 1968, *75,* 335–346.

Gordon, D. A. The relation between the thresholds of form, motion and displacement in parafoveal and peripheral vision at a scotopic level of illumination. *American Journal of Psychology,* 1947, *60,* 202–225.

Graham, C. H. Depth and movement. *American Psychologist,* 1968, *23,* 18–26.

Grüsser-Cornehls, U., Grüsser, O., & Bullock, T. H. Unit responses in the frog's tectum to moving and non-moving stimuli. *Science,* 1963, *141,* 820–822.

Hallett, P. E., Marriott, F. H. L., & Rodger, F. C. The relationship of visual threshold to retinal position and area. *Journal of Physiology,* 1962, *160,* 364–373.

Hartline, H. K. The response of a single optic nerve fiber of the vertebrate eye to illumination of the retina. *American Journal of Physiology,* 1938, *121,* 400–415.

Hubel, D. H., & Wiesel, T. N. Receptive fields, binocular interaction and functional architecture in the cat's visual cortex. *Journal of Physiology,* 1962, *160,* 106–154.

James, W. *The principles of psychology.* New York: Dover Publications, 1950.

Johnson, C. A. *Practice and feedback effects on peripheral movement thresholds.* Paper presented at the Eastern Psychological Association Convention. Philadelphia, Pennsylvania, 1973.

Johnson, C. A., & Leibowitz, H. W. Velocity–time reciprocity in the perception of motion: Foveal and peripheral determinations. *Vision Research,* 1976, *16,* 177–180.

Klein, G. S. The relation between motion and form acuity in parafoveal and peripheral vision and related phenomena. *Archives of Psychology* (New York), 1942, *275,* 1–70.

Leibowitz, H. W. Effect of reference lines on the discrimination of movement. *Journal of the Optical Society of America,* 1955, *45,* 829–830.

Lettvin, J. Y., Maturama, H. R., Pitts, W. H., & McCullough, W. S. Two remarks on the visual system of the frog. In W. A. Rosenblith (Ed.), *Sensory communications.* New York: Wiley, 1961.

Matin, L., Pearce, D. G., Matin, E., & Kibler, G. B. Visual perception of direction in the dark: Role of local sign, eye movements and ocular proprioception. *Vision Research,* 1966, *6,* 453–469.

McGolgin, F. H. Movement thresholds in peripheral vision. *Journal of the Optical Society of America,* 1960, *50,* 774–779.

Michael, C. R. Retinal processing of visual images. *Scientific American,* 1969, *220,* 105–114.

Riggs, L. A. Visual acuity. In C. H. Graham (Ed.), *Vision and visual perception.* New York: Wiley, 1965. (a)

Riggs, L. A. Electrophysiology of vision. In C. H. Graham (Ed.), *Vision and visual perception.* New York: Wiley, 1965. (b)

Ruch, T. C. Vision. In T. C. Ruch & H. D. Patton (Eds.), *Physiology and biophysics*. Philadelphia: Saunders, 1965.

Salvatore, S. *The effect of stimulus size, stimulus complexity and retinal complexity and retinal eccentricity on the absolute threshold of motion at a photopic level and at a scotopic level of background illumination*. Unpublished doctoral dissertation, Brown University, 1974.

Stratton, G. M. Visible motion and the space threshold. *Psychological Review,* 1902, *9,* 433–447.

Sugarman, R. C., & Cohen, W. Perceived target displacement as a function of field movement and asymmetry. *Perception & Psychophysics,* 1968, *3,* 169–173.

Teichner, W. H., & Krebs, M. J. Estimating the detectability of target luminances. *Human Factors,* 1972, *14,* 511–519.

von Kries, J. Notes on Chapter 29. In H. von Helmholtz & J. P. C. Southall (Eds.), *Physiological optics* (Vol. 3). New York: Optical Society of America, 1925.

Wertheim, T. Uber die indirekte Sehssharfe. *Zeitshrift Psychologie Physiologie Sinnesorganne,* 1894, *7,* 172–183.

33. Apparent Motion and the Motion Detector[1]

Oliver Braddick and Alan Adlard

Ever since Riggs, Ratliff, Cornsweet, and Cornsweet (1953) and Ditchburn and Ginsborg (1952) first described the effects of image stabilization, it has been clear that the human visual system is primarily responsive to dynamic, rather than static stimuli. Electrophysiological studies of other species support this view. In particular, neurons responding selectively to movement in the image have been found to be very pervasive in a wide range of visual systems. In the analysis of the properties of these neurons, discontinuous stimulation has proved a powerful tool (Barlow & Levick, 1965; Bishop, Dreher, & Henry, 1972; Emerson & Gerstein, 1977). The response evoked by movement can also be generated by the successive exposure of stationary stimuli that are separated in space, and the use of such stimuli allows the temporal and spatial organization of the motion-detecting mechanisms to be deciphered.

The attraction of discontinuous stimulation lies not only in the analytical possibilities that it opens up, but also in the analogy with a famous perceptual phenomenon. This has been variously called the phi phenomenon, beta apparent motion, and stroboscopic motion, but what it amounts to is the appearance of smooth and continuous motion that can be generated by a succession of stationary, displaced images. It is of course the phenomenon responsible for the effectiveness of movie films, television, and many advertising signs. It was also one of the jumping off points for the Gestalt movement in perceptual psychology (Wertheimer, 1912). If motion detectors respond similarly to discontinuous and continuous motion, does this mean that we have identified the physiological substrate of the perception of stroboscopic movement?

On looking into the perceptual literature on stroboscopic movement, one finds that this assertion does not seem a very promising one. Rather, one finds reports that

[1]We thank the Medical Research Council for support.

the critical parameter is not retinal separation but apparent separation (Attneave & Block, 1973), apparent movement over much greater distances than any plausible receptive field dimension (Smith, 1948), and apparent motions in depth between plane figures (Kolers, 1972). Further, one finds that the occurrence or direction of apparent motion depends on the subject's attitude (Neuhaus, 1930), past experience (Neff, 1936), and interpretations of the pattern as an object (Sigman & Rock, 1974). All this suggests that apparent motion ought perhaps to be pursued within an approach that considers perception as an interpretive process rather than one that relates elementary psychophysical data to understood neurophysiological mechanisms. This impression may be confirmed by anyone who has looked at a simple stroboscopic motion display as the parameters of temporal and spatial intervals were adjusted, and experienced the frustrating slipperiness of the textbook transitions from the perception of simultaneity to optimal motion, to jerky motion, to succession.

The criteria for the limits of apparent motion are not easy to use and even less easy to maintain stably when the stimulus is the classic one of a single-element figure exposed successively in two positions. However, if one uses a display containing a very large number of pattern elements, a new criterion becomes possible. The display is what Julesz (1971) has called a "random-dot kinematogram": In a matrix of random black and white square elements, the elements in a central area are all displaced through the same distance on successive exposures, while the elements in the surrounding area remain in the same positions. The dots in the central area appear to move as a coherent object, and the boundary between this moving zone and the stationary surround appears clearly defined. Now in any single exposure the elements form a homogeneous random field within which no boundary is defined. If the presentation of successive exposures is sufficiently separated, a succession of homogeneous fields is what is perceived. The appearance of the boundary segregating the moving from the stationary area, therefore, can only occur by virtue of some visual mechanism that detects the spatiotemporal relationship between elements in successive exposures. That relationship is what underlies stroboscopic apparent motion. However, it is considerably easier for a subject to report the presence or absence of a perceived boundary than it is for him to reliably distinguish apparent motion from a discontinuous appearance.

When the perception of this boundary, or "perceptual segregation," is used as the criterion for apparent motion, one finds rather different properties and parameters from those obtained in studies of classic apparent movement using isolated stimulus elements (Braddick, 1973, 1974). Table 33.1 summarizes some of the important differences. Generally, the constraints on the occurrence of perceptual segregation from discontinuous displacement are considerably more severe than those on the perception of classic apparent motion; for example, the limits on spatial and temporal discontinuity are stricter, and dichoptic stimulation is ineffective in the case of segregation as compared with the classic criterion.

It has been suggested that these differences arise because the two types of performance depend on two distinct processes extracting information about visual dis-

TABLE 33.1

Determinants of Apparent Motion Found with Two Perceptual Criteria

Criterion of segregation in random-dot array	Criterion of appearance of smooth motion for isolated element
Spatial displacement must be 15 min or less	Spatial displacement may be many degrees
Interstimulus interval must be less than 70–100 msec (with 100-msec stimulus exposure)	Interstimulus interval may be up to at least 300 msec
Segregation abolished by bright uniform field exposed in interstimulus interval	Motion perceived whether interstimulus interval is bright or dark
Successive stimuli must be delivered to the same eye (or both binocularly)	Successive stimuli may be delivered to the same or different eyes

placement (Braddick, 1974). If this suggestion is correct, the process that determines segregation in random-dot displays would appear to be the lower-level process in the visual system in light of the following: its short spatial and temporal range over which it can combine information; its vulnerability to interference from an input (bright uniform field) that is likely to have little effect on high-level pattern-processing mechanisms; and its failure to operate dichoptically. This low-level "short-range" process may plausibly be identified with the response of directionally selective neurons in the visual pathway to discontinuous stimulation, while the higher-level longer range process responsible for classic apparent motion seems to be of a more interpretive nature. This interpretation is supported by the observation of Regan and Spekreijse (1970) that 10-min displacements of an area within a random-dot pattern, but not 20 min and larger displacements, yield a characteristic visually evoked cortical potential. It may also be relevant that the spatial limit found for the short-range process (about 15 min) is similar to the size found for motion-detecting subunits in neurons in the rabbit (Barlow & Levick, 1965) and cat (Emerson & Gerstein, 1977) visual pathways.

This is not to assert that the higher-level process is inoperative in random-dot displays. Indeed, it is notable that in cases where perceptual segregation of the displaced area does not occur, such as with a bright interstimulus interval (ISI) or with ISIs of greater than 120 msec, the motion of individual pattern elements or clusters of elements may still be visible. This may be attributed to the higher-level process, which can yield the perception of motion, but not that of segregation.

Similarly, one would not expect the short-range process to act only in random-dot patterns. The classic type of display consisting of isolated elements ought to activate this process if spatial and temporal displacements are within the appropriate range. It would be surprising if its action was not reflected in some way in the perception of these stimuli: One would expect that apparent movement with short temporal and spatial discontinuities would show different perceptual properties from that outside the range of the low-level process. One such difference has been reported by Petersik (1975) and Pantle and Picciano (1976). They used a display first described by Ternus (1926), similar to that shown in Figure 33.1A. In this display a set of

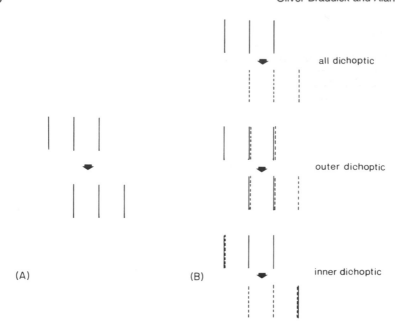

Figure 33.1. (A) The basic display sequence yielding group-movement and element-movement reports. In this and other figures, patterns appearing coincidentally in space but successively in time are drawn vertically displaced. A complete display sequence consisted of the upper pattern followed by the lower, with the upper then reappearing. (B) Three dichoptic conditions of presentation. Lines presented to the left eye are shown as solid; those presented to the right eye as broken. In the actual displays all lines were solid. Versions of these displays in which left- and right-eye images were interchanged were used on half the trials.

three elements is shown alternately in two positions and so arranged that the positions of the two rightmost elements in one exposure coincide with the positions of the two leftmost elements in the alternating exposure. Ternus reported that, even though two of the three elements remain individually in constant positions, the group of three elements was perceived as moving to and fro as a whole. He regarded this as a Gestalt phenomenon; that is, the perception was determined by the overall organization of the stimulus rather than by its local properties. Petersik showed that the occurrence of this group-movement phenomenon depends on the temporal parameters. Group movement was perceived for relatively long ISIs (80 msec) but when the ISI was short (20 msec), the predominant perception was of "element motion"; that is, the outer element was perceived as moving to and fro around or across two stationary central elements. Pantle and Picciano (1976) replicated this finding and also showed that element rather than group movement was perceived when the presentation was dichoptic, with the two stimulus patterns being displayed to different eyes. These authors suggest that element and group movement result from two distinct mechanisms and explicitly identify the mechanisms yielding element movements with that involved in the segregation of random-dot patterns.

This identification is supported by the effects of varying the ISI [segregation of random-dot patterns by apparent motion disappears in the range 70–100 msec (Braddick, 1973)] and of dichoptic presentation [ineffective for segregation (Braddick, 1974) and element movement (Pantle & Picciano, 1976)]. We have extended this list of analogies by studying the effects of luminance in the ISI on the transition from element to group movement perception. Braddick (1973) showed that if during the ISI a uniform field comparable in luminance to the space-average luminance of the random-dot patterns was presented, the maximum ISI for segregation fell from the value of 70–100 msec found with a dark ISI to 20–30 msec. In contrast, such a uniform field in the ISI had little or no effect on the appearance of motion in the classic display where a single isolated element is displaced.

We used the display of Figure 33.1A, where the elements are lines 1.5° long and are separated by 1.1°. The pattern shown in the upper half of the figure was initially displayed and the subject was instructed to fixate between the two right-hand lines. The subject initiated the display sequence, which consisted of a variable ISI, 200-msec exposure of the pattern illustrated in the lower half of the figure, a repetition of the ISI, and finally reappearance of the initial pattern. Thus the subject saw a single displacement and its reversal in a rapid sequence. He was required to report whether he saw a uniform displacement of the whole group of lines (group movement) or a displacement of the outer line with the others remaining stationary (element movement). (Other responses were permitted but were rarely used.) Trials in which the field during the ISI was either dark or uniformly bright with the same background luminance as the pattern were randomly interleaved, as were values of the ISI duration ranging from 20 to 120 msec.

Figure 33.2 shows the results for four subjects, each receiving 20 presentations in each condition. With dark ISI, the data show the transition from element to group

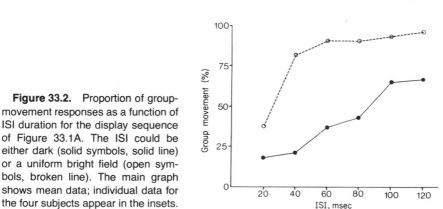

Figure 33.2. Proportion of group-movement responses as a function of ISI duration for the display sequence of Figure 33.1A. The ISI could be either dark (solid symbols, solid line) or a uniform bright field (open symbols, broken line). The main graph shows mean data; individual data for the four subjects appear in the insets.

movements as the ISI duration is increased. These data are comparable to those of Petersik (1975). With the bright ISI, there is a fair proportion of element-movement reports for the shortest ISI (20 msec), but the proportion of group-movement reports is always greater than for the dark ISI and rises close to 100% at intermediate ISI durations. The bright intervening field thus seems to be strongly promoting group movement relative to element movement over the same range of ISI durations (30 msec and above) in which it abolishes the segregation effect in random-dot arrays, thus supporting the idea that the process promoting element-movement perception is that responsible for segregation.

However, this identification is difficult to maintain because of a conspicuous apparent inconsistency in the spatial parameters involved. For effective segregation in random-dot patterns, the discontinuity has to be small in space as well as in time. Yet the spatial displacement that is perceived in element movement in the line display is by no means small. It is three times the interelement separation, that is, over 3°. Thus the perceptual effect ascribed to the short-range process involves a range of movement 3 times greater than that ascirbed to the long-range process, and about 10 times greater than the spatial limit implied by the segregation experiments (Braddick, 1974).

It does not seem possible to maintain that the short-range process is responsible for the perceived motion of the outermost element. However, this element is not the only one involved in the difference between element and group movement. In the element-movement percept, the two inner elements are seen as stationary, while in group movement they appear to move with the group. Perhaps, then, the short-range process acts in the case of element movement, not by generating a signal that the outer element moves, but by generating a signal that the inner elements remain stationary. Any system of directionally selective detectors must have a characteristic null response when no movement occurs.

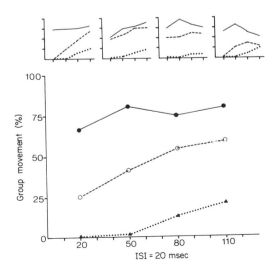

Figure 33.3. Proportion of group-movement responses as a function of ISI duration for the three dichoptic display sequences illustrated in Figure 33.1B. The main graph shows mean data; individual data for the four subjects appear in the insets. (●——), all dichoptic; (○--), inner dichoptic; (▲···), outer dichoptic.

This possibility can be tested by using some of the variables that affect the short-range and longer-range processes differentially, and applying them selectively to the different elements of the pattern. One way of doing this is illustrated in Figure 33.1B. The whole display can be presented dichoptically (top), which is known to favor group movement (Pantle & Picciano, 1976). Alternatively, dichoptic presentation can be restricted to the outer elements (middle), or to the inner elements (lower), with the other elements being presented to both eyes together. In other respects the procedure was similar to that of the previous experiment, with the field being dark during the ISI.

The results are presented in Figure 33.3. With dichoptic viewing of the whole pattern, the proportion of group-movement responses was uniformly high, confirming the result of Pantle and Picciano. A good proportion of group-movement responses also occurs when the inner lines are dichoptic, but there are very few, especially for short ISIs, when the outer lines are dichoptic. Thus the effect of dichoptic presentation in reducing element movement seems to depend on the dichoptic presentation not of the element that apparently moves, but of the elements that are apparently stationary.

The manipulation of ISI duration shows a similar effect. With the use of display sequences of the type illustrated in Figure 33.4, the ISIs for the inner and outer elements can be dissociated: In the sequence labeled A, 120 msec (most of which is light) elapse between the disappearance of the outer line on the left and its reappearance on the right, while only 20-msec (dark) ISI separates the disappearance and

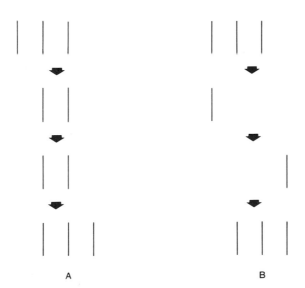

A   B

Figure 33.4. Two display sequences dissociating ISI for the "inner" and "outer" elements of the display. In each case, the temporal sequence was as follows: first row exposed at onset of trial, second row exposed for 50 msec, 20 msec dark ISI, third row exposed for 50 msec, fourth row exposed for 200 msec. The sequence is then repeated in reverse order.

reappearance of the inner lines. In sequence B, the reverse is true. The proportions of group-movement responses for these stimulus sequences are shown in Figure 33.5. Effectively no group movement is reported for sequence A, while it is reported on nearly 100% of trials for sequence B. With the basic sequence of Figure 33.1A, 120-msec light ISI favored group movement strongly while 20-msec dark ISI favored element movement. These results follow the same pattern if the ISI for the *inner elements* is taken as the critical variable. This result is striking in that a simple analysis might well have predicted the opposite: It would seem reasonable that the apparent motion from one outer position to the other (element motion) should occur most readily when these positions follow one another directly in time rather than when another stimulus (the inner lines in sequence A) intervenes.

Our conclusion, then, is that element movement is indeed perceived under those conditions of presentation in which the low-level, short-range process is activated. However, that process is not activated by the spatiotemporal sequence involved in the element that appears to move. Rather, the conditions for the apparently stationary elements are those appropriate for activating the short-range process. The spatial displacement of those elements is zero, so presumably what the short-range process signals is "no movement." Now, these conditions (short, dark ISI, binocular presentation) do not rule out the higher-level, longer-range process. This process, we have suggested, is more interpretive in nature; that is, the perceived movement that the process generates may be selected from among alternatives on the basis of complex information about the overall configuration, past experience, and so on. With the spatial arrangement of these displays, it can select either group or element motion. But if the low-level process—hypothetically, activity of directional detectors quite early in the visual pathway—is signaling that the inner two lines are stationary, that information constrains the interpretation that the higher-level pro-

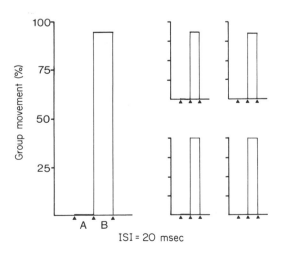

Figure 33.5. Proportion of group-movement responses for the two display sequences illustrated in Figure 33.4. The left-hand diagram shows mean data; individual data for the four subjects appear in the insets on right.

cess can select. If the inner elements have to be seen as stationary, then the third element must be seen to move between the two outer positions. In the conditions of long or bright ISI, or dichoptic presentation, the low-level process is inactive and there is therefore no such constraint on the interpretation selected by the higher-level process. The higher-level process is free to behave like a good Gestaltist and select its interpretation in light of the overall configuration, that is, the group movement that is generally perceived under these conditions.

These experiments, apart from their specific conclusions about the role of two processes in the perception of apparent motion, may perhaps yield some general lessons about the interpretation of perceptual phenomena in terms of neural mechanisms. First, perceptual processes, such as the organization of movement perception in multielement patterns, that appear too complex and unpredictable for analysis in terms of understood physiological mechanisms, nonetheless at least receive their input information via the basic machinery of the visual pathway. Therefore an understanding of the input that the basic machinery provides may be essential for any attempt at understanding the more complex processes.

Second, it is characteristic of the higher processes that they operate with a good deal of freedom: The phenomena of multistable or reversible figures yield many examples where a variety of perceptions is possible with the same input. The action of the lower-level mechanisms wired into the visual pathway is likely to be more closely determined by the stimulus, and the role of this determinate action in the overall process is to constrain the freedom available to the higher-level "interpretive" processes.

Third, the perceptual consequences of physiological processes in the visual pathway depend on how the information coming up the visual pathway is used by higher processes. As in the case considered here, the answer to this question is not always obvious; we might not have supposed that, with certain stimuli, the role of motion detectors would be to signal which parts of the display were stationary rather than which parts were moving. To take another example, it is evident from the facts of stereoscopic vision that the visual pathway transmits information concerning which eye received a particular stimulus. However, it turns out not to be the case that this information can be used to discriminate which eye received a monocular flash (Templeton & Green, 1968). So if we attempt to draw inferences about physiological mechanisms from perceptual experiments, we must recognize that these inferences depend on particular hypotheses about how sensory information is used. It is fairly obvious that this is an issue in the study of phenomena such as alternative perceptions of apparent movement. It is less obvious, but may not be less true, in the case of basic psychophysical experiments on detection, color and brightness vision, and spatial and temporal properties of the visual system. No psychophysicist can employ a preparation consisting of the isolated front end of the visual pathway, or route nerve impulses directly from the ganglion cell to the finger on the response key without an intervening perceptual process. That process is not necessarily interested in the same aspects of the neural signal as the psychophysicist.

REFERENCES

Attneave, F., & Block, G. Apparent movement in tridimensional space. *Perception & Psychophysics,* 1973, *13,* 301–307.

Barlow, H. B., & Levick, W. R. The mechanism of directionally selective units in rabbit's retina. *Journal of Physiology,* 1965, *178,* 477–504.

Bishop, P. O., Dreher, B., & Henry, G. H. Simple striate cells: Comparison of responses to stationary and moving stimuli. *Journal of Physiology,* 1972, *227,* 15P–17P.

Braddick, O. The masking of apparent motion in random-dot patterns. *Vision Research,* 1973, *13,* 355–369.

Braddick, O. A short range process in apparent motion. *Vision Research,* 1974, *14,* 519–527.

Ditchburn, R. W., & Ginsborg, B. L. Vision with a stabilised retinal image. *Nature,* 1952, *170,* 36–37.

Emerson, R. C., & Gerstein, G. L. Simple striate neurons in the cat. II. Underlying directional asymmetry and directional selectivity. *Journal of Neurophysiology,* 1977, *40,* 136–155.

Julesz, B. *Foundations of cyclopean perception.* Chicago: University of Chicago Press, 1971.

Kolers, P. A. *Aspects of motion perception.* Oxford: Pergamon Press, 1972.

Neff, W. S. A critical investigation of the visual apprehension of movement. *American Journal of Psychology,* 1936, *48,* 1–42.

Neuhaus, W. Experimentelle Untersuchung der Scheinbewegung. *Archiv für die Gesamte Psychologie,* 1930, *75,* 315–458.

Pantle, A. J., & Picciano, L. A multistable movement display: Evidence for two separate motion systems in human vision. *Science,* 1976, *193,* 500–502.

Petersik, J. T. Two types of apparent movement in the same visual display. Paper presented at the 16th annual meeting of the Psychonomic Society, Denver, Colorado, 1975.

Regan, D., & Spekreijse, H. Electrophysiological correlate of binocular depth perception in man. *Nature,* 1970, *225,* 92–94.

Riggs, L. A., Ratliff, F., Cornsweet, J. C., & Cornsweet, T. N. The disappearance of steadily fixated visual test objects. *Journal of the Optical Society of America,* 1953, *43,* 495–501.

Sigman, E., & Rock, I. Stroboscopic movement based on perceptual intelligence. *Perception,* 1974, *3,* 9–28.

Smith, K. R. Visual apparent movement in the absence of neural interaction. *American Journal of Psychology,* 1948, *61,* 73–78.

Templeton, W. B., & Green, F. A. Chance results in utrocular discrimination. *Quarterly Journal of Experimental Psychology,* 1968, *20,* 200–203.

Ternus, J. Experimentelle Untersuchungen über phänomenale Identität. *Psychologische Forschung,* 1926, *7,* 81–136.

Wertheimer, M. Experimentelle Studien über das Sehen von Bewegung. *Zeitschrift für Psychologie,* 1912, *61,* 161–265.

34. Visual Sensitivity to Moving Stimuli: Data and Theory

P. Ewen King-Smith

I. Introduction

A basic principle of visual physiology is that conscious responses are usually generated by some *change* in the image falling on the retina; cortical neurons generally respond best to changes in both the temporal and spatial distribution of the image, since temporal changes alone (e.g., flashes of diffuse light) or spatial variations alone (a stationary pattern) cause little or no response (e.g., Hubel & Wiesel, 1962). Under normal circumstances, the spatiotemporal changes that stimulate vision are provided by motion of patterned stimuli across the retina; this motion may correspond either to the motion of objects within the visual field or to the motion of the visual image across the retina during eye movements. The importance of this motion is emphasized by the demonstration that an image which is "stabilized" (stationary) on the retina fades away, largely or completely, within the first few seconds of viewing (Ditchburn & Ginsburg, 1952; Riggs, Ratliff, Cornsweet, & Cornsweet, 1953).

To aid in understanding the role of retinal image motion in visual detection, we have made measurements of visual sensitivity in response to controlled motion of the retinal image; that is, the moving stimulus was viewed through an image stabilization system (King-Smith & Riggs, 1978) to eliminate (or greatly reduce) any retinal image motion generated by eye movements. A single vertical line or edge was generated electronically on an oscilloscope (Schade, 1956) and was viewed foveally as it moved laterally within the display area of 4° (horizontally) by 2° (vertically). In most experiments, the subject's task was to adjust the contrast of the stimulus to the detection threshold—he was not required to see the motion per se; standard errors of the contrast thresholds ranged between 9 and 15% of the plotted values. Measurements with these localized stimuli are complimentary to those using sinusoidal gratings (e.g., Sekuler & Levinson, 1974; Tolhurst, 1973; van

427

Nes, 1968). Both types of stimuli have advantages; for example, the sensitivity to a moving line or edge may be conceptually easier to relate to the detection of everyday objects, while sinusoidal gratings of high and low spatial frequencies can be used to selectively isolate parallel mechanisms responding to fine and coarse details.

II. Sensitivity to Moving Stimuli—Data

A. Dependence on Amplitude and Velocity

Contrasting thresholds for the detection of a 3-min-wide dark line are plotted in Figure 34.1 as a function of amplitude of motion for 1-Hz triangular wave (△) and square-wave (□) motion. For triangular-wave motion, the line moves back and forth across the fixation point at constant speed, while square-wave motion corresponds to sudden jumps back and forth between symmetrically opposite positions; thus these motions mimic, respectively, the "drift" and "saccadic" types of eye movement (Ditchburn, 1973, Ch. 4). Amplitude is defined as the peak displacement from the mean position and is thus half the peak-to-peak motion. The dotted line represents the contrast threshold for a line that is switched on and off at 1 Hz (.5 sec on, .5 sec off) without altering the mean illumination of the screen.

It is seen that the lowest threshold (highest sensitivity) occurs for triangular-wave motion of 16-min amplitude, that is, a velocity of about 1 deg sec^{-1}; this is close to the velocities for optimum "visibility" (i.e., percentage of time for which a stimulus is visible) of a line found by Ditchburn, Fender, and Mayne (1959), Drysdale (1975), and Sharpe (1972). The minimum threshold for square-wave motion is for 4-min amplitude (i.e., 8-min jumps in position) and this threshold is about 1.5 times higher than for optimum triangular-wave motion. The threshold for on–off presentation is a further factor of about 1.5 times higher than for optimum square-wave motion. Thus, for these measurements, smooth motion yields the highest sensitivity, but it should not be concluded that drifts are necessarily more

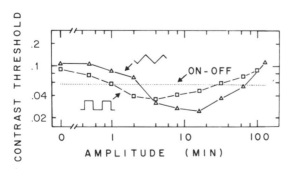

Figure 34.1. Comparison of contrast thresholds for a 3-min dark line as a function of amplitude of 1-Hz triangular- (△) and square- (□) wave motion; the dotted line is the threshold for on–off presentation. For all experimental data in this chapter, stimuli were viewed through an image stabilizor and the subject was LAR; retinal illumination was 90 trolands. Contrast thresholds were determined by the method of adjustments using a 20-sec viewing period (except for some data in Figure 34.3). Contrast was defined at $\Delta L/L$ where L was the mean luminance of the screen and ΔL was the difference in luminance between the line and the screen.

effective than saccades for generating visual responses. Some comparable data for
the detection of a moving edge are given by King-Smith and Riggs (1978); the most
significant observation is that the optimum amplitude of motion for edge detection
is generally about twice that for line detection.

In a number of ways, the visual response to motion was found to be quite
different from our expectations. For example, it might be imagined that the 1-Hz
triangular-wave measurements of Figure 34.1 simply represent contrast thresholds
for lines moving at different velocities; that is, velocity is the important parameter
determining sensitivity in this case, and given this, other parameters (amplitude and
frequency) are unimportant. It is therefore surprising that when the measurements
were repeated at the lower frequency of .125 Hz, the contrast thresholds were found
to be different when plotted as a function of velocity [Figure 34.2 (▼)]. The
agreement between the data at the two frequencies is good at velocities above 16
min sec^{-1}; for small amplitudes, however, better correspondence occurs when the
results are plotted as a function of amplitude (King-Smith & Riggs, 1978). It seems
that, for small amplitude motion, threshold is mainly determined by amplitude of
motion while velocity is the main factor for rapid motion; further evidence for this
proposition is presented by King-Smith and Riggs (1978).

B. Sensitivity at Different Frequencies

The proposition that amplitude, not velocity, is the most important factor in
determining sensitivity to small movements is supported by the data of Figure 34.3
(from King-Smith, Riggs, Moore, & Butler, 1977) where contrast thresholds have
been measured as a function of frequency of sinusoidal motion. The results are
expressed as detection threshold relative to that for a stationary (stabilized) line;
circles correspond to the thresholds set at the end of 20 sec of viewing while the
triangles were determined from a separate experiment and correspond to the means
of settings after 20, 40, 60, and 80 sec—this allowed time for at least one cycle of
motion at the lowest frequency used. The results again conflicted with our expectations. Contrast threshold is seen to be nearly constant in the range of $^{1}/_{16}$-8 Hz despite the fact that velocity increases by a factor of 128 over this range. This supports

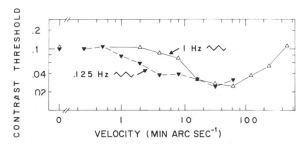

Figure 34.2.   Contrast thresholds for 1 (△) and .125 Hz (▼) triangular-wave motion of a 3-min
dark line plotted as a function of velocity.

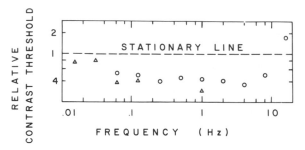

Figure 34.3. Contrast thresholds for a 3-min dark line as a function of frequency of sinusoidal oscillation with 3-min amplitude. The dashed line corresponds to the threshold for a stationary (stabilized) line. (○), Thresholds derived from 20-sec viewing time; (△), 80-sec viewing time (see text). [From King-Smith et al. (1977).]

the proposition that the visual response to small amplitude motion is mainly dependent on amplitude rather than velocity.

The other main conclusion from Figure 34.3 is that the mechanisms responding to low-amplitude motion behave like a band pass filter responding over about 7 octaves, down to remarkably low frequencies. Below $1/16$ Hz, the threshold increases toward the value for a stationary line; at a high frequency (16 Hz), the threshold increases above that for a stationary line because the motion is too rapid to be visible at threshold and it simply has the effect of blurring the line. The results of Figure 34.3 are roughly in agreement with Krauskopf's (1957) observation that small amplitude (2 min) sinusoidal oscillations of 1–5 Hz lower the threshold about equally while oscillations of 10 Hz or more raise the threshold.

C. Time Course of Response to Motion

If the visual mechanisms responding to small amplitude motion behave like a broad band pass filter with a response extending to relatively low frequencies, one would correspondingly expect a relatively prolonged response to step type stimuli; for example, a capacitor-coupled circuit with a low-frequency f_0 of $1/16$ Hz (cf. Figure 34.3) would respond to a step input with an exponential decay having a time constant of $1/(2\pi f_0)$, that is, about 2.5 sec.

To test this prediction, the subject viewed a near-threshold dark line that jumped back and forth through 4 min (i.e., square-wave motion of 2-min amplitude) at a low frequency (.06 Hz). An image stabilization system was again used. Whenever the stimulus was visible, the subject pushed a button, thus applying a steady voltage to the input of an averaging computer that was triggered by each leftward jump of the line. Thus the computer accumulated a response proportional to the probability of seeing the line at any time during the cycle. A typical probability histogram, derived from 24 stimulus cycles, is shown in Figure 34.4A. Probability increases rapidly at about .5 sec after a jump, reaches a maximum after about 2 sec, and decays to near zero in the next 4–5 sec. A quantitative analysis, taking account of the nonlinearity

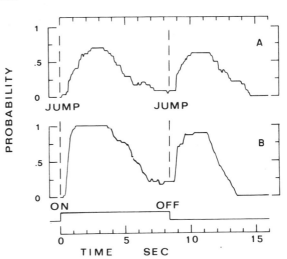

Figure 34.4. Probability histograms recording how the probability of seeing a line varies during a stimulus cycle. In (A), the line jumped back and forth through 4 min at the times indicated while in (B), the line was switched on and off. The method of recording the histograms is described in the text. The 3-min dark line had a contrast of 10%.

of the probability of seeing curve (King-Smith *et al.*, 1977), indicates that the decay phase may be fitted by an exponential with a time constant of 2.5 sec—in agreement with the value previously derived from consideration of the low-frequency limit.

A corresponding histogram derived from on–off presentation (Figure 34.4B) adds support to the suggestion that the visual response mechanisms behave like a capacitor-coupled circuit. The most striking observation is the response occurring at "off," that is, when the dark line is replaced by a uniform screen. This off response is a type of negative afterimage of the line and, apart from its reversed polarity, it is similar in strength, duration, and appearance to the original on response. [Similar off responses have been described by Keesey (1969) and Koenderink (1972).] This off response is reminiscent of the behavior of a capacitor-coupled circuit where the response to switching off a steady voltage input is approximately equal and opposite to the response when the voltage is originally applied. The analogy of the capacitor-coupled circuit will be extended in the following section.

III. Theory of Detection of a Moving Line

A. General Model of Line Detection

A moving line is a stimulus whose intensity varies as a function of both space and time; one may therefore ask whether visual sensitivity to a moving line can be derived from a knowledge of the spatial and temporal properties of line detection or whether it depends on more complex spatiotemporal interactions. To answer this question, we have tested a simple model based on psychophysical measurements of the spatial and temporal properties of line detection. The model incorporates the suggestion that there are parallel mechanisms responding to detailed "pattern" and

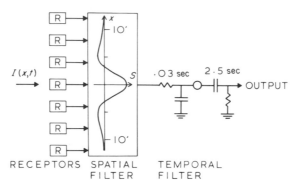

Figure 34.5. Model of the spatial and temporal properties of the pattern system responding to a fine line. A similar model is proposed for the flicker system. See text for details.

"flicker" information, respectively (Keesey, 1972; King-Smith & Kulikowski, 1975; Kulikowski & Tolhurst, 1973; Tolhurst, 1973). These may be related to a similar dichotomy found by electrophysiologists (Enroth-Cugell & Robson, 1966; Gouras, 1968). A more detailed description of the model is given in King-Smith (1978).

The model of one of these mechanisms—the pattern system—is represented in Figure 34.5; the flicker system was modeled in a similar way but with quantitative differences. The receptors R respond to the intensity distribution $I(x, t)$ and their outputs are summated by a linear "spatial filter" having a central excitatory and surround inhibitory region. The filter's sensitivity or weighting function S, as a function of horizontal position x, is taken from the subthreshold summation measurements of Kulikowski and King-Smith (1973); a broader weighting function is used for the flicker system, and is derived from measurements with a line flickering at 8 Hz (King-Smith & Kulikowski, 1975). The output from the spatial filter passes through a two-stage temporal filter. The first stage is an integration resistor–capacitor (RC) circuit whose time constant, .03 sec, has been derived from high-frequency attenuation of pattern detection sensitivity for sinusoidal modulation of a line (Keesey, 1972; King-Smith & Kulikowski, 1975). From these same references, a time constant of .017 sec was derived for the flicker system.[1] The output from the integration RC circuit then passes via an isolation stage (circle, Figure 34.5) to a capacitor-coupled RC circuit whose time constant of 2.5 sec for the pattern system is taken from the discussion in Section II,C. For the flicker system, the corresponding value of .1 sec is derived from low-frequency attenuation of flicker modulation

---

[1] A single RC stage is considerably too simple to explain the high-frequency attenuation of the visual system (de Lange, 1958; Kelly, 1971; Veringa & Roelofs, 1966); however, the present model is not intended as a precise description, but is meant to give insight, in a simple and reasonably quantitative way, into the mechanisms detecting a moving line. In view of the differences between subjects and conditions for the various data used, a more complex model does not seem justified.

sensitivity (Keesey, 1972; King-Smith & Kulikowski, 1975). The assumption that spatial filtering occurs before temporal filtering is made simply for convenience of calculation; identical predictions would have been made if all or part of the temporal filtering occurred before the spatial filter, for example, in the receptors. The present model has a number of features in common with the electrophysiological model of Rodieck (1965).

B. Some Predictions of the Model

Figure 34.6 illustrates some computer plots of the response of the pattern system to a line moving from left to right at the constant velocities indicated; the thick curve corresponds to the output of the spatial filter before attenuation by the temporal filter and thus corresponds to the weighting function of the spatial filter (peak response set to unity). At low velocities, the response is limited by the capacitor-coupled RC circuit and is approximately the differential of the weighting function; at high velocities, the response is limited by the integration RC circuit and it approximates an integral of the weighting function. At intermediate velocities (4–16 min sec^{-1}) the response is a good approximation to the weighting function and the strongest response occurs for a velocity of about 8 min sec^{-1}; the corresponding optimum velocity for the flicker system is about 2 deg sec^{-1}.

The peak responses of the two systems at different velocities are plotted as the continuous curves in Figure 34.7. The pattern system responds well to a wide range of velocities; the response exceeds half maximum over the velocity range .6 min sec^{-1} to 2 deg sec^{-1}. The flicker system responds well over a relatively narrower range. For triangular-wave motion of low amplitude, the line moves through only a restricted region of the receptive field, rather than the whole region, as in Figure 34.6. The peak response may therefore be reduced, and the dashed curves in Figure 34.7 show the peak response obtainable from the pattern system at .125 and 1 Hz; for each calculated value, the central position of the movement was optimized and the response was calculated after any initial transient from presenting the moving line had decayed. No corresponding corrections were needed for the flicker system at these frequencies.

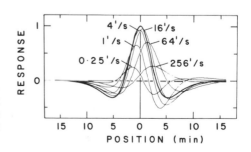

Figure 34.6. Response of the pattern system to a line moving from left to right through the receptive field at the velocities indicated; the thick line is the output from the spatial filter (Figure 34.5).

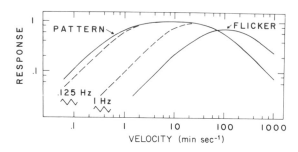

Figure 34.7. Peak response of the pattern and flicker system as a function of line velocity. The dashed curves correspond to triangular-wave motion of .125 and 1 Hz.

C. Tests of the Model

The data of Figures 34.3 and 34.4 have been partially incorporated in the model so the independent data of Figures 34.1 and 34.2 will be used to test the predictions of the model.

Consider first the observation from Figure 34.1 that the sensitivity to optimum triangular-wave motion of 1 Hz is about twice that for on–off presentation. Is the response of the model (Figure 34.5) correspondingly greater for triangular-wave motion? The maximum response of the pattern system to 1-Hz triangular-wave motion may be seen from Figure 34.7 to be about .90 unit, where 1 unit corresponds to the peak unattenuated output from the spatial filter. For on–off presentation, maximum response will evidently occur when the line is presented at the center of the receptive field; the output from the spatial filter will then alternate between 0 and 1 unit in a square-wave manner. However, the effect of the capacitative-coupling circuit (Figure 34.5) is to convert this signal to a waveform that alternates about the zero output level, that is, between about $-.5$ and $.5$; detailed calculations give a peak response of .52. Thus the maximum response of the pattern system to 1-Hz triangular-wave motion is about 1.7 times that for 1-Hz on–off presentation—in reasonable agreement with the corresponding sensitivity ratios of 2.3 and 1.6 for the two subjects of King-Smith and Riggs (1978). Calculations show that the flicker system should be about equally sensitive to optimum triangular-wave motion and on–off presentation; however, the prolonged time course of response to on–off presentation (Figure 34.4B) indicates that the pattern system dominates in this response, although it is suggested later (Figures 34.8 and 34.9) that the flicker system may contribute significantly to the optimum response to triangular-wave motion.

Why is the response to optimum square-wave motion also greater than that for on–off presentation (Figure 34.1)? Here it may be shown that the optimum response of, say, the pattern system to square-wave motion occurs when the line jumps back and forth between regions of peak inhibition and peak excitation of the spatial filter; as the line jumps to the excitatory peak, the direct excitatory response is added to a postinhibitory "rebound" response. The size of these optimum jumps would be 5 min (i.e., 2.5-min amplitude) for the pattern system and 10 min (5-min amplitude) for the flicker system; these figures are in reasonable agreement with the observed

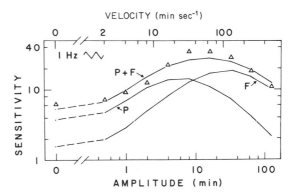

Figure 34.8. Comparison of experimental sensitivity data (△) with the predictions of the model (curve marked P + F) assuming linear addition of the responses from pattern and flicker systems; triangular-wave motion of 1 Hz was used. P and F are the contributions of the pattern and flicker systems, respectively. See text for details.

optimum amplitude of about 4 min (Figure 34.1) and would be consistent with a contribution from both systems to the square-wave movement response. As a quantitative example, the peak inhibition of the pattern system is 32% of the peak excitation (Figure 34.6). Thus, as the line jumps from one peak position to the other, the output of the spatial filter is a square wave alternating between 1 and $-.32$, that is, a peak-to-peak response of 1.32. The output from the capacitative-coupling circuit depends only on this peak-to-peak response, and so it will be 1.32 times greater than the output for on–off presentation. If we also take into account probability summation from the units centered at the two positions of the line for square-wave motion (cf. one position for on–off presentation), much of the difference between the sensitivities for optimum square-wave motion and on–off presentation can be explained. A more detailed consideration of the sensitivity to square-wave motion is given in King-Smith (1978).

Turning to the data of Figure 34.2 for two frequencies of triangular-wave motion, one may correlate the reduced threshold for low-velocity motion at .125 Hz compared with 1 Hz with a corresponding higher sensitivity calculated for the pattern system in Figure 34.7; in both Figures 34.2 and 34.7, the curves for the two frequencies merge at a velocity of about 16 min sec^{-1}.

We have attempted to fit sensitivity (reciprocal threshold) data at both frequencies of triangular-wave motion using two further assumptions:

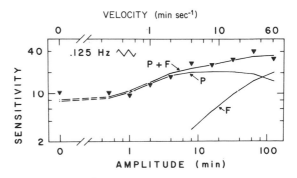

Figure 34.9. Comparison of experimental data with the predictions of the model, as in Figure 34.8, but for a frequency of .125 Hz.

1. The response to a stationary line is due to motion of the image generated by contact lens slippage, etc. This response may be expressed in terms of an amplitude A_0, that is, the amplitude of triangular-wave motion that would cause the same response. When a triangular-wave motion of amplitude A is superimposed, the two motions are equally likely to be in phase or out of phase at any moment; for this reason, we have not assumed that the responses to the two types of motion add linearly, but we assume that the total response is given by an effective amplitude $(A^2 + A_0^2)^{1/2}$. The precise form of this equation is significant only when A is about equal to A_0; the important point is that, for very small amplitude, response is determined by the slippage A_0 while it is determined by the amplitude, A, of superimposed line motion when this is large. The slippage amplitude assumed—$A_0 = 0.62$ min for 1-Hz motion—is in reasonable agreement with direct determinations (Riggs & Schick, 1968). However, our calculations do not rule out the alternative possibility of a genuine sustained response to a perfectly stabilized line.

2. We assume, for simplicity, that the responses of pattern and flicker systems to triangular-wave motion are added linearly; other types of interaction are, of course, not excluded.

Experimental data are compared with theory for a frequency of 1 Hz in Figure 34.8 and for .125 Hz in Figure 34.9; the triangles are the experimental data from Figure 34.2 replotted in terms of sensitivity, while the upper curve, labeled P + F, is the predicted sensitivity assuming linear summation of responses of the pattern and flicker systems. The curves labeled P and F are the contributions of the pattern and flicker systems, respectively; the relative contributions of these two systems were adjusted to provide a least squares fit to the data. The standard deviations of the data points from the graphs are .08 and .07 log unit at 1 and .125 Hz, respectively (7 deg of freedom); this is not much greater than the standard errors of measurement for the data points (about .05 log unit). Although there may be some systematic deviations between theory and data—for example, for the medium amplitude range of Figure 34.8—the agreement indicates that the present model may prove a useful starting point for the analysis of visual sensitivity to a moving line.

IV. Summary

To account for the visual response to a moving line, we proposed a model consisting of parallel pattern and flicker systems, each consisting of a spatial filter followed by a temporal filter (Figure 34.5). Although the model is not intended to be exact, it provides a reasonably quantitative fit to the data of relative sensitivities to triangular- and square-wave motion and on–off presentation (Figure 34.1) and to sensitivity data for different frequencies of triangular-wave motion as a function of amplitude (Figure 34.2). The responses of pattern and flicker systems predominate at low and high velocities, respectively. The model is also compatible with frequency response measurements for small amplitude motion (Figure 34.3) and with the time course of visual response to a sudden jump in line position (Figure 34.4).

ACKNOWLEDGMENTS

Lorrin Riggs acted as subject and provided invaluable help with the construction of the apparatus and design of the experiments. Robert K. Moore provided expert assistance. This work was supported by an S.R.C. Senior Visiting Fellowship and U.S.P.H.S. National Eye Institute Grant 5RO1-EY00744.

REFERENCES

Ditchburn, R.W. *Eye movements and visual perception.* Oxford: Clarendon Press, 1973.

Ditchburn, R.W., Fender, D.H., & Mayne, S. Vision with controlled movements of the retinal image. *Journal of Physiology,* 1959, *145,* 98–107.

Ditchburn, R. W., & Ginsburg, B. L. Vision with a stabilised retinal image. *Nature (London),* 1952, *170,* 36–37.

Drysdale, A.E. The visibility of retinal blood vessels. *Vision Research,* 1975, *15,* 813–818.

Enroth-Cugell, C., & Robson, J.G. The contrast sensitivity of retinal ganglion cells of the cat. *Journal of Physiology,* 1966, *187,* 517–552.

Gouras, P. Identification of cone mechanisms in monkey ganglion cells. *Journal of Physiology,* 1968, *199,* 533–547.

Hubel, D.H., & Wiesel, T.N. Receptive fields, binocular interaction and functional architecture in the cat's visual cortex. *Journal of Physiology,* 1962, *160,* 106–154.

Keesey, U.T. Visibility of a stabilised target as a function of frequency and amplitude of luminance variation. *Journal of the Optical Society of America,* 1969, *59,* 604–610.

Keesey, U.T. Flicker and pattern detection: A comparison of thresholds. *Journal of the Optical Society of America,* 1972, *62,* 446–44ι.

Kelly, D.H. Theory of flicker and transient responses. I. Uniform fields. *Journal of the Optical Society of America,* 1971, *61,* 537–546.

King-Smith, P. E. Analysis of the detection of a moving line. *Perception,* 1978 (in press).

King-Smith, P.E., & Kulikowski, J.J. Pattern and flicker detection analysed by subthreshold summation. *Journal of Physiology,* 1975, *249,* 519–548.

King-Smith, P.E., & Riggs, L. A. Visual sensitivity to controlled motion of a line or edge. *Vision Research,* 1978 (in press).

King-Smith, P.E., Riggs, L.A., Moore, R.K., & Butler, T.W. Temporal properties of the human visual nervous system. *Vision Research,* 1977, *17,* 1101–1106.

Koenderink, J.J. Contrast enhancement and the negative afterimage. *Journal of the Optical Society of America,* 1972, *62,* 685–689.

Krauskopf, J. Effect of retinal image motion on contrast thresholds for maintained vision. *Journal of the Optical Society of America,* 1957, *47,* 740–744.

Kulikowski, J.J., & King-Smith, P.E. Spatial arrangement of the line, edge and grating detectors revealed by subthreshold summation. *Vision Research,* 1973, *13,* 1455–1478.

Kulikowski, J.J., & Tolhurst, D.J. Psychophysical evidence for sustained and transient detectors in human vision. *Journal of Physiology,* 1973, *232,* 149–162.

de Lange, H. Research into the dynamic nature of the human fovea-cortex systems with intermittent and modulated light. I. Attenuation characteristics with white and coloured light. *Journal of the Optical Society of America,* 1958, *48,* 777–784.

Riggs, L.A., Ratliff, F., Cornsweet, J.C. & Cornsweet, T.N. The disappearance of steadily fixated test objects. *Journal of the Optical Society of America,* 1953, *49,* 495–501.

Riggs, L.A., & Schick, A.M.L. Accuracy of retinal image stabilization achieved with a plane mirror on a tightly fitting contact lens. *Vision Research,* 1968, *8,* 159–169.

Rodieck, R.W. Quantitative analysis of cat retinal ganglion cell response to visual stimuli. *Vision Research,* 1965, *5,* 583–601.

Schade, O.H. Optical and photoelectric analog of the eye. *Journal of the Optical Society of America,* 1956, *46,* 721–739.

Sekuler, R., & Levinson, E. Mechanisms of motion perception. *Psychologia*, 1974, *17*, 38–49.

Sharpe, C.R. The visibility and fading of thin lines visualised by their controlled movement across the retina. *Journal of Physiology (London)*, 1972, *222*, 113–134.

Tolhurst, D.J. Separate channels for the analysis of the shape and the movement of a moving visual stimulus. *Journal of Physiology (London)*, 1973, *231*, 385–402.

van Nes, F.L. Enhanced visibility by regular motion of retinal images. *American Journal of Psychology*, 1968, *81*, 367–374.

Veringa, F., & Roelofs, J. Electro-optical interactions in the retina. *Nature (London)*, 1966, *211*, 321–322.

Applied Topics

35. Effect of the Aberrations of the Eye on Visual Perception

Michel Millodot

The human eye is not perfect. This simple fact was known in the last century, and Helmholtz humorously said that if an optician were to manufacture an optical system as defective as the eye he would surely go bankrupt. Indeed the eye suffers from various imperfections. The basic treatise on these aberrations has been masterfully produced by LeGrand (1967). In this chapter, I propose to review briefly some of the well-established facts, to add some new knowledge, and hopefully to integrate this information in order to emerge with some views, however ephemerous, on the importance of aberrations in visual perception.

I. Spherical Aberration

Spherical optical surfaces refract light rays differently near the optical axis (this is in the domain of paraxial or Gaussian optics) than away from the axis. Light rays penetrating into the eye near the edge of the pupil are refracted differently than paraxial rays. Consequently, the retinal image formed by a system with a large pupil is a blurred patch and is said to be affected by spherical aberration. There are two types of spherical aberrations: positive (or undercorrected) and negative (or overcorrected). These depend upon whether the marginal rays are focused in front of, or behind, the paraxial rays, respectively.

Calculations obtained by simple ray tracing procedures yield considerable amounts of positive spherical aberration: .5D at 1 mm, 2D at 2 mm, and 4D at 4 mm off the optical axis (Ivanoff, 1953; Jenkins, 1963). However, actual measurements of the spherical aberration of the human eye do not usually exceed 1D even with the most dilated pupil. The average value is about .5D of positive spherical aberration. With accommodation, it changes to a slightly smaller amount of spherical aberration, which in many cases is of the negative type.

The reason for this discrepancy between theory and practice has been attributed to the unusual topography of the cornea. The human cornea is, to the regret of contact lens practitioners, aspherical. It is flatter toward its periphery, is thus less powerful, and is thereby able to correct (perhaps only partially) its otherwise large positive spherical aberration. Obviously nature most likely devised the human eye so as to correct its spherical aberration rather than to make contact lens fitting irksome. Variations in the refractive index of the crystalline lens in various meridians (Nakao, Ono, Nagata, & Iwata, 1969) may assist in further reducing this aberration, although these can only be self-correcting to the lens.

A. Corneal Contribution

The respective contributions of lens and cornea to aberration reduction still remain uncertain. One interesting approach to this problem is to study the effect of contact lenses with spherical front surfaces on the spherical aberration of the eye. These reintroduce a spherical cornea. Bonnet (1964) found that in an aphakic eye (i.e., lacking a crystalline lens) corrected by a contact lens, the aberration was almost equal to its theoretical value, that is, about 2D, 2 mm away from the optical axis. With spectacle correction, however, the aberration amounted to less than half this value, and that is practically what one finds in a normal eye. Consistent with these findings are measurements by Millodot (1969), who showed that visual acuity

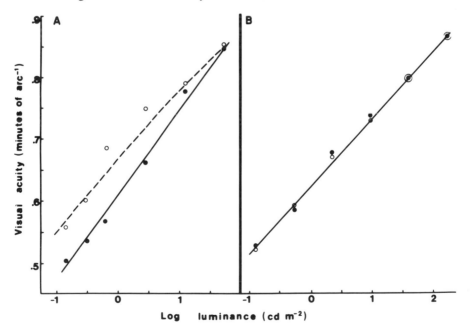

Figure 35.1. Variation of visual acuity as a function of luminance with (A) hard contact lenses (●) and glasses (○) and (B) soft contact lenses (○) and glasses (●).

with contact lenses deteriorated more rapidly in the dark when the pupil was dilated than with spectacles (Figure 35.1A). This has been attributed to the reintroduction of some spherical aberration by the contact lens which manifests itself at low luminances. The finding was further confirmed by similar measurements of visual acuity with an artificial pupil. More evidence in support of this view was provided by Kerns (1974), who compared visual acuity with spherical and aspherical front surface contact lenses, thus simulating the human cornea. He found that visual acuity was better with aspherical lenses. In addition, Millodot (1975) further demonstrated that visual acuity with soft contact lenses conforming to the natural corneal topography was not reduced relative to spectacles (see Figure 35.1B).

All these experiments seem to indicate that the absence of any significant spherical aberration in the eye may be essentially attributed to the asphericity of the cornea, and visual perception is not usually interfered with by this aberration. When the pupils are large, visual performance is diminished, as Krauskopf (1964) has noted. Even under these circumstances spherical aberration is not very significant because of the salutary effect of the Stiles–Crawford phenomenon.

II. Chromatic Aberration

The refractive index of the media of the eye varies with the wavelength of light. This general phenomenon is called dispersion. As a rule the refractive index increases when the wavelength decreases. It follows that in blue light the eye becomes more refractive, that is, myopic, than in red light. This phenomenon has long been known and was observed by Isaac Newton.

Longitudinal chromatic aberration in the human eye has been found to amount to about 1D between the F and C lines (486.1 and 656.3 nm, respectively) and to be of the order of 2D over the whole visible spectrum (see Figure 35.2). Most investigators seem to be in good agreement (see review by LeGrand, 1967) about these values and the data obtained electrophysiologically (Ronchi & Millodot, 1974). (In the following discussion allusion will only be made to the longitudinal chromatic aberration, that is, the dioptric distance along the optical axis.)

A. Age and Chromatic Aberration

It seems that all previous measurements of chromatic aberration have been made on young adults. But what is the influence of age on this defect? In a study by Millodot (1976a) chromatic aberration was measured on 58 people of various ages. The results are illustrated in Figure 35.3 and indicate a remarkable decline in chromatic aberration with age, especially after the fifth decade of life. Beyond the sixth decade, chromatic aberration was found to be equal to a third of its value in young adults. In the human eye such achromatization is possible if the difference in refractive indices of the lens and of the vitreous in blue and red light ($n_F - n_C$) changes with age. Millodot and Newton (1976) measured the brightness of photo-

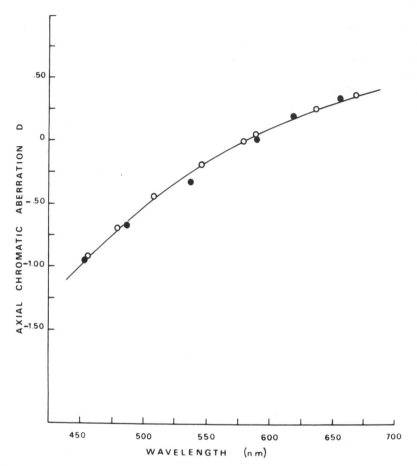

Figure 35.2. Axial chromatic aberration as a function of wavelength in young adults. The open circles are the data of Bedford and Wyszecki (1957) and the closed circles the data of Millodot (1976a). [From Millodot (1976a). Reprinted with permission.]

graphs of Purkinje–Sanson images in red and blue light in two groups of subjects, young and old. The brightness of these images depends upon the values of the indices of the media on both sides of an optical surface. The results of this experiment suggest that the refractive indices of the lens and of the vitreous for blue and red light change with age in a manner compatible with the results of Millodot (1976a).

B. Contribution of Lens and Cornea

The chromatic aberration of the human eye is equal to the sum of the dispersion induced by various optical surfaces. The older literature seems to assume that the lens is more dispersive than the cornea (see LeGrand, 1967).

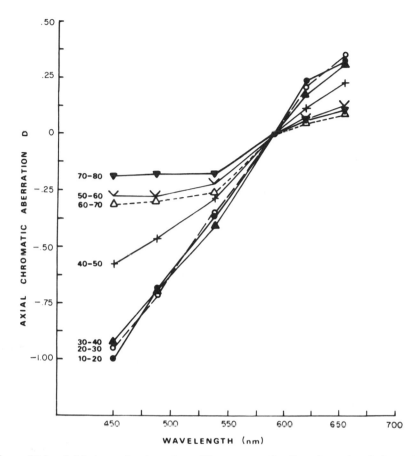

Figure 35.3. Axial chromatic aberration of the eye as a function of wavelength for various age groups indicated beside each curve. [From Millodot (1976a). Reprinted with permission.]

However, there is some evidence showing that the involvement of the lens is in fact more or less proportional to its refractive importance. Ivanoff (1953) found that chromatic aberration of an aphakic eye amounted to .75D (between 483 and 712 nm). This finding was corroborated by Millodot (1976a). Calculations [based on a formula derived by Millodot and Newton (1976)] of the chromatic aberration of the cornea between lines F and C give a value of .79D, that is, 74% of the chromatic aberration of the whole eye.

Sivak and Millodot (1975) measured chromatic aberration of the eye while the cornea was virtually neutralized by being immersed in water. They found that the chromatic aberration of the lens contributed 28.5% of the aberration of the whole eye (see Figure 35.4). This result is in good agreement with the calculations previously reported and with the data on aphakic eyes. Thus the lens appears to have approximately the same dispersive effect as the cornea in spite of its heterogeneity.

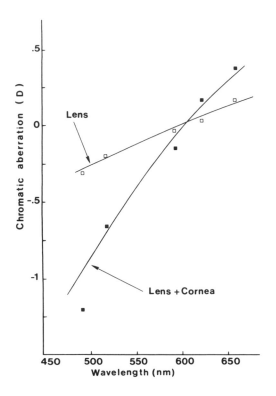

Figure 35.4. Axial chromatic aberration of the whole eye and of the lens alone. The curves were drawn by inspection. [Modified from Sivak & Millodot (1975).]

C. Effect of Accommodation

Calculations by Ivanoff (1953) point to an increase of about 2.1% per diopter of accommodation. Using a different formula derived by Millodot and Newton (1976) one arrives at an increase of .24D (or 23% of the total amount of chromatic aberration between lines F and C) for 10D of accommodation. Empirical determinations of chromatic aberration with accommodation are sparse. Nutting (1914) noted that chromatic aberration increases when viewing at 25 cm compared to viewing at infinity. On the other hand, Jenkins (1963) reported that chromatic aberration decreases when looking at near objects (tested at 33 cm). However, Jenkins' results are not in good accord with either the theory or results of other authors; Jenkins found more chromatic aberration at distance, especially beyond 600 nm, while his measurements for near vision reflect a barely appreciable difference with, say, the data of Figure 35.2.

Other measurements by Millodot and Sivak (1973) present no significant change in chromatic aberration with observation distance. Yet, in a subsequent experiment in which most of the chromatic aberration was eliminated by an achromatizing lens, Sivak and Millodot (1974) obtained a significant increase in the residual chromatic aberration with 7D of accommodation. This finding may be attributed to the fact that "noise" was reduced by the introduction of the achromatizing lens. Nevertheless, for moderate accommodative efforts chromatic aberration can be regarded as somewhat independent of accommodation.

D. Wavelength Focused on the Retina

It has been traditionally accepted that there is a single wavelength focused on the retina at all times. Helmholtz (1909) assumed that the retina was situated halfway between the red and violet focal points, that is, around 500 nm; for Emsley (1955) it was 555 nm; for Wald and Griffin (1947) and Bedford and Wyszecki (1957) it was 578 nm; for Hartridge (1918) and Lapicque (1937) it was 580 nm. Many other authors have assumed that the eye is in focus for the bright sodium light at 589 nm.

What evidence is there? Polack (1905) observed that the eye was not focused for the same wavelength at all observation distances. He found that long wavelengths were in focus for distance vision and short wavelengths for near vision. This result was confirmed by Ivanoff (1953), Kellershohn, Chatelain, and Roubault (1957), Jenkins (1963), and Millodot and Sivak (1973) whether the target was illuminated in white light or with independent wavelengths.

Millodot and Sivak (1973) extended these observations to 8.3D of accommodation, whereas Ivanoff had used a maximum accommodative stimulus of 2.5D. These two sets of measurements are shown in Figure 35.5.

It is clear from these results that the eye is focused for the long wavelengths (685 nm according to Ivanoff) when the stimulus to accommodation is nil. The eye is focused on radiation at 589 nm when the eye accommodates .7D, according to Ivanoff, and .8D according to Millodot and Sivak (1973). And as accommodation increases (i.e., the viewing object is brought closer), the eye is focused for shorter and shorter wavelengths. However, if the wavelength of the target being viewed is changed but not its distance from the eye, the accommodative stance appears to remain unaltered, as evinced by monitoring the nonfixing eye with a refractometer (Millodot & Bobier, 1976). Interestingly if one wears colored filters (with narrow band pass) for some 4 hr, the accommodative mechanism is found to alter (Millodot, 1976b). The cause of this shift in wavelength has been regarded by Ivanoff (1953) and LeGrand (1967) to be a physiological response of the eye to spare its accommodation by focusing on the shorter wavelengths when viewing near objects. It must be a learned response since attempts to disturb the phenomenon by paralyzing accommodation (Millodot & Sivak, 1973) or minimizing the aberration with an achromatizing lens (Sivak & Millodot, 1974) did not prevent the shift from occurring.

This shift may have some effects on visual phenomena, as specified in the following:

1. It offers a means of extending the range of accommodation by 1–2D beyond that afforded by mechanical properties of the lens.
2. It may explain the residual accommodation of as much as 1D in young aphakics.

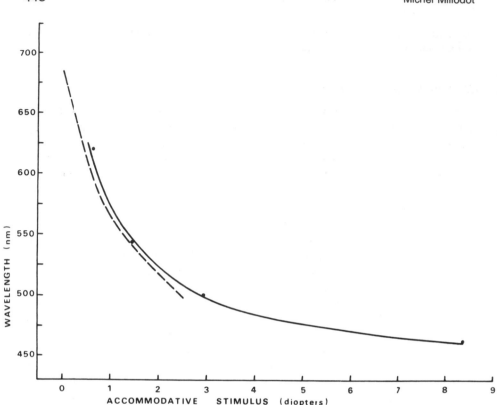

Figure 35.5. Wavelength in focus on the retina as a function of the accommodative stimulus. The dashed line represents the results of Ivanoff (1953) and the continuous curve those of Millodot and Sivak (1973). [From Millodot & Sivak (1973). Reprinted with permission.]

3. The perception of colors does not remain the same at all distances, but varies in brightness.
4. Tritanopia (blue blindness) observed in the fovea may be caused in part by a reduction of the blue response for distant objects due to the enlargement of the blur circle on the retina which may be absent for stimulation at very close range.

III. Comment

Does chromatic aberration obtrude on visual perception? Visual acuity, for example, is not better when chromatic aberration is eliminated (Hartridge, 1947). This phenomenon is due partly to the fact that the focus of the eye is not steady because of the microfluctuations of accommodation (Arnulf, Dupuy, & Flamant, 1951). Evidence of acuity deficits can be demonstrated when observation time is limited and chromatic aberration is eliminated (Millodot, 1968). Campbell and

Gubisch (1967) showed that contrast sensitivity rather than visual acuity is affected by the presence of chromatic aberration. Nonetheless, chromatic aberration is regarded in general (at high luminance and small pupil) as not intruding very much onto visual perception. This is believed to be partially due to (*a*) yellow filtering of the lens, (*b*) absorption of macular pigment, and (*c*) sharp spectral sensitivity of cone vision toward long wavelengths. In addition, it has been suggested that separate red- and green-sensitive channels exist (Regan, 1975); therefore, the most sharply focused image is seen at any given moment independently of its color. Such a system would be compatible with the shift in wavelength as a function of observation distance, as previously described.

IV. Oblique Astigmatism

The peripheral dioptrics of the eye displays a considerable error of refraction due primarily to the presence of oblique ray astigmatism (e.g., Ferree, Rand, & Hardy, 1931; Millodot & Lamont, 1974). Naturally this aberration leads one to predict that it may contribute to poor visual acuity in the periphery.

A study of acuity with and without correction of the peripheral refractive error was carried out by Millodot, Johnson, Lamont, and Leibowitz (1975) using Landolt rings and sinusoidal gratings: Their results are summarized in Figure 35.6. These clearly show that the refractive error of the periphery of the eye does not limit visual acuity. They are in good agreement with observations of some parts of the retina by Weale (1956) and Green (1970) and were again confirmed throughout the horizontal visual field by Rempt, Hoogerheide, and Hoogenboom (1976). However, correc-

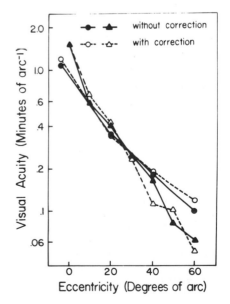

Figure 35.6. Visual acuity as a function of stimulus eccentricity with and without correction of peripheral refractive error for sinusoidal gratings (circles) and Landolt rings (triangles). [From Johnson *et al.* (1976). Reprinted with permission.]

tion of all aberrations by means of an interferometric technique (Frizen & Glansholm, 1975) leads to some improvement in acuity in the periphery, at least beyond 20–30° eccentricity.

On the other hand, peripheral correction leads to a difference in motion threshold (Johnson & Leibowitz, 1974), in peripheral increment threshold (Frankhauser & Enoch, 1962), and in absolute threshold (Ronchi, 1971). This has been interpreted by Johnson, Leibowitz, Millodot, and Lamont (1976) as further evidence of the existence of two modes of visual processing pertaining to identification ("what") and localization ("where") of visual stimuli. Specifically, the function for discrimination of detail associated with the identification system might be expected to be sensitive to blur in central vision but not necessarily in the periphery. In contrast, the localization system would be sensitive to image quality over most of the visual field, thus making motion and abrupt luminance changes appropriate stimuli for peripheral vision.

V. Conclusion

This review of the most significant aberrations of the eye implies that under most normal conditions of vision, the performance of the eye is not limited by its aberrations. In fact, the dioptrics of the eye are as good as deemed necesssary, and whatever limits visual performance lies in the retina–brain pathways. If aberrations do not significantly affect visual perception, then why has nature allowed such large amounts of some aberrations while minimizing others (spherical aberration)? The speculative answer to this question proposed here is that aberrations of the eye (whatever the eye tolerates of these), rather than interfering with vision, may play a positive role in visual perception. This has been illustrated by pointing out, for example, the facilitative effect of chromatic aberration on accommodation and the degrading result of peripheral dioptrics aimed at letting the localization mode of processing predominate outside central vision. In brief, aberrations of the eye may be regarded as optical filters aimed at enhancing visual perception and not as defects causing a degradation of the retinal image.

REFERENCES

Arnulf, A., Dupuy, D., & Flamant, F. Les microfluctuations d'accommodation de l'oeil et l'acuité visuelle pour les diamètres pupillaires naturels. *Comptes Rendus hebdomadaires des séances de l'Académie des Sciences,* 1951, *231,* 349.

Bedford, R.E., & Wyszecki, G. Axial chromatic aberration of the eye. *Journal of the Optical Society of America,* 1957, *47,* 564–565.

Bonnet, R. *La topographie cornéenne.* Paris: N. Desroches Editeur, 1964.

Campbell, F.W., & Gubisch, R.W. The effect of chromatic aberration on visual acuity. *Journal of Physiology,* 1967, *192,* 345–358.

Emsley, H.H. *Visual optics* (5th ed). London: Hatton Press, 1955.

Ferree, C.E., Rand, G., & Hardy, C. Refraction for the peripheral field of vision. *Archives of Ophthalmology,* 1931, *5,* 717-731.

Frankhauser, F., & Enoch, J.M. The effects of blur on perimetric thresholds. *Archives of Ophthalmology,* 1962, *68,* 240-251.

Frisen, L., & Glansholm, A. Optical and neural resolution in peripheral vision. *Investigative Ophthalmology,* 1975, *14,* 528-536.

Green, D.G. Regional variations in the visual acuity for interference fringes on the retina. *Journal of Physiology,* 1970, *207,* 351-356.

Hartridge, H. Chromatic aberration and resolving power of the eye. *Journal of Physiology,* 1918, *52,* 175-246.

Hartridge, H. The visual perception of fine detail. *Philosophical Transactions of the Royal Society, Ser. B,* 1947, *232,* 519-671.

Helmholtz, H. *Handbuch der physiologischen Optik* (3rd ed., Vol. 1). Hamburg: Vos, 1909.

Ivanoff, A., *Les aberrations de l'oeil.* Paris: Masson, 1953.

Jenkins, T.C.A. Aberrations of the eye and their effects on vision, II. *The British Journal of Physiological Optics,* 1963, *20,* 161-201.

Johnson, C.A., & Leibowitz, H.W. Practice, refractive error and feedback as factors influencing peripheral motion thresholds. *Perception & Psychophysics,* 1974, *15,* 276-280.

Johnson, C.A., Leibowitz, H.W., Millodot, M., & Lamont, A. Peripheral visual acuity and refractive error: Evidence for 'two visual systems'? *Perception & Psychophysics,* 1976, *20,* 460-464.

Kellershohn, C., Chatelain, P., & Roubault, H. Répartition spectrale d'une source lumineuse et accommodation de l'oeil. *Comptes Rendus de la Societé de Biologie,* 1957, *151,* 985-987.

Kerns, R.L. Clinical evaluation of the merits of an aspheric front-surface contact lens for patients manifesting residual astigmatism. *American Journal of Optometry,* 1974, *51,* 750-757.

Krauskopf, J. Further measurements of human retinal images. *Journal of the Optical Society of America,* 1964, *54,* 715-716.

Lapicque, C. *La formation des images retiniennes.* Paris: Revue d'Optique, 1937.

LeGrand, Y. *[Form and space vision]* (M. Millodot, & G.G. Heath, trans.). Bloomington: Indiana University Press, 1967.

Millodot, M. Effet des microfluctuations de l'accommodation sur l'acuité visuelle. *Vision Research,* 1968, *8,* 73-80.

Millodot, M. Variation of visual acuity with contact lenses. *Archives of Ophthalmology,* 1969, *82,* 461-465.

Millodot, M. Variation of visual acuity with soft contact lenses: A function of luminance. *American Journal of Optometry,* 1975, *52,* 541-544.

Millodot, M. The influence of age on the chromatic aberration of the eye. *Albrecht v. Graefes Archives for Clinical and Experimental Ophthalmology,* 1976, *198,* 235-243. (a)

Millodot, M. L'effet de filtres colorés sur la réfraction de l'oeil. *Annales d'Oculistique,* 1976, *209,* 605-608. (b)

Millodot, M., & Bobier, C. The state of accommodation during the measurement of axial chromatic aberration of the eye. *American Journal of Optometry,* 1976, *53,* 168-172.

Millodot, M., Johnson, C.A., Lamont, A., & Leibowitz, H.W. Effect of dioptrics on peripheral visual acuity. *Vision Research,* 1975, *15,* 1357-1362.

Millodot, M., & Lamont, A. Refraction of the periphery of the eye. *Journal of the Optical Society of America,* 1974, *64,* 110-111.

Millodot, M., & Newton, I.A. A possible change of refractive index with age and its relevance to chromatic aberration. *Albrecht v. Graefes Archives for Clinical and Experimental Ophthalmology,* 1976, *201,* 159-167.

Millodot, M., & Sivak, J.G. Influence of accommodation on the chromatic aberration of the eye. *British Journal of Physiological Optics,* 1973, *28,* 169-174.

Nakao, S., Ono, T., Nagata, R., & Iwata, K. The distribution of refractive indices in the human crystalline lens. *Japanese Journal of Clinical Ophthalmology,* 1969, *23,* 903-906.

Nutting, P.G. The axial chromatic aberration of the human eye. *Proceedings of the Royal Society, Ser. A,* 1914, *90,* 440-443.

Polack, A. Optotypes en couleurs complémentaires. *Bulletin de la Societé d'Ophtalmologie de France,* 1905, *22,* 334–341.

Regan, D. Recent advances in electrical recording from the human brain. *Nature,* 1975, *253,* 401–407.

Rempt, F., Hoogerheide, J., & Hoogenboom, W.P.H. Influence of correction of peripheral refractive errors on peripheral static vision. *Ophthalmologica,* 1976, *173,* 128–135.

Ronchi, L. Absolute threshold before and after correction of oblique-ray astigmatism. *Journal of the Optical Society of America,* 1971, *61,* 1705–1709.

Ronchi, L., & Millodot, M. The cortical counterpart of the chromatic aberration of the eye. *American Journal of Optometry,* 1974, *51,* 635–641.

Sivak, J.G., & Millodot, M. Axial chromatic aberration of the eye with achromatizing lens. *Journal of the Optical Society of America,* 1974, *64,* 1724–1725.

Sivak, J.G., & Millodot, M. Axial chromatic aberration of the crystalline lens. *Atti della Fondazione Giorgio Ronchi,* 1975, *30,* 173–177.

Wald, G., & Griffin, D.R. The change in refractive power of the human eye in dim and bright light. *Journal of the Optical Society of America,* 1947, *37,* 321–336.

Weale, R.A. Problems of peripheral vision. *British Journal of Ophthalmology,* 1956, *40,* 392–415.

36. Patterned Elicited ERGs and VECPs in Amblyopia and Infant Vision[1]

Samuel Sokol,

I. Introduction

The human electroretinogram (ERG) and visually evoked cortical potential (VECP) have grown steadily during the past 35 years in their usefulness for detecting, diagnosing, and investigating a wide variety of visual disorders. This era of development began with the introduction of the scleral contact lens electrode, a viable and comfortable means of maintaining the electrical contact required for recording ERG over long periods of time (Riggs, 1941). The contact lens electrode was soon used to record ERGs from humans with congenital night blindness and retinitis pigmentosa (Riggs, 1954) and was later used in conjunction with the stimulus technique of phase alternation (Caldwell, Howard, & Riggs, 1971) to record ERGs from a group of patients with hereditary optic atrophy. Visually evoked cortical potentials were also examined in this latter study. With the many advances in computer technology and the availability of simpler stimulus generators, for example, TV monitors, the application of electrophysiology to ophthalmology and neurology has entered a new period of expansion and development. The ERG and the VECP can now be recorded in response to patterned stimuli. This may provide a means of more accurately investigating disorders of the eye that involve photopic mechanisms such as macular degeneration. In fact, VECP, in response to patterned stimuli, has been valuable in the detection of amblyopia, optic neuritis, multiple sclerosis, field defects, and in the measurement of visual acuity in infants and nonverbal patients (Sokol, 1976). The purpose of this chapter is to review some recent electrophysiological findings in two areas of ophthalmology that have benefited greatly from the use of alternating patterned

[1]This work was supported by National Institutes of Health Research Grant EY-00926 and Career Development Award EY-70275-01A1.

453

stimuli: the detection and investigation of amblyopia in adults and children and the measurement of visual acuity and maturation of the visual system in normal infants and infants with suspected visual defects.

II. Amblyopia

A. Childhood

Amblyopia is generally defined as a reduction in visual acuity in one or both eyes that cannot be corrected by refractive means and in which no obvious pathology can be detected (Burian & Von Noorden, 1974). Also, it is now known that the pattern VECP, particularly when elicited by checks subtending 30 min of arc or less, can easily detect the presence of amblyopia (Dawson, Perry, & Childers, 1972; Sokol & Bloom, 1973; Sokol & Shaterian, 1976, pp. 59–67; Sokol, 1977, pp. 410–417; Lombroso, Duffy, & Robb, 1969; Arden, Barnard, & Mushin, 1974). Figure 36.1 shows the amplitude as a function of check size for VECPs obtained from a child with normal vision and three children with amblyopia. These records were obtained with a sinusoidally alternating pattern stimulus (12 alternations sec^{-1}) of high contrast. The results of the subject with normal vision show that a peak VECP occurs in

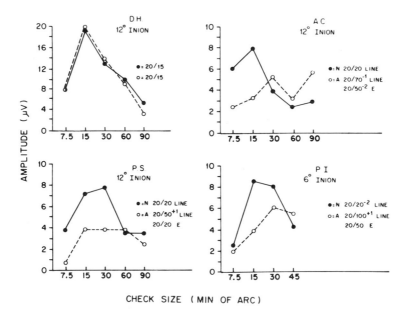

Figure 36.1. Amplitude of pattern VECP as a function of check size for one child (DH) with normal vision and three amblyopic children. (●) VECP from normal eye. (○) VECP from amblyopic eye. N = normal, A = amblyopic. Line refers to acuity measured by Snellen line chart. E refers to acuity measured by using E letters shown singularly.

both eyes with checks subtending 15 min of visual angle. Amblyopic subject AC shows a peak at 15 min for the normal eye, reduced amplitudes at 7.5 and 15 min for the amblyopic eye, and larger signals at 30, 60, and 90 min. Subject PS shows a peak between 15 and 30 min for the normal eye, and no difference in amplitude for 15, 30, and 60 min in the amblyopic eye. Even though the acuity improves to 20/20 with separate E testing, the VECP amplitudes remain reduced. Subject PI viewed a smaller field and gives results similar to those obtained with a 12° field: a peak at 15 min for the normal eye and significantly reduced amplitudes for 15 and 30 min in the amblyopic eye. Any type of pattern presentation, that is, transient or steady-state pattern reversal or pattern onset–offset, will detect amblyopia.

B. Adult

1. VISUALLY EVOKED CORTICAL POTENTIALS

The pattern VECP is particularly valuable for the clinical detection of amblyopia in children but adult amblyopes have little to gain since they read eye charts reliably. The importance of the VECP in adult amblyopia lies in its value for research. A variety of stimulus conditions can be presented to adults and long testing sessions are possible.

One disadvantage of using fast alternation rates is that component waveform analysis is lost; but since signals can be recorded in less time with rapid alternation,

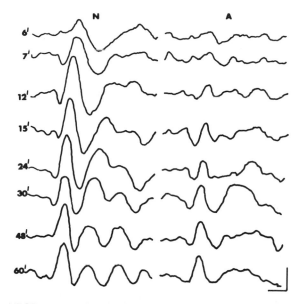

Figure 36.2. VECP waves obtained from an adult with an anisometropic amblyopia. Acuity in normal eye (N) was 20/20, in the amblyopic eye (A) 20/300. Check sizes in minutes of arc are shown to the left. The vertical line = 5 μV; horizontal line = 50 msec.

it can be valuable in the clinical testing of young children. Adults, on the other hand, can be presented with pattern reversal at slow rates, and the component analysis of amplitude and implicit time can be accomplished. For example, Figure 36.2 shows VECP waveforms obtained from the normal and amblyopic eyes of a 32-year-old woman with a refractive amblyopia. The checkerboard stimulus was generated by a TV monitor, the rate of alternation of the checks was 1.88 sec^{-1}, and the contrast was 85%. The waveform of the VECP obtained with stimulation of the normal eye consisted of a prominent negative component at approximately 80 msec for checks subtending 7–30 min of arc (N_1), a positive component (P_1) for all check sizes from 100 to 125 msec, and a second negative component (N_2) between 130 and 175 msec. There is an orderly shift in the implicit time of the P_1 component from 125 msec for 6-min checks to 100 msec for 60-min checks. The second negative component, like P_1, demonstrates a shift in implicit time with longer implicit times for 6-min checks. The waveform of the VECP from the normal eye changes considerably with changes in check size. Specifically, the number of waves that follow the N_2 component increases with check size. The VECP recorded from stimulation of the amblyopic eye presents a different picture. The amplitudes of all components are smaller, particularly with small checks. There is little change in the implicit times of the P_1 component as check size changes, nor is there a change in the complexity of the waveform as the checks become larger.

2. ELECTRORETINOGRAM

An even more important aspect of studying the electrophysiology of adult amblyopes is that it is possible to record their ERGs. There have been no published studies to date measuring the pattern ERG in an amblyope. In previous studies (Burian & Lawwill, 1966; Nawratzki, Auerbach, & Rowe, 1966), ERGs were recorded with unpatterned flashing lights, and no difference in the ERG amplitudes or implicit times was found when normal and amblyopic eyes were compared.

Figure 36.3 shows records of the ERG[2] and VECPs recorded simultaneously from the adult amblyope whose VECP records are shown in Figure 36.2. The amplitude of the VECP is smaller in the amblyopic eye than in the normal eye for 24- and 48-min checks. Also, the ERG amplitudes are smaller in the amblyopic eye; both the b-wave and the afterpotential (Armington, Corwin, & Marsetta, 1971) are reduced. In order to be certain that the reduction in the ERG was not the result of optical distortions by the contact lens electrode and since it is known that the VECP is sensitive to optical distortion and refractive errors (Millodot & Riggs, 1970), the VECP was recorded with the contact lens removed. Figure 36.3 shows that the amplitude of the VECP is unchanged with and without the contact lens. Even though it has been reported that the human retina does not exhibit sharp spatial tuning properties (Armington et al., 1971; Spekreijse, Van der Tweel, & Zuidema, 1973), this does not rule out the possibility that there is some other type of defect in the photopic mechanisms of the retina of an amblyope.

---

[2] See Bloom and Sokol (1977) for details of the contact lens electrode used to record the pattern ERG.

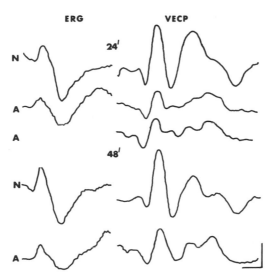

Figure 36.3. Pattern reversal ERGs and VECPs simultaneously recorded from an adult amblyope. N (normal eye), A (amblyopic eye). ERGs are shown in left column, VECPs in right. Records for two check sizes (24 and 48 min) are also shown. Note absence of a second ERG with 24 min in the amblyopic eye. In this condition the contact lens electrode was removed and only the VECP was recorded. Horizontal line = 50 msec. Vertical line = 5 μV for the VECP and 2.5 μV for the ERG.

III. Infant VECPs

A. Measurement of Acuity

For many years ophthalmologists have read that infant acuity was very poor and that it was not until 3 years of age that acuity reached adult levels (Newman, 1975, pp. 500–528). Recently, however, a number of behavioral (see Dobson and Teller, this volume, Chapter 31) and electrophysiological studies have shown that infant acuity develops rapidly and that by 6 months of age infants have acuity equivalent to 20/20 Snellen.

Sokol and Dobson (1976) measured the pattern reversal VECPs in infants between the ages of 2 and 6 months. The stimulus was a checkerboard pattern alternating at 12 reversals sec^{-1}. Signals were recorded from infants using check sizes between 7.5 and 30 min of visual arc. During the first 6 months the amplitude–check size function showed a shift in the location of the peak amplitude from large checks to small checks; by 6 months of age the infants peaked between 7.5 and 15 min of arc, and the descending slopes of the amplitude–check size function were similar to those obtained with adults. These data indicated that by 6 months infants had acuity similar to adult levels. Sokol (1978) extrapolated the amplitude–check size function to 0 μV (Campbell & Maffei, 1970) to estimate acuity in infants from

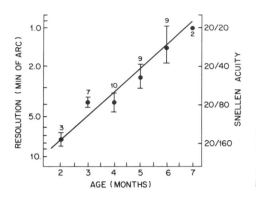

Figure 36.4. VECP acuity for infants from 2 to 7 months. Closed circles are the mean acuities, and the vertical line indicates ±1 *SE* of the mean. The number of infants tested is shown for each age group. [From Sokol, (1978).]

2 to 7 months of age. Figure 36.4 shows the VECP acuity data from these infants: At 2 months mean VECP acuity is 20/160, and by 6 months it has increased to nearly 20/20. Marg *et al.* (1976) found similar VECP acuity using a 20° field of patterned appearance–disappearance bar gratings of different spatial frequencies. Even though there are considerable differences in the design of the Sokol and Marg studies, that is, field size, type of pattern stimulus, method of stimulus presentation, and criterion for VECP thresholds, the data closely agree.

B. Maturation of the Visual System

Several investigators have measured the amplitude of the patterned elicited VECP in infants as a function of changes in check size (Harter & Suitt, 1970; Karmel, Hoffman, & Fegy, 1974; Sokol & Dobson, 1976; Marg *et al.,* 1976; Sokol, 1978). In addition, there have been a number of studies concerned with the effects of maturation on the amplitude and implicit time of the unpatterned flash-elicited VECP (Maurer, 1976). However, little attention has been paid to the maturation of the amplitude and implicit time of patterned elicited VECP at slow reversal rates. There have been some reports of changes in implicit time with flash-elicited pattern VECPs (Harter & Suitt, 1970; Karmel *et al.,* 1974), but it has been suggested that there is a nonlinear interaction of luminance and spatial frequency with this type of stimulus (Spekreijse, Khoe, & van der Tweel, 1973, pp. 141–156; Regan, 1972). Therefore, a pattern stimulus of constant mean luminance is more appropriate for a study of the development of the human visual system's capacity to process spatial information.

We have recently studied the maturation of the human visual system as reflected by changes in the pattern reversal VECP in a group of infants between the ages of 4 and 24 weeks. Figure 36.5 shows waveforms from two infants obtained with a pattern reversal checkerboard (1.88 alternations sec^{-1}). The checks subtended 15 min of visual angle. It was not until 100 days of age that signals in response to 15-min checks were distinguishable from noise. The most prominent component between 105 and 119 days is a positive wave at 145–150 msec. Between 126 and 133 days the positive component is increased in amplitude and occurs at 140–150

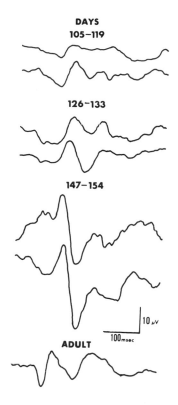

Figure 36.5. Pattern reversal VECP (1.88 alternations sec^{-1}) obtained for 15-min checks from two infants between the ages of 105 and 154 days. Subject O's records are the top record of each pair, Subject D's the lower. Also shown is the VECP obtained from an adult under identical stimulus conditions.

msec. A negative component has emerged between 185 and 200 msec, and a second positive component is seen at 230 msec. At 147–154 days a small negative component is present at 105 msec; P_1 is now between 125 and 133 msec. N_2 is much larger in amplitude, and the implicit time has decreased to between 170 and 180 msec. We find that in comparison to a group of normal adults the N_1–P_1–N_2–P_2 complex is still as much as 25 msec longer in the 24-week-old infant. For example, the P_1 adult implicit time occurs at 107 msec with a standard deviation of 2.9 msec, while the mean infant value for P_1 is 130 msec. Therefore, if the implicit time can be considered to be a reflection of neural transmission of the visual system then it appears that the infant visual system is not completely matured by 24 weeks. When the infant implicit time reaches the adult level remains to be determined.

C. Clinical Value

Often the clinician is unable to be certain if an infant sees well. The mother may report that the child does not pick up small objects, does not recognize faces across the room, or that one eye occasionally turns in or out. If the presence of a refractive error is eliminated and the ophthalmologist cannot find any definitive evidence of retinal or optic nerve pathology, a VECP can be used to determine if the defect is

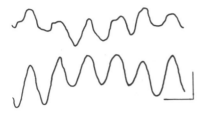

Figure 36.6. Rapid pattern reversal VECP (15 alternations sec⁻¹) recorded from a 7-month-old infant with a congenital cataract in her right eye. Upper record is the VECP recorded from the cataractous eye, lower record the VECP from the normal eye. Horizontal line = 75 msec. Vertical line = 10 μV.

further along the visual pathways. For example, early detection of amblyopia may be achieved with the pattern VECP by recording signals from each eye. If the signals are equal then the ophthalmologist has a quantitative index to use for future reference (see Figure 36.1). Another example is shown in Figure 36.6: VECPs were recorded from a 7-month-old child with a congenital cataract in the lens of the right eye. The cataract was very small (1 mm in diameter) but was located in the center of the pupil. The amplitude of the VECP recorded with stimulation of the right eye was smaller. Two possibilities may account for the reduced VECP: There is a mild amblyopia because the cataract is located in the center of the pupil and/or the cataract is blocking the stimulus from reaching what still may be a normal fovea. In any case, the VECP can be used to monitor the child's visual development and provide a quantitative measure for the ophthalmologist until the child is old enough to read visual acuity charts.

A final example of the use of patterned VECPs is in pediatric ophthalmology where they are valuable in following the visual development of premature infants, particularly those who have received oxygen at birth for life support and may have acquired the unwanted side effects of retinal damage due to high oxygen levels. Figure 36.7 shows VECP records from two infants with a chronological age of 22 weeks. The records indicated by P were recorded from an infant born 8 weeks prematurely. The records marked N were recorded from an infant born at full term. The signals obtained with 60-min checks are similar both in amplitude and in implicit times. However, the records from 15-min checks are significantly different. The signal obtained from the premature infant has smaller amplitude components and the implicit times are longer. The waveform is more like a full-term infant at 18 weeks (see Figure 36.5, second pair of records).

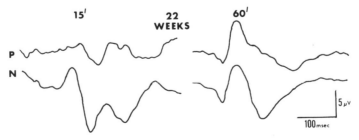

Figure 36.7. Pattern reversal VECPs recorded at 22 weeks of age from a normal (N) and a premature infant (P). Checks subtended 15 min (left column) and 60 min (right column).

ACKNOWLEDGMENTS

I thank Kathleen Jones and Daniel Nadler for their help in data collection.

REFERENCES

Arden, G.B., Barnard, W.M., & Mushin, A.S. Visually evoked response in amblyopia. *British Journal of Ophthalmology*, 1974, *58*, 183–192.

Armington, J.C., Corwin, T.R., & Marsetta, R. Simultaneously recorded retinal and cortical responses to patterned stimuli. *Journal of the Optical Society of America*, 1971, *61*, 1514–1521.

Bloom, B.H., & Sokol, S. A corneal electrode for patterned stimulus electroretinography. *American Journal of Ophthalmology*, 1977, *83*, 272–275.

Burian, H.M., & Lawwill, T. Electroretinographic studies in strabismic amblyopia. *American Journal of Ophthalmology*, 1966, *61*, 422–430.

Burian, H.J., and Von Noorden, G.K. *Binocular vision and ocular motility: Theory and management of strabismus.* St. Louis: C.V. Mosby, 1974.

Caldwell, J.B.H., Howard, R.O., & Riggs, L.A. Dominant juvenile optic atrophy. *Archives of Ophthalmology*, 1971, *85*, 133–147.

Campbell, F.W., & Maffei, L. Electrophysiological evidence for the existence of orientation and size detectors in the human visual system. *Journal of Physiology*, 1970, *207*, 635–652.

Dawson, W.W., Perry, N.W., & Childers, D.G. Variations in human cortical response to patterns and image quality. *Investigative Ophthalmology*, 1972, *11*, 789–799.

Harter, M., & Suitt, C. Visually-evoked cortical responses and pattern vision in the infant: A longitudinal study. *Psychonomic Science*, 1970, *18*, 235–237.

Karmel, B.Z., Hoffmann, R.F., & Fegy, M.J. Processing of contour information by human infants evidenced by pattern-dependent evoked potentials. *Child Development*, 1974, *45*, 39–48.

Lombroso, C., Duffy, F., & Robb, R. Selective suppression of cerebral-evoked potentials to patterned light in amblyopia ex anopsia. *Electroencephalography and Clinical Neurophysiology*, 1969, *27*, 238–247.

Marg, E., Freeman, D.N., Peltzman, P., & Goldstein, P. Visual acuity development in human infants: Evoked potential measurements. *Investigative Ophthalmology*, 1976, *15*, 150–153.

Maurer, D. Infant visual perception: Methods of study. In L.B. Cohen & P. Salapatek (Eds.), *Infant perception: From sensation to cognition* (Vol. 1): *Basic visual processes.* New York: Academic Press, 1975.

Millodot, M., & Riggs, L.A. Refraction determined electrophysiologically: Responses to alternation of visual contours. *Archives of Ophthalmology*, 1970, *84*, 272–278.

Nawratzki, I., Auerbach, E., & Rowe, H. The electrical response in retina and occipital cortex following photic stimulation of normal and amblyopic eyes. *American Journal of Ophthalmology*, 1966, *61*, 430–434.

Newman, M. Visual acuity. In R.A. Moses (Ed.), *Adler's physiology of the eye.* St. Louis: C.V. Mosby, 1975.

Regan, D. *Evoked potentials in psychology, sensory physiology and clinical medicine.* New York: Wiley, 1972.

Riggs, L.A. Continuous and reproducible records of the electrical activity of the human retina. *Proceeding of the Society of Experimental Biology of New York*, 1941, *48*, 204–207.

Riggs, L.A. Electroretinography in cases of night blindness. *American Journal of Ophthalmology*, 1954, *38*, 70–78.

Riggs, L.A., Johnson, E.P., & Schick, A.M.L. Electrical responses of the human eye to changes in wavelength of the stimulating light. *Journal of the Optical Society of America*, 1966, *56*, 1621–1627.

Sokol, S. Visually evoked potentials: Theory, techniques and clinical applications. *Survey of Ophthalmology,* 1976, *21,* 18–44.

Sokol, S. Visual evoked potentials to checkerboard pattern stimuli in strabismic amblyopia. In J.E. Desmedt (Ed.), *Visual evoked potentials in man: New developments.* Oxford: Clarendon Press, 1977.

Sokol, S. Measurement of infant visual acuity from pattern reversal evoked potentials. *Vision Research,* 1978, *18,* 33–39.

Sokol, S., & Bloom, B.H. Visually evoked cortical responses of amblyopes to a spatially alternating stimulus. *Investigative Ophthalmology,* 1973, *12,* 936–939.

Sokol, S., & Dobson, V. Pattern reversal visually evoked potentials in infants. *Investigative Ophthalmology,* 1976, *15,* 58–62.

Sokol, S., & Shaterian, E.T. The pattern-evoked cortical potential in amblyopia as an index of visual function. In S. Moore, J. Mein, & L. Stockbridge (Eds.), *Orthoptics: Past, present and future.* Miami, Florida: Symposia Specialists, 1976.

Spekreijse, H., Khoe, L.H., & van der Tweel, L.H. A case of amblyopia; electrophysiology and psychophysics of luminance and contrast. In G.B. Arden (Ed.), *The visual system: Neurophysiology, biophysics and their clinical application* (Vol. 24): *Recent advances in experimental biology and medicine.* New York: Plenum Press, 1972.

Spekreijse, H., van der Tweel, L.H., & Zuidema, Th. Contrast evoked responses in man. *Vision Research,* 1973, *13,* 1577–1601.

37. Visually Evoked Cortical Potentials in Children with Hereditary Macular Degenerations[1]

Michael A. Sandberg and Marc H. Effron

I. Introduction

Attempts to demonstrate abnormal visually evoked cortical potentials (VECPs) in children with reduced acuity and macular disease have depended on either a normal fellow eye for comparison (Copenhaver & Beinhocker, 1963; Copenhaver, Beinhocker, & Perry, 1964; Copenhaver & Perry, 1964; Fishman & Copenhaver, 1967) or on extensive involvement of the posterior pole (Copenhaver & Beinhocker, 1963). This approach has limited value in children with hereditary macular degenerations where the disease is typically bilateral and the area of involvement is initially small.

A recent study has shown that a two-channel stimulator-ophthalmoscope may be used to detect abnormal central foveal function in the VECP from all 24 patients tested (ages 11–56) with visual acuity 20/25 or less and hereditary macular degenerations (Sandberg, Berson, & Ariel, 1977). Furthermore, the sensitivity of the technique was demonstrated in the detection of a 30-min foveolar cyst in a patient with visual acuity 20/25. The present investigation extends this work to show the usefulness of this procedure in additional cases of children with hereditary macular degenerations.

II. Methods

A hand-held, two-channel, Maxwellian-view stimulator-ophthalmoscope (Sandberg & Ariel, 1977) was used to present a white, 1.5° stimulus flickering at 5 Hz

[1]This work was supported in part by Specialized Research Center Grant IP50EYU2014 from the National Eye Institute and in part by the National Retinitis Pigmentosa Foundation, Baltimore, Maryland, and the George Gund Foundation, Cleveland, Ohio.

with retinal illuminances of 5.6 (Stimulus I) or 7 log trolands (Stimulus II). Either stimulus was centrally superimposed on a white, 10° steady background of 5 log trolands. With this instrument, the examiner was able to visualize and focus the stimulus on the patient's fundus through a dilated pupil and position the stimulus on the anatomical foveola throughout testing. The background was used not only to visualize retinal landmarks, but also to minimize possible effects of stray light from the stimulus.

Scalp potentials were recorded between the vertex and 1 cm above the inion, differentially amplified at a gain of 100,000 with respect to an earground, further amplified at a gain of 16 by a spike filter tuned to 5 Hz ($Q = 4$), and summed ($N = 64$; analysis time = 512 msec) by a signal-averaging computer. An upward deflection denoted an increasing positivity of the electrode near the inion. Averaged waveforms were displayed on an oscilloscope and photographed. Under these conditions, VECPs for normal observers (ages 6–52) are .7–3.8 μV in peak-to-peak amplitude and 90–148 msec in implicit time to the first positive peak for Stimulus I, and 1.4–6.3 μV in amplitude and 88–145 msec in implicit time for Stimulus II (Sandberg, Berson, & Ariel, 1977).

Four normal observers (ages 6–15) with V_A 20/20 or better and nine patients (ages 5–14) with V_A 20/25 to 20/400 and hereditary macular degenerations, not previously reported, were included in this study. Patients had macular changes visible on ophthalmoscopy, including granularity, with or without a foveal reflex, a "beaten mallet" appearance to the macula, and/or areas of depigmentation or atrophy in the macula. Full-field ERGs under dark-adapted conditions to white light were characteristically at least 300 μV. All patients had clear media and no evidence of nystagmus.

III. Results

All four normal observers gave VECPs that fell within the previously established normal range with respect to both amplitude and implicit time (Section II). All nine patients with hereditary macular degenerations gave abnormal VECPs to Stimulus I. Figure 37.1 illustrates recordings from a normal observer and three representative patients (P_1, P_2, and P_3). Abnormal VECPs were either out of phase or so reduced in amplitude as to be indistinguishable from noise.

Figure 37.2 presents recordings from a normal observer and four siblings (P.Co., K.Co., B.Co., and G.Co.) in a family where some of the members have juvenile macular degeneration. P.Co. and K.Co. with normal acuities and normal fundi gave normal VECPs. B.Co. and G.Co. with reduced acuities and macular granularity gave VECPs that were indistinguishable from noise.

Three of the nine patients with hereditary macular degenerations found abnormal with Stimulus I gave normal VECPs to the more intense test light of Stimulus II. Figure 37.3 shows responses to Stimuli I and II from two representative patients

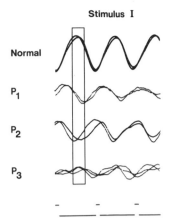

Figure 37.1. VECPs from a normal observer and three patients with juvenile macular degeneration in response to a flickering 1.5°, 5.6 log-troland stimulus centrally superimposed on a steady 10°, 5 log-troland background and positioned on the anatomical foveola. Patient visual acuities were 20/30 (P₁), 20/25 (P₂), and 20/400 (P₃). At least two traces are superimposed for each case. Vertical lines designate normal range of implicit time to first positive peak. Calibration markers (bottom trace) denote onset and duration of 20 msec stimulus, horizontally, and .5 µV, vertically.

with hereditary macular degenerations who were normal to Stimulus II but abnormal to Stimulus I.

IV. Discussion

The present report extends a previous study of hereditary macular degenerations (Sandberg, Berson, & Ariel, 1977) to show that in children abnormal central foveal function can be detected in the VECP elicited with a two-channel stimulator-ophthalmoscope with the stimulus focused and positioned on the anatomical foveola throughout testing. All patients tested with V_A 20/25 or less and an abnormal appearance to the macula gave abnormal VECPs. Patients could be distinguished

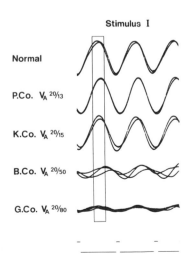

Figure 37.2. VECPs from a normal observer and four siblings aged 15 (P.Co.), 13 (K.Co.), 12 (B.Co.), and 14 (G.Co.) from a family with juvenile macular degeneration. Stimulus conditions, vertical lines, and calibration same as Figure 37.1.

Stimulus II   Stimulus I

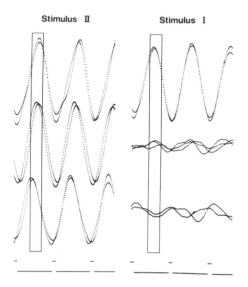

Figure 37.3. VECPs from a normal observer (top row), a patient with V_A 20/400 and macular degeneration (middle row), and a patient with V_A 20/100 and macular degeneration (lower row). Recordings were elicited by a flickering 1.5° stimulus centrally superimposed on a steady 10°, 5 log-troland background and positioned on the anatomical foveola. Stimulus intensity was 7 log trolands (Stimulus II) or 5.6 log trolands (Stimulus I). Calibration same as Figure 37.1.

from the normal population on the basis of shifts in phase, reductions in amplitude, or both. This approach is particularly applicable to individuals with bilateral hereditary macular degenerations where a normal fellow eye is not available for comparison.

Sensitivity of the technique depended on a precise adjustment of stimulus and background retinal illuminances, an adjustment that could be made with the stimulator-ophthalmoscope because both light beams were presented in Maxwellian view. This study, as well as a previous investigation (Sandberg, Berson, & Ariel, 1977), has shown that some patients with hereditary macular degenerations have normal function with a bright stimulus increment but abnormal function with a weak stimulus increment.

The present technique proved to be valuable for evaluating children with short attention spans and some variations in fixation. The examiner could easily compensate for slight changes in eye position with the hand-held stimulator-ophthalmoscope to maintain the stimulus on the anatomical foveola. A spike filter tuned to the stimulus frequency permitted recording in an open room without a copper cage enclosure. Reproducible responses could be obtained within a few minutes for a given patient.

REFERENCES

Copenhaver, R., & Beinhocker, G. Evoked occipital potentials recorded from scalp electrodes in response to focal visual illumination. *Investigative Ophthalmology,* 1963, *2,* 393–406.

Copenhaver, R., Beinhocker, G., & Perry, N., Jr. Visual evoked retinal and occipital potentials. *Documenta Ophthalmologica,* 1964, *18,* 473–482.

Copenhaver, R., & Perry, N., Jr. Factors affecting visually evoked cortical potentials such as impaired vision of varying etiology. *Investigative Ophthalmology*, 1964, *3*, 665–675.

Fishman, R., & Copenhaver, R. Macular disease and amblyopia: The visual-evoked response. *Archives of Ophthalmology*, 1967, *77*, 718–725.

Sandberg, M., & Ariel, M. A hand-held two-channel stimulator-ophthalmoscope. *Archives of Ophthalmology*, 1977, *95*, 1881–1882.

Sandberg, M., Berson, E., & Ariel, M. Visually evoked response testing with a stimulator-ophthalmoscope: Macular scars, hereditary macular degenerations, and retinitis pigmentosa. *Archives of Ophthalmology*, 1977, *95*, 1805–1808.

38. On the Road to Specific Information in Evoked Potentials[1]

Robert M. Chapman

I. Introduction

Lorrin Riggs pioneered the study of the correlation between electrophysiological measures and psychophysical facts. He invented and inventively used the contact lens electrode for recording the electroretinogram (Riggs, 1941) and later was one of the first to use averaging methods to study visually evoked potentials. Various physical parameters of the stimuli, such as light intensity, wavelength, spatial characteristics, and so on, have been related to evoked potential measures (for review, see Riggs & Wooten, 1972, pp. 690–731; Riggs, 1974). The method of stimulating the eye with counterphase alternation of various stripe patterns (Riggs, Johnson, & Schick, 1964) has been extensively used with evoked potential recording and has been useful for studying not only spatial problems, but also color problems. The relations of evoked potentials to various psychophysical parameters are discussed in several other chapters in this volume.

This chapter will concentrate on the relations between general state and cognitive factors and evoked potentials. It is apparent that the waveform of the evoked potential is dependent on many factors in addition to the physical aspects of the stimulus. One example comes from an experiment in which subjects were presented with visual stimuli (luminous numbers and letters), only some of which were relevant to a numerical comparison task (Chapman & Bragdon, 1964). The evoked potentials tended to be larger to the task-relevant stimuli. Stimulus luminance only weakly controlled the overall amplitude of the evoked potential, which did not decrease appreciably with lower luminance stimuli until the recognition threshold was reached (Figure 38.1). Furthermore, the size of the evoked potentials to identical sequences of number and letter stimuli was found to depend on whether the

[1]Supported in part by NIH Research Grant 5 R01 EY1593 from the National Eye Institute.

stimuli were relevant to the tasks, which were either numerical or alphabetic comparisons (Chapman, 1965). Task-relevant stimuli (whether numbers or letters) produced larger evoked potentials than when the same stimuli were irrelevant. That basic finding has been subsequently amplified in considerably more detailed and sophisticated ways, including randomized sequences (Figure 38.2) (Chapman, 1966), evoked potential differences for different kinds of processing (Chapman, 1969, pp. 262–275), using auditory stimuli (Sheatz & Chapman, 1969), evoked potential measures at various time points (Chapman, 1973, pp. 69–108), and latent components analyses (Chapman, 1974a, pp. 38–42; Chapman, McCrary, Bragdon, & Chapman, in press). The major evoked potential effect appeared to be a higher positive elevation approximately 300–500 msec after a task-relevant stimulus. A similar evoked potential effect has since been extensively reported and has been variously referred to as P300, P3, late positive component, and so on. We shall return to this P300 component in a moment.

It is often suggested that the earlier components of the evoked potential are more related to the physical parameters of the stimuli and the later components are more

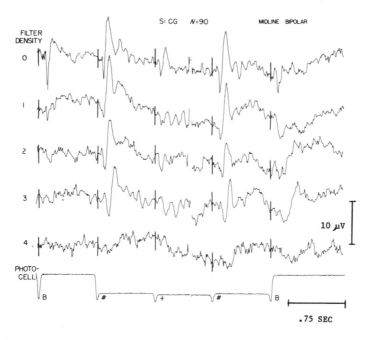

Figure 38.1. Averaged evoked potentials to relevant numbers (# = randomly selected digits 1–9) and irrelevant control stimuli (B for blank square, + for plus sign). Subject's task was to say which of the two numbers was numerically smaller. Relative luminances inversely related to filter density. With neutral filters from 0 down to 3, this subject answered 100% of the problems correctly; the 4 neutral density filter brought the luminance down to threshold for number recognition with attendant performance decrement. Records were bipolar on the scalp midline between CPZ (site between Cz and Pz) and Oz with the ground electrode over the mastoid; positive at the central-parietal electrode is up. Experiment described by Chapman and Bragdon (1964).

RANDOMIZED ORDER   S:PH
N=1920

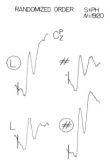

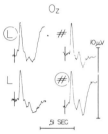

Figure 38.2. Averaged evoked potentials to letters (L) and numbers (#) when task relevant (circled) and when irrelevant (not circled). The letter or number stimuli were made task relevant by alphabetic or numeric comparison tasks. Order of letter and number stimuli, as well as the particular letters and numbers, were randomized. Only responses to stimuli whose relevance could not be anticipated were averaged. Recordings are monopolar from central-parietal (CPZ) and occipital (OZ) midline sites; ground electrode over mastoid. Positive up. [From R. M. Chapman, Human evoked responses to meaningful stimuli. *Seventeenth International Congress of Psychology, Moscow*, 1966, 6, 53–59.]

related to the psychological parameters. Although this appears to be a reasonable first-order approximation, there is increasing evidence of temporal overlap and early appearance in evoked potentials of psychological effects. For example, significant effects of task relevance were found in a number–letter experiment when the evoked potential amplitude was measured at 105 msec after the stimulus (Chapman, 1973).

II. Measuring Evoked Potential Components

If there are several superimposed effects contributing to the recorded evoked potentials, then how may these effects be sorted out? In addition to manipulating systematically experimental variables, it seems desirable to have a system of evoked potential measurement that identifies and measures evoked potential components which may overlap in time. The observed evoked potential is influenced by many factors. A model is needed to determine the effect of these factors. For example, we have assumed that the response to a stimulus is the linear sum of a number of independent components. Each component has a fixed time course. Some variables affect the magnitude of one component more than another. The resultant waveform under any circumstance is the weighted sum of a set of basis functions:

$$R(t) = S_1 f(t) + S_2 g(t) + \cdots + S_k p(t) + C(t),$$

where $S_1, S_2, \ldots$, are the weights determined by the experimental conditions, and $f(t)$, $g(t), \ldots$, are the basis functions (as functions of time). Note that $C(t)$ is the centroid and has a fixed weight; this part of the evoked potential is that which is common to all of the responses that have been measured. This general approach includes a set of analytical methods of which Fourier analysis is but one member. In the method that we have applied, we do not use as basis functions expressions such as $\sin(t)$ and $\cos(t)$, but rather we derived the basis functions from the responses themselves. In essence, we assume that an experimental variable, say, stimulus relevance, affects the weights of certain of the basis functions (which weights may be positive or negative). The differences in waveform with variations of stimulus relevance reveal these components. The actual method of analysis, varimaxed principal components analysis, is related to factor analysis. Specifically, we measured evoked potentials, having 102 time points spaced 5 msec apart, under a variety of experimental conditions. The basic analytical operation is the correlation of the responses at each time point and the factoring of the resulting correlation matrix. The details may be found in Chapman, McCrary, Bragdon, and Chapman (in press) and Dixon (1975, program BMDP4M).

A varimaxed principal components analysis was applied to evoked potential data obtained in the number–letter experiment (Chapman, 1974a; Chapman, McCrary, Bragdon, & Chapman, in press). Eight latent components, accounting for 96% of the total evoked potential variance, were extracted. Example plots of the latent components as they contributed to evoked potentials are shown in Figure 38.3. Each of the components was significantly related to various experimental conditions.

We feel that this approach has advantages over the traditional one of looking for prominent bumps with certain latencies in the evoked potentials (e.g., P300 or N100) and then examining the variation of the size of the potentials with experimental conditions. The size and latency of a certain promontory may vary with irrelevant variables. In fact, the landmark may be completely submerged under some conditions that fill in neighboring valleys with additional hills. The P300 is a positive promontory peaking about 300–500 msec poststimulus which is elicited by task-relevant, target, or rare stimuli (Chapman & Bragdon, 1964; Sutton, Braren, & Zubin, 1965). However, there is not always a positive peak precisely at 300 msec (peaks near 400 msec are often reported). Compare this kind of bump analysis with the analysis of the variation of our Component 2 with experimental conditions illustrated in Figure 38.4. This component is reliably related to stimulus relevance. Component scores are more stable than amplitude measures at one time point, since a component score is based on a number of time points. It can be evaluated even at small values, and can have negative as well as positive weights. It is unlikely by standard methods that one would follow a component's variations from positive through small values to negative values. Moreover, once a basis function has been derived from one set of data, it can be transformed and used as a template to measure other sets of evoked potential data by a cross-product procedure.

In both time course and amplitude variation with experimental conditions, Component 2 in Figure 38.4 is similar to what has been called P300 in the traditional bump analysis literature. The method used provides both component waveform (basis functions) and component score (weight) information. Component 2 (Figure 38.4) had a maximum at 410 msec and reached half of this maximum at 260 msec.

Figure 38.3. Evoked potentials reproduced for 2 of 16 conditions in number–letter experiment to illustrate their composition. Components' resultant waveforms (rows B through I) are shown scaled appropriately, that is, the fundamental time course of each component (basis functions = rotated component loadings multiplied by standard deviations) was multiplied by the mean of 12 subjects' component scores for each condition (weights). The resultant waveforms in two columns differ only by their weights, that is, component scores $(S_1, S_2, \ldots, S_8)$, which are measures of the contribution of each component to the evoked potentials. The basis functions, $f(t), g(t), \ldots, m(t)$, and therefore the shapes of the waveforms in the two columns are the same. The centroid (row A) is the mean evoked potential for the entire set. The reproduced evoked potential is obtained by the simple sum of rows A–I. Monopolar CPZ data (positive up) for 12 subjects. Experimental conditions: Left column, number stimuli when relevant and evoked

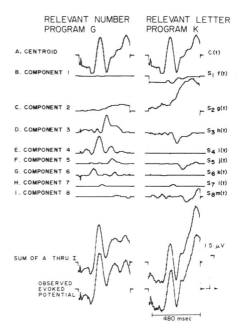

potential collected by program G (first intratrial position when subject perceives and stores stimulus information); right column, letter stimuli when relevant and evoked potential collected by program K (fourth intratrial position when subject perceives a relevant stimulus, expected with 100% certainty, and uses that information for alphabetic comparison). The 5-μV standard applies to the entire figure. The 510-msec records include 30-msec prestimulus and 480-msec poststimulus periods. [From analysis reported by Chapman (1974a) and Chapman, McCrary, Bragdon, & Chapman (in press).]

The amount of this evoked potential component differed significantly for relevant and irrelevant stimuli (circled versus uncircled data in Figure 38.4). Since the stimulus sequence was randomized, this component is associated with poststimulus processing rather than representing a general state existing prior to the visual stimuli. Rather than being related to general arousal or general attention, this component may be related to selective arousal or selective attention that is conditioned by the stimulus information relevant to the subject's task (Chapman, 1969).

III. Specific Cognitive Factors

Thus, the evoked potential depends on the sensory aspects of the stimulus and its task relevance. In addition, the newest and smallest area of investigation concerns the dependence of the evoked potential on specific cognitive factors, for example, semantic meanings (Chapman, 1974b, pp. 43–45; Chapman, 1978a,b; Chapman, Bragdon, Chapman, & McCrary, 1977, pp. 36–47; Chapman, 1976; Chapman, McCrary, Chapman, & Bragdon, 1978), letter encoding, alphabetic comparison,

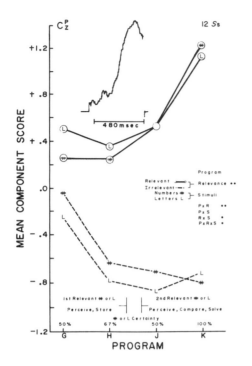

Figure 38.4. Scores (mean of 12 subjects) for evoked potential latent Component 2 obtained for 16 information-processing conditions. Programs G, H, J, and K are arbitrary designations for subsets of intratrial positions 1, 2, 3, and 4, respectively (details in Chapman, 1973); the experimental conditions relating to these programs when the stimuli are task relevant are indicated above the abscissa. Component 2 behaves like P300 of other studies. The component scores are Ss in the general equation given in the text and are in standard score units. Three-way factorial analysis of variance summarized for program × relevance × stimulus design; statistically significant effects indicated by · for $p < .05$ and ·· for $p < .01$. Inset illustrates Component 2's resultant waveform for one condition: Program K, relevant numbers; the height of this waveform is approximately 5 μV, positive up. [From Chapman, McCrary, Bragdon, & Chapman (in press).]

expected stimulus relevance, and storage of information in short-term memory (Chapman, 1974a; Chapman, McCrary, Bragdon, & Chapman, in press).

A. Semantic Meaning

We tested the hypothesis that evoked potentials depend on semantic meaning by applying an old and reliable recipe of Osgood's (1952). Osgood's analysis of connotative meaning has shown that subjects' judgments of words on semantic differential scales are based largely on three dimensions: evaluation (E), potency (P), and activity (A) (Osgood, 1971). By selecting words that scored high or low on one of the dimensions and relatively neutral on the other two (Heise, 1971), we obtained six classes of words (E+, E−, P+, P−, A+, A−) representing the positive and negative extremes of the evaluation, potency, and activity dimensions. Twenty words from each of the six semantic classes were randomly assigned to a list. Two such lists were constructed with different words except for the P− class where the same words were used. The words belonging to these semantic classes were flashed and the average evoked potentials for these classes were analyzed. The principle involved in this approach (Chapman, 1974b; Chapman, Bradgon, Chapman, & McCrary, 1977) is that while the background EEG is being averaged to obtain evoked potentials, the physical characteristics of the words are being averaged to control for their effects and the meanings of the words are being averaged to provide a common core of connotative meaning. The words within each list were given in different random orders from run to run so that the subjects could not anticipate either a semantic class or a particular word. Thus, differences in the evoked potentials to these semantic categories can be associated with poststimulus processing of semantic information, with the comparison of responses to the two lists aiding in the establishment of the reliability and generality of the effects.

Coping with the large individual differences in evoked potential waveforms was a problem. It was solved by standardizing the evoked potentials for each subject separately before proceeding with the analysis. The evoked potential amplitudes at each time point were converted to z scores (mean = 0, variance = 1). For a group of 10 subjects the average responses to the six semantic classes before and after standardization are shown in Figure 38.5. The differences were reliable enough to discriminate the semantic classes on the basis of the brain responses (Chapman, McCrary, Chapman, & Bragdon, 1978).

The standardized potentials to the six semantic classes for two lists for 10 subjects were entered into a varimaxed principal components analysis (Dixon, 1975, BMDP4M program). The component scores that resulted were the evoked potential measures used in multiple discriminant analyses (Dixon, 1975, BMDP7M program). When the evoked potentials were classified to word classes from opposite

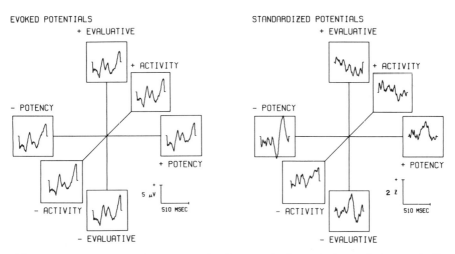

Figure 38.5. Average brain responses for six semantic classes before and after standardization. The semantic classes are based on Osgood's evaluation, potency, and activity dimensions that define a three-dimensional semantic space, represented schematically here. The evoked potentials cover 510 msec (102 time points × 5 msec) along the horizontal axis, beginning at the time the words were flashed. The vertical axes for the evoked potentials are in microvolts, in the left panel, and are in standard units z in the right panel. For the standardized potentials each subject's data at each time point were transformed to z scores (means = 0 and variances = 1). Averages include data for 2 lists and 10 subjects. Monopolar recordings (bandpass: .1 to 70 Hz) from a scalp location one-third of the distance from Cz to Pz. [From Chapman *et al.* (1978).]

ends of each semantic dimension (E+ versus E−, P+ versus P−, A+ versus A−), the success rates expected by chance were 50%. The overall success rate obtained in developing the discriminant functions was 97%. This was cross-validated by a jackknifed procedure in which each evoked potential in turn was left out of the development of the discriminant functions and then classified; the overall jackknifed cross-validation success rate was 90%. When the same classification functions for one word list were applied to the evoked potential data obtained from the other word list, the overall success rate was 73%. In addition to these analyses of one dimension at a time, functions were developed to discriminate simultaneously among all six semantic classes, in which case the success rates expected by chance would be 16.7%. The jackknifed success rates were 42% for List 1 and 43% for List 2 data, some 2.5 times better than chance. The applications to the "other-list" data averaged 40%. These analyses mean that evoked potentials contain information that is reliably related to connotative meaning of words and that these evoked potential effects generalize across different word lists.

All of these success rates were obtained across subjects; that is, the same classification functions were used for all 10 subjects. There were no significant individual differences in success rates. This is evidence that not only can evoked potential effects be found that relate to connotative semantic meaning, but also these evoked potential effects tend to be similar in different individuals.

Thus some components of evoked potentials seem to depend on meaning. They were not directly tied to the physical parameters of the stimuli, since each semantic class was represented by a number of words with similar distributions of letters and the effects generalized across lists of words. Nor can the components be explained by general states. Since (a) there were six semantic classes, (b) the subjects could not anticipate which semantic class might occur on any trial, and (c) these evoked potential effects occurred within 510 msec, the different effects did not seem sufficiently pervasive or long-lived to be explained by some general state such as arousal or attention. On the other hand, combinations of evoked potential components were reliably related to the semantic classes of the stimulus words.

B. Cognitive Operators

Other aspects of the response seem to depend on cognitive operators (Chapman, 1974a; Chapman, McCrary, Bragdon, & Chapman, in press). Let us briefly look at one of these, namely, one that appears to be related to storage of information in short-term memory. In the number–letter information-processing experiment, previously discussed, the first relevant stimulus must be stored in the subject's memory in order to be compared with the second relevant stimulus occurring later in the trial. The principal components analysis of the evoked potentials uncovered a component that was related to these information storage conditions. The scores for this latent component are shown in Figure 38.6 (upper left panel). They are relatively high when the subject is storing the information from the first relevant stimulus, which

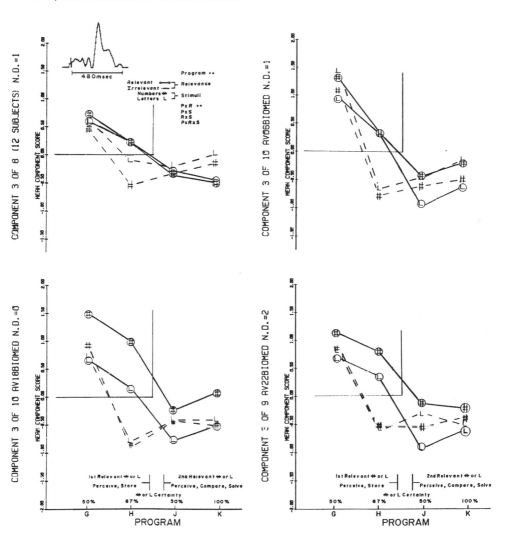

Figure 38.6. Storage component of evoked potentials in number–letter experiment. Component score plotted as function of 16 experimental conditions in each panel (similar to Figure 38.4). Upper left panel: Mean data from 12 subjects. Upper right and lower panels: Data from one subject at three luminance levels (neutral density = 1, 0, and 2). Inset (upper left) shows waveform when stimulus information is being stored. Monopolar recording from scalp site between Cz and Pz.

occurs randomly in either the first or second intratrial position (program G or H). The "storage" component scores are also relatively high when the first stimulus is irrelevant (program G), suggesting that irrelevant information may be stored when there is no previous short-term memory load at that time in the trial. The latent evoked potential component associated with these experimental conditions has a maximum amplitude about 250 msec after the stimulus (Figure 38.6, inset) and is orthogonal to the other latent components identified in the analysis, for example, P300, CNV-resolution, and so on (Figure 38.3). This storage component is not dependent on particular parameters of the physical stimuli, since with identical letter and number stimuli it varied with specific information-processing conditions. Nor did it relate to a general state carrying across the trial; of special note is that it was not associated with the second relevant stimulus (program J or K) to which attention also must be paid to solve the number or letter comparison tasks. Thus, this storage evoked potential component does not depend on specific sensory aspects of the stimulus, the general state of the subject, or general stimulus relevance.

This was tested further in experiments that varied the stimulus luminance (Chapman, 1977). Data from one subject were obtained at three luminance levels spaced 1 log unit apart, one higher and one lower than that previously reported (Chapman, 1974a; Chapman, McCrary, Bragdon, & Chapman, in press). Separate varimaxed principal component analyses were done at each luminance level. In each analysis a latent evoked potential component was found that was similar to the storage component. The component scores were related to the experimental conditions in a similar way, as may be seen by the similar patterns of scores in the four panels of Figure 38.6. Furthermore, the waveforms of this latent evoked potential component were similar, with maximum loadings at about 250 msec. For the previous experiment the maximum was at 250 msec; for the new data the maxima are at 245 msec, 250 msec, and 255 msec for neutral densities of 0, 1, and 2, respectively (high to low luminance). Thus, varying the luminance by a ratio of 100:1, which altered the overall evoked potential, did not interfere with detecting this latent evoked potential component. This component appears to be related to the specific cognitive operation of storing information in short-term memory.

IV. Conclusion

Evoked potentials have been studied in relation to psychophysical properties of stimuli, general states of subjects, and cognitive processes. A pervasive question is how specific are the functional relationships that may be established between experimental variables and evoked potential effects. It is suggested that finding such specificity may be aided by applying multivariate data analysis techniques, such as varimaxed principal components analysis, to evoked potentials. This approach has been illustrated with sample data from information-processing and semantic meaning research. The evidence bears out the idea that evoked potential components have rather specific functional relations. Of course, data analysis alone is helpless without careful manipulation of experimental conditions. A start has been made to trace the processing of stimulus information within the nervous system past analyses of psychophysical stimulus parameters, beyond the modulating influence of general states, and into the domain of specific cognitive processing.

ACKNOWLEDGMENTS

John W. McCrary, John A. Chapman, and Henry R. Bragdon contributed greatly to this research. Deep appreciation is extended to Lorrin A. Riggs for his help and his example.

REFERENCES

Chapman, R. M. Evoked responses to relevant and irrelevant visual stimuli while problem solving. *Proceedings of the American Psychological Association,* 1965, 177–178.

Chapman, R. M. Human evoked responses to meaningful stimuli. *Seventeenth International Congress of Psychology, Moscow,* 1966, *6,* 53–59.

Chapman, R. M. Definition and measurement of "psychological" independent variables in an average evoked potential experiment. In E. Donchin & D.B. Lindsley (Eds.), *Average evoked potentials: Methods, results, and evaluations* (NASA SP-191). Washington, D.C.: U.S. Government Printing Office, 1969. Pp. 262–275.

Chapman, R. M. Evoked potentials of the brain related to thinking. In F. J. McGuigan & R. Schoonover (Eds.), *Psychophysiology of thinking.* New York: Academic Press, 1973. Pp. 69–108.

Chapman, R. M. Latent components of average evoked brain responses functionally related to information processing. In *International Symposium on Cerebral Evoked Potentials in Man* (pre-circulated abstracts). Brussels: Presses Universitaires de Bruxelles, 1974. Pp. 38–42. (a)

Chapman, R. M. Semantic meaning of words and average evoked potentials. In *International Symposium on Cerebral Evoked Potentials in Man* (pre-circulated abstracts). Brussels: Presses Universitaires de Bruxelles, 1974. Pp. 43–45. (b)

Chapman, R. M. (Chair). ERPs and language. In David A. Otto (Program Chair), *Transcript of panel at 4th International Congress on Event Related Slow Potentials of the Brain (EPIC IV).* Hendersonville, North Carolina, 1976.

Chapman, R. M. Light intensity and the "storage" component in visual evoked potentials. *Electroencephalography and Clinical Neurophysiology,* 1977, *43,* 778.

Chapman, R. M. Language and evoked potentials. In David A. Otto (Ed.), *Multidisciplinary perspectives in event-related brain potential research* (EPA-600/9-77-043). Washington, D.C.: U.S. Government Printing Office, 1978 (in press). (a)

Chapman, R. M. Connotative meaning and averaged evoked potentials. In H. Begleiter (Ed.), *Evoked brain potentials and behavior.* New York: Plenum Press, 1978 (in press). (b)

Chapman, R. M., & Bragdon, H. R. Evoked responses to numerical and non-numerical visual stimuli while problem solving. *Nature,* 1964, *203,* 1155–1157.

Chapman, R. M., Bragdon, H. R., Chapman, J. A., & McCrary, J. W. Semantic meaning of words and average evoked potentials. In J.E. Desmedt (Ed.), *Progress in clinical neurophysiology,* (Vol. 3): *Language and hemispheric specialization in man: Cerebral event-related potentials.* Basel: Karger, 1977, Pp. 36–47.

Chapman, R. M., McCrary, J. W., Bragdon, H. R., & Chapman, J. A. Latent components of event-related potentials functionally related to information processing. In J.E. Desmedt (Ed.), *Progress in clinical neurophysiology* (Vol. 6); *Cognitive components in cerebral event-related potentials and selective attention.* Basel: Karger (in press).

Chapman, R. M., McCrary, J. W., Chapman, J. A., & Bragdon, H. R. Brain responses related to semantic meaning. *Brain and Language,* 1978, *5,* 195–205.

Dixon, W. J. (Ed.) *BMDP biomedical computer programs.* Berkeley: University of California Press, 1975.

Heise, D. R. Evaluation, potency, and activity scores for 1551 words: A merging of three published lists. Chapel Hill, North Carolina: University of North Carolina, Department of Sociology, 1971.

Osgood, C. R. The nature and measurement of meaning. *Psychological Bulletin,* 1952, *49,* 197–237.

Osgood, C. E. Exploration in semantic space: A personal diary. *Journal of Social Issues,* 1971, *27,* 5–63.

Riggs, L. A. Continuous and reproducible records of the electrical activity ot the human retina. *Proceedings of the Society for Experimental Biology and Medicine,* 1941, *48,* 204–207.

Riggs, L. A. Responses of the visual system to fluctuating patterns. *American Journal of Optometry and Physiological Optics,* 1974, *51,* 725–735.

Riggs, L. A., Johnson, E. P., & Schick, A. M. L. Electrical responses of the human eye to moving stimulus patterns. *Science,* 1964, *144,* 567.

Riggs, L. A., & Wooten, B. R. Electrical measures and psychophysical data on human vision. In D. Jameson & L.M. Hurvich (Eds.), *Handbook of sensory physiology* (Vol. VII/4): *Visual psychophysics.* New York: Springer-Verlag, 1972. Pp. 690–731.

Sheatz, G. C., & Chapman, R. M. Task relevance and auditory evoked responses. *Electroencephalography and Clinical Neurophysiology,* 1969, *26,* 468–475.

Sutton, S., Braren, M., & Zubin, J. Evoked potential correlates of stimulus uncertainty. *Science,* 1965, *150,* 1177–1188.

Subject Index

A
B
C 8
D 9
E 0
F 1
G 2
H 3
I 4
J 5